To the many conscientious, responsible health professionals who know that being a personal trainer means more than perkily chirping, "I'm Mindy! Lift your leg."

SECOND EDITION

The Personal Trainer's Handbook

Teri S. O'Brien, MS, JD

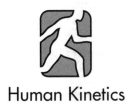

Human Kinetics

Library of Congress Cataloging-in-Publication Data

O'Brien, Teri S., 1955-
  The personal trainer's handbook / Teri S. O'Brien.--2nd ed.
    p.   cm.
  Includes bibliographical references (p.   ) and index.
    ISBN 0-7360-4501-5 (Soft Cover)
    1. Personal trainers--Handbooks, manuals, etc.   2. Personal
  trainers--Vocational guidance--Handbooks, manuals, etc.   I. Title.
    GV428.7 .O37   2003
    613.7'1--dc21

                                                    2002153987
ISBN: 0-7360-4501-5

The Web addresses cited in this text were current as of March 7, 2003, unless otherwise noted.

Acquisitions Editor: Michael S. Bahrke, PhD
Developmental Editor: Elaine H. Mustain
Assistant Editor: Maggie Schwarzentraub
Copyeditor: Barbara Juhas Walsh
Proofreader: Sue Fetters
Indexer: Susan Danzi Hernandez
Permission Manager: Dalene Reeder
Graphic Designer: Nancy Rasmus
Graphic Artist: Francine Hamerski
Photo Manager: Leslie A. Woodrum
Cover Designer: Jack W. Davis
Photographer (cover): Leslie A. Woodrum
Photographer (interior): Leslie A. Woodrum
Art Manager: Kelly Hendren
Illustrator: Argosy and Marge Pavich
Printer: Versa Press

Printed in the United States of America   10 9 8 7 6 5 4 3 2 1

Human Kinetics
Web site: www.HumanKinetics.com

United States: Human Kinetics
P.O. Box 5076
Champaign, IL 61825-5076
800-747-4457
e-mail: humank@hkusa.com

Canada: Human Kinetics
475 Devonshire Road Unit 100
Windsor, ON N8Y 2L5
800-465-7301 (in Canada only)
e-mail: orders@hkcanada.com

Europe: Human Kinetics
107 Bradford Road
Stanningley
Leeds LS28 6AT, United Kingdom
+44 (0) 113 255 5665
e-mail: hk@hkeurope.com

Australia: Human Kinetics
57A Price Avenue
Lower Mitcham, South Australia 5062
08 8277 1555
e-mail: liahka@senet.com.au

New Zealand: Human Kinetics
P.O. Box 105-231, Auckland Central
09-523-3462
e-mail: hkp@ihug.co.nz

CONTENTS

PREFACE

Since the publication of the first edition of *The Personal Trainer's Handbook*, the personal training industry has enjoyed robust growth. No doubt part of the increased interest in hiring qualified trainers has been fueled by news about the dramatic and life-changing impact that exercise and lifestyle choices can have on health, especially later in life. An eager public, swelled by the ranks of aging baby boomers, has clamored for specifics on how they can live longer and, more important, live stronger. The International Health, Racquet and Sportsclub Association (IHRSA) American Sports Data Health Club Trend Report shows that from 1999 to 2000, the number of Americans who used a personal fitness trainer grew by approximately 32% to just over five million (IHRSA press release, October 10, 2001). In addition, improving public health by doubling the percentage of Americans who maintain a healthful weight and who are physically active on a regular basis is an official goal of federal government policy (United States Department of Health and Human Services 2000).

The market has responded. Consider this statistic provided by one of the leading continuing-education organizations in the industry, IDEA Health and Fitness Association. In 1992, IDEA had 782 members in its personal training category. Today there are more than 8,000 (Ideafit.org). It's difficult to know precisely how many people are actively involved in personal training, but estimates are all over the board, ranging from 40,000 (Davis 2002) to 55,000 (IDEA Personal Trainer 2000) to over 100,000 (Helliker 1999). In addition to the increasing numbers of adults who want to get fit and healthy and stay that way, another factor appears to have contributed to the burgeoning numbers of people entering the profession. Personal training offers practitioners the chance to make a difference in people's lives, and that can go a long way toward career satisfaction. In fact, even educated professionals such as dentists and attorneys have entered the field, enticed by what they could only have dreamed of before—happy clients who are actually glad to see them (Helliker 1999)!

As the industry has grown, it has seen improved standards, new specialties within the broader frame-work of personal training, and hundreds of organizations claiming to certify professionals as qualified. The premier certifying agencies, American College of Sports Medicine (ACSM), American Council on Exercise (ACE), and National Strength and Conditioning Association (NSCA), have revised their standards and devised several new certifications. For all these reasons, it's an exciting time to be part of this dynamic, life-changing profession.

The news is not all good, though. At the same time that all these dramatic changes have occurred, some things have stayed depressingly the same. A visit to any large health club might feature the following all-too-common sights: The inarticulate size-3-hat, size-17-shirt type runs amok, barking like a drill instructor, demanding that unfortunate clients execute his poorly conceived program. The glorified rep counter with the glassy-eyed stare, masquerading as a "personal trainer" (that's what her shirt says, anyway), robotically drones on with her numeric mantra, oblivious as her client serves as a living, breathing example of how *not* to do an exercise. Increasing numbers of lawsuits have been filed against fitness professionals, with most experts predicting more on the way (Herbert 2000). Some experts note that doctors, many of whom would like to see their patients exercise consistently, are sometimes reluctant to refer them to personal trainers due to their public image. Legitimate concerns about legal liability and referrals to unqualified personal trainers discourage the medical community from doing so (Physican and Sports Medicine 2000). Clearly, our work is not done.

What's New in This Edition

Like all great professionals, great personal trainers are constantly striving to stay on the cutting edge. They want to learn the results of the latest scientific research and apply it when working with their clients. In short, they know that in a dynamic world, you can't be your best by standing still. Many readers of the first edition of this book have told me how terrific and information-packed it is. They've also shared ideas about how to make a good book even better. I listened and added tons of useful stuff that they (and you) can begin using *today* to vault you to the top of the profession. Speaking of cutting edge, I'm very excited about the CD-ROM accompanying this book. For details on this exciting addition, please read on.

• **Business and legal issues.** When I spoke to personal trainers about updating this book, they all mentioned a desire for more information about setting up a business. Consumers have become more sophisticated about personal training, so to be successful today, it's not enough to be a good personal trainer. More than ever, personal trainers need to think and act as businesspeople. To help, I've added a sample business/marketing plan, as well as a detailed explanation of the differences among types of business organizations. To help you get new clients, I've included new information on selling your program through effective communication. Though it's true that the threat of litigation against personal trainers looms larger now than ever before, there are ways to minimize the risk of a lawsuit. I've revised the waiver form to address some recent litigation and included a new form to use for conducting home workouts. Because being an ethical professional is the best protection against being sued, I've included new information on the American College of Sports Medicine's Code of Ethics.

• **Customer service.** It's more important to keep clients than to get them, so I've included new material about customer service, including details about the surefire technique to make clients love you: active listening.

• **Program design.** Even though most professional personal trainers have studied anatomy and physiology, either formally or on their own to prepare for certification exams, I include a brief primer on the basics of exercise physiology, the science behind the art of personal training. To make your program design even more effective, I've improved an extremely useful and popular feature of the first book, the Resistance Workout Guide—the fully illustrated key to teaching clients perfect form for the most common resistance training exercises. The new and improved version not only tells you how to do these exercises right (and the typical ways people do them wrong), it also lists the specific muscles that each exercise targets.

• **The top ten.** So you can avoid the top 10 mistakes personal trainers make, I've included a list of these mistakes and the reasons trainers make them. You'll find this in chapter 9.

The Art of Exercise Prescription

The art of exercise prescription is the successful integration of exercise science with behavior techniques that result in long-term program compliance and attainment of the individual's goals. This new edition will equip you with what you need to achieve that successful integration.

• **Advanced matters.** The best personal trainers realize that the key to both their own satisfaction and their clients' success is to go beyond the merely physical. They strive to be more than trainers. They want to be coaches as well. Coaching is a process that happens inside the cranium, so I've included some important information on the stages of change that people go through when they modify their lifestyles. This information will help you become that indispensable partner your client needs to reach his or her goals.

• **More new stuff!** This edition takes what was already an invaluable resource for the fitness professional to a whole new level by including even more information that you can use immediately.

- A glossary of terms common in the fitness field. If you've ever wondered what "steady state," "syncope," or "standard of care" means, we've got your answer right here, and lots more.

- A new section on handling emergencies. I hope you'll never have to deal with these types of situations, but just in case, I've provided some suggestions to help you handle injuries and accidents.

- Information on selling and dealing with commonly raised client objections.

- The CD-ROM. When I wrote the first edition of *The Personal Trainer's Handbook,* I knew that personal trainers and other fitness professionals would appreciate my including sample versions of all the essential forms needed to establish and run a successful personal training business. Based on feedback I've gotten from readers, I was right: Personal trainers *love* this feature. That's why I'm so excited about the CD-ROM that accompanies this edition of the book. It contains reproducible versions of these forms that you and your attorney can modify to suit the needs of your business and your state law. And there's even more on the CD. Pop it in your computer and you'll find case studies that illustrate program design and execution concepts in a way that even a beginner can use to be a personal training superstar. In addition, the CD provides excerpts from several Human kinetics books that will take you to the next level off expertise. These include field-based tests for muscular imbalance; charts describing the actions of major muscles and the joints on which they act; material on customizing your client's eating plan, periodization, working with clients who have bad backs and chronic conditions; and much more.

What Hasn't Changed

One thing that hasn't changed is the original mission of *The Personal Trainer's Handbook*: to teach personal trainers the practical information they need to be genuine health professionals who have and effectively use expertise to change individual lives and the overall health and wellness of their communities, while at the same time having fun, rewarding careers. In short, to do well by doing good.

Several years ago I had the pleasure of seeing the amazing IMAX movie made during the dramatic 1996 climb up Mount Everest that was the subject of the book *Into Thin Air*, and it got me to thinking about Sir Edmund Hillary and Sherpas and personal trainers. The 1996 climb ended in tragedy, but Hillary's was triumphant. On May 29, 1953, he became one of the first of two humans ever to reach the summit of Mount Everest. I say "two" because his Sherpa, Tenzing Norgay, accompanied Hillary. Neither man would say who reached the summit first. Both men always said they reached the summit together: "We climbed as a team." Neither man was willing to claim the credit, each knowing that without the other, he would not have made it.

Their achievement highlighted the indispensable contribution of Sherpas in Everest expeditions. Commentators have noted that the Sherpas not only are extremely talented climbers, but also seem to possess a unique attitude that enables them to perform their tasks with competence as well as with alacrity. (That's one of my favorite words. It means "cheerful enthusiasm.") The Sherpas performed with alacrity even in the severe conditions of Everest. Some have suggested that this attitude may be due to the way that they view the mountain, and therefore their work. To the Sherpas, the mountain is a spiritual entity, and therefore their work is not a job but a calling. Though they were originally employed as porters and assistants to haul the gear up the mountain, their burning determination and their indomitable spirit so impressed everyone who employed them that they became respected full partners, sharing in the shining moment at the top of the world.

I think that good personal trainers are like Sherpas. They must be strong. They must be reliable. They must be determined. And, like Sherpas, they must be attracted to the challenge and achievement of their work. The pay is good, but they aren't in it just for the money. They delight in being in the fortunate position of making money doing something they really love. Like Sherpas, though, we personal trainers cannot do the long, hard climb for our clients. We can only guide and support them. As the client reaches the summit of his personal fitness goal, he should be able to truly say to you, "I can't do it without you, but you can't do it for me." If you think of the trust and responsibility that is reflected in the work of Sherpas and the respect they inspire in those they support, you'll have a good start in thinking of yourself as a personal trainer in a position of trust and responsibility. I hope that this book helps you in that mission.

ACKNOWLEDGMENTS

I would like to thank some of the individuals who helped produce this book you now hold in your hands.

The invaluable ideas of Mike Bahrke, acquisitions editor at Human Kinetics, inspired me to create the new content that makes this second edition unique. Elaine Mustain, developmental editor, edited this second edition and made a good book even better with her excellent suggestions. Maggie Schwarzentraub, an assistant editor by title and an all-around troubleshooter, made sure I stayed on track.

Thanks also go to the folks at the Lakeshore Athletic Club who generously opened their fine facilities to us; Les Woodrum, Human Kinetics photographer extraordinaire; Lizette Badillo, a model of fitness and a fine fitness model; and Santos Rodriguez, who looks terrific in sweats.

Dr. Wayne Westcott, one of the country's most renowned authorities on strength training, took the time to read the manuscript of an enthusiastic but unknown author and then wrote a glowing letter endorsing its publication. He exemplifies the observation that the bigger they are, the more they help others.

Dr. Thomas Sattler, my academic mentor and a bright, funny, energetic dynamo, has been an inspiration to his students and a joy to his friends.

Ellen Mandarino, a talented and creative graphic designer, never gave up her faith that this project would be completed (no matter how many times I changed things around). Her faith and encouragement sustained me on many a day.

Marge Pavich, who created the original drawings in the Resistance Workout Guide, maintained her sunny disposition in the face of the prodigious numbers of photographs I gave her as models for drawings ("Teri, I can't put your head on this guy's body!").

Steve Dahl, my friend and client, told me to relax and let it happen. Although it was not what I wanted to hear, it was exactly what I needed to hear.

Judy Tullis, of clear mind and thick skin and proprietor of the world's greatest secretarial service, somehow managed to keep me organized and otherwise saved my bacon on a regular basis. Someone was looking out for me on the day she became my friend. She's also got some dynamite lats.

Jay Nickleski, Mary Beckley, and Jo Cozzi helped with the pictures for the Resistance Workout Guide.

Barb Nevoral, Maryse Jerich, Kapila Anand, and Pramod Anand gave valued encouragement along the way.

Ron Lilek, my husband, my partner, and my friend—words are not enough.

Core Beliefs Behind Excellence in Personal Training

This book began with a vision and a set of core beliefs that preceded my entry into the personal training business and that I hope will become clear to you as you read on.

I used to close my eyes and visualize working as a knowledgeable, well-educated health professional. I imagined myself designing customized fitness programs that take into account the unique physical, psychological, and personal situations of a variety of individuals and groups, with clients who were excited about the empowering benefits of exercise and inspired to achieve their personal best. I aspired to be a member of a well-respected profession in which all practitioners perform their duties with the degree of skill and competence expected of health professionals, providing the finest quality of service to their clients with enthusiasm and care.

A Worst-Case Scenario

Some time after I started my business, when I was spending less time daydreaming and more time in the real world, I gradually discovered that my dream, though certainly possible for me to achieve, was at variance with the reality of my profession. The following story, told to me by a young woman I know, illustrates the point.

A client went to a health club for her first (and last, as it turned out) workout with a personal trainer. She tingled with excitement as she prepared to meet with her personal trainer for the first time. Even though she had been going to the health club for some time, she envisioned working with a professional personal trainer as the key to kicking her program into high gear and achieving that lean, sculpted look that entices most people into exercise in the first place. "This will be the way to get skinny," she thought gleefully. Leaving aside whether you think "getting skinny" is a laudable goal, you'll probably agree that it's preferable to thinking, *This will be the way to end up in the emergency room.* Her trainer was the club's manager and claimed to have a college degree in kinesiology. He looked the part, fit and lean with an enthusiastic manner. Not only that, he was a man with a plan. The primary objective for the workout—no, the be-all and end-all of this *first session*—was to keep her heart rate elevated, even during the resistance portion. Yes, he said, you will get dizzy. Yes, you will be winded. That's how we know you're getting a quality workout, he explained.

How did he plan to accomplish this quickened pulse and increased respiration? He decided that she should run. Not walk briskly, but embark on a flat-out, heart-pounding, sweat-pouring run through the club, dodging pieces of equipment and her fellow fitness enthusiasts.

They began the workout/obstacle course. In short order, it was obvious that this workout would not disappoint. Within only a few minutes, the client was winded, weak, and woozy. Her arms had turned to quivering jelly. He kept exhorting her to go faster, all the while saying, "Look at me; don't look down!" She followed his instructions well—so well, in fact, that she didn't notice the small platform surrounding one machine until she was sprawled on the floor with her face resting on it. She had turned her ankle and tripped. As she had fallen forward, she'd tried to brace herself with her now useless, exhausted arms, which barely cushioned her slide into what can best be described as a face skate. She said, "When I asked my trainer if my nose was bleeding, he said he thought I had a scratch."

Her trainer's attitude could charitably be described as unconcerned. In fact, he was completely blase but seemed grateful that it was winter. "When you get out to your car, just put some snow on your face to keep the swelling down," he said casually before sending her on her way. "What swelling? I thought it was just a scratch," the client thought as she walked shakily out to her car, her weakness and vertigo increasing with every step.

Somehow she was able to drive herself home. She stumbled into the house and lay down, hoping that soon she would feel if not normal, at least well enough to sit up. Several hours later, the excrutiating pain emanating from the center of her face convinced her that she had endured something more than just a scratch. She noted, "When I got to the emergency room, the staff informed me that I was lucky to have only a broken nose. They thought I had broken my cheekbone, too." Her trainer's reaction? He never even called to see if she was OK. In fact, she never heard from him again. (Her lawyer, however, did have several opportunities to talk to him and to the owners of the club.)

Learning From Others' Mistakes

The moral of the story is that there is a very wrong way to do personal training, and that plenty of people are doing it the wrong way. This incident is an illustration of a universal truth: As important and valuable as formal education is, without experience and common sense, it doesn't qualify you to do anything.

Another lesson: Just because someone wears the uniform and looks the part doesn't mean she can actually do the job. Think of that goofy old commercial where a popular soap opera actor hawked over-the-counter medication with the line, "I'm not a doctor, but I play one on TV." Looking fit doesn't qualify a person to design safe, effective exercise programs.

Finally, an undertaking started with poorly designed objectives and executed with poorly designed plans yields poor results. Raw enthusiasm and good intentions without careful thought behind them are a dangerous combination, especially where heavy objects are involved.

I hope that you take something else from this story. Remember how the client was looking forward to working with a trainer? How horribly disappointed this experience must have left her. I don't think the trainer understood the emotional investment she had in this session. The client viewed his expertise, support, and encouragement as the keys to transforming her body, and therefore her life. Perhaps to him, this session that she had eagerly anticipated for days was just another hour on the job. Perhaps he had good intentions but no common sense, a potentially dangerous combination. Whatever the case, he just didn't get it.

I want you to "get it," to understand what being a professional personal trainer is all about. My vision, though a little more realistic now, remains uncompromised: I want every trainer to understand what an important job she is doing and take seriously the responsibility to uphold the high standards that elevate our professional standing among the public. I want you to be the best you can be.

Core Beliefs: A Firm Foundation

As I thought more about my vision, I realized that it had developed from a collection of values. Without these core beliefs I would not have been able to put into words what being a personal trainer should be. They are the foundation on which the vision is built, so it's important that you know something about them.

Core Belief One: A Personal Trainer Is a Health Professional

It seems so obvious, but this point is too easily lost. Exercise is a powerful therapy. Administered correctly, it can dramatically improve most of the major indicators of good health (heart rate, blood pressure, endurance, strength, body composition). Conversely, administered incorrectly or negligently, exercise can be downright dangerous! A professional personal trainer must have a working knowledge of anatomy, physiology, and biomechanics so that he will know how to deal with each client's particular needs and limitations. How should you modify a shoulder press so your client can do it without pain? Should she be doing a shoulder press at all? How should the program of a 60-year-old diabetic differ from the program of a 30-year-old recreational athlete? Are there exercises that no one should do under any circumstances, or that this particular client shouldn't do? A professional personal trainer must be able to answer these questions.

Core Belief Two: Personal Trainers Are in a Position of Trust and Responsibility

We do a very important job, and therefore have a responsibility to do our work with professionalism rather than just go through the motions. We help people transform themselves from weak supplicants of whatever cards life deals them ("I used to like to work in my garden, but now my back hurts whenever I do") to fully functional, vigorous creatures who are in command of their own lives and excited about every new day and new possibility. Because we often detect silent diseases such as high blood pressure through our monitoring and screening, we are sometimes a person's first introduction to needed medical attention. This responsibility is of the utmost importance.

Perhaps it is because of the seriousness with which I regard this issue that I am astounded by the attitude of many in the fitness field. I don't mean the many fine, conscientious trainers who have great credentials and attitudes. I also don't mean you. The very fact that you're reading this book demonstrates that you have the commitment to be the best that separates you from the people I'm about to describe. I mean people like club owners who pay fit but unqualified people $10 an hour and call them "trainers." Or the muscular guy who's lifted weights for 12 years and has 20-inch biceps, but doesn't know a rotator cuff from a pant cuff.

As a personal trainer, you are in a position to have a dramatic, lifelong impact on the health of your clients. If you do a good job, your clients will be eternally grateful, and they will show it. As a person with the ability to profoundly change people's lives, you are in a unique position of trust and responsibility. Your clients will take your advice and suggestions very seriously. They will tell you personal things about their lives, their hopes, their dreams. They will let you see their real feelings, not just the happy public face that they put on the rest of the day. You must be worthy of their trust.

Core Belief Three: A Personal Trainer Is a Teacher

Recently, a client, knowing about my passion for rubber stamps, gave me one for my collection. It says, "To Teach Is to Touch Someone's Life Forever." At first I was confused. Why is this for me? I haven't stood at a chalkboard since I completed the required semester of teaching in my master's program, and to this day I have trouble operating an overhead projector. Then it hit me. Of course, a personal trainer must, in addition to all other roles, be a teacher. Our overall objective must be independence for our clients. We must empower them so that they are confident enough to exercise on their own, not just when we're cracking the whip behind them. To paraphrase an old saying, "Give a man a dumbbell and you work him for a day; teach him to train and you make him fit for a lifetime." It's not enough to just show your clients how to do their workouts correctly while you're there watching them. You have to teach them and help them master the important form points of each exercise, the things you look for when you watch them, the fine adjustments that you make to improve the effectiveness of the workout.

Core Belief Four: Any Important Endeavor Must Begin With Agreed-Upon, Specific Goals and Objectives

Everything in life, including exercise, should be about goals and objectives. Your programs, from the selection of each exercise, to the number of sets and repetitions, to the overall yearly plan for each client, should be designed with specific short-term, intermediate, and long-term objectives in mind. Similarly, you should understand the specific objective of each exercise you recommend. What muscles or muscle groups are you trying to work? Why? Making these decisions requires a lot of thought. Think back to the broken nose story. That was a great, albeit extreme, example of a poorly formulated objective leading to a really bad result. The law of unintended consequences strikes again.

Goals are more specific than general objectives. They provide landmarks on your client's journey to reaching her ultimate objective. As important as they are, designing a program with specific short-term, intermediate, and long-term goals is only the first part of the process. You've got to get your client to buy into the plan. If you can convince her that there is a logical thought process and sound planning behind what you're asking her to do, you'll have a much better chance of getting her to stick to the program over the long run. Specific, measurable, agreed-upon goals plus commitment to the process equals results!

A final but very significant point about the importance of goals and objectives: One of the most important things you will do for your clients is to encourage and motivate them, especially during times when they are experiencing plateaus, injuries, or other periods when they don't see any progress. During these times, your job is to encourage your client to keep his eyes on the prize and remember why it's important to work out consistently and stick to a healthy diet. You must be the voice that answers the question "What's the point?" when his enthusiasm for the program flags by reminding him about his overall goals and how terrific he will feel when he achieves them. In short, motivation comes from mutual understanding and agreement about agreed-upon long- and short-term objectives. You must be able to explain the objective of every exercise, every set, and every rep you ask your client to do. Here's something really cool to think about: After your client has worked with you awhile, he will actually hear your voice inside his head, encouraging him, telling him how to do it right. Think about that: It's almost like immortality.

Core Belief Five: Never Run From the Truth

Recently, one of those horror-story-of-the-night network television magazine shows featured a piece on the overprescription of antibiotics. They did the usual ambush, hidden-camera thing that has become a TV cliché. An anonymous producer, working undercover, visited several doctors' offices, feigning flulike symptoms and requesting antibiotics. Two out of three of the doctors wrote prescriptions for antibiotics, even though these drugs are worthless against viruses. The next day the reporter returned to the office of one of the prescribing physicians to ask her why she would give a patient who wasn't even sick a prescription that would have no effect even if she were. The doctor explained that it wasn't her fault that patients demand antibiotics, and besides, "Medicine is a business and if I don't give them what they want they'll go somewhere else." This attitude reflects a shirking of professional responsibility that you should avoid at all costs.

Even if ethics aren't enough to convince you, here's another reason. The doctor couldn't be more wrong: This kind of thinking isn't good for business. The day will come when you have to tell a client something she doesn't want to hear. Let's face it: We'd all like to be told, "Nah, you don't need to stop eating hot fudge sundaes and French fries four

or five times a day. You can eat what you want and still have a body like a *Sports Illustrated* swimsuit model. Exercise? Only when you feel like it." No, you aren't the food police, but you are going to have to tell your clients that, if they want to achieve their goals, there are certain foods and beverages that they need to consume only in moderation, if not eliminate.

Furthermore, there are going to be days when they are going to have to push themselves (with your help, of course) to get their workouts in even when they'd rather be watching TV. You, like the doctor, may think that such frankness is no way to win friends and influence people. You may be especially reluctant to say these things to someone who is paying you. Trust me: Your clients will respect you for telling them the truth. They know that they can't reach their goals without enduring a little D & D (discomfort and deprivation), and they don't really expect you to say anything different. In fact, they'd be horribly disappointed if you spared them the challenges you have planned for them. You can't blame them for trying, though.

Core Belief Six: They Say the Devil Is in the Details, but That's Not All You'll Find There

In my 10-plus years of personal training, I have observed that something else is also in the details: the difference between excellence and mediocrity, between achievement and failure, between progress and stagnation. Being professional means more than the obvious things like looking the part, showing up on time, and not dropping a dumbbell on the client's foot. The differences between the qualified health professional and the glorified spotter might not be obvious at first glance. They might even be invisible, but the difference in the effect on clients is anything but. It is dramatic. Your background in anatomy and physiology, not to mention your knowledge and understanding of your client's unique needs, marks you for all the world as a caring, knowledgeable professional. Your attentiveness to every detail, and especially to your client, distinguishes you from the casual hit-or-miss gym rat providing an occasional tip or spot, or the distracted club employee who may be called away at any moment to answer a phone or help someone at the counter.

Core Belief Seven: Individuals Have More Control Over Their Health Than a Health Professional Does

We have a responsibility to educate our clients about how much control they have over their own health and independence. Many of us have accepted as inevitable the loss of strength and independence that people often suffer as they get older, but we know now that our bodies don't have to tumble into an accelerating decline if we are prepared to do something about it. With your help, your client will realize the control he has over his own health, and this feeling of power and positive energy will carry over into every aspect of life.

Core Belief Eight: A Business, No Matter How Small, Should Be Run Like a Business

Some trainers seem to believe that because they are one-person businesses (or maybe because they don't have to wear suits, nylons, and dress shoes to work) they are somehow exempt from all the irritating paperwork that torments other small-business people. To remain clueless about these things is not only unprofessional, it's risky.

Taxes aren't the only thing to worry about. Potential liability for injuries is a serious issue for personal trainers, whether they realize it or not. It's ironic that the trainer most likely to injure someone is the one least likely to have any insurance or any assets to compensate the victims of his negligence. Even though the best protection is careful planning and program design, a practicing health professional should maintain adequate insurance coverage and provide his clients with informed consents and waivers to sign before beginning a program.

The Moral of the Story

Recently, I received a note from a longtime client. In part, she wrote, "As one gets older, it is too easy to accept and believe in a lot of self-imposed limitations. I was fortunate enough to meet you before much damage was done. You have a unique and nurturing approach that I'm sure is natural, not cultivated. It stems from a high degree of intelligence, sensitivity, and generosity. Simply stated, thanks to me for finding you. Thanks to you for being there." My vision for you is to receive notes like this from your many satisfied clients and to glow with satisfaction and pride the way I'm glowing as I write these words and relive the feeling I had when I read that note.

Establishing Your Personal Training Business

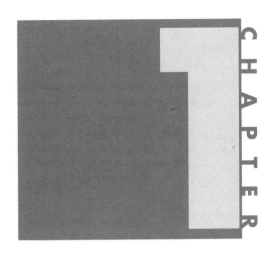

CHAPTER 1

Standing on the Threshold

Questions we'll answer in this chapter:

- How do I know whether personal training is for me?

- What do I need to get started?

- Does it matter which certification I get?

- Should I start my own business or work for someone else?

- Is it better to work in a gym or health club, or in people's homes?

You're considering a career in personal training. After all, you've always loved working out. Unlike many of your friends, who sometimes say you're becoming a little bit of a bore talking about the benefits of exercise and a healthy lifestyle, you view your time in the gym as the best hour of the day. By becoming a personal trainer, you can do what you love and make money. The more you think about it, the more you realize that this idea is a win-win. Now what?

Threshold Question 1: Is It Right for Me?

In every career there are trade-offs, and personal training is no exception. The question you have to answer is whether the trade-offs add up to a good deal for you.

The Bad Part

Despite what you may be tempted to think when you listen to your friends describe their glamorous, high-paying gigs, there is no perfect occupation, and personal training is no exception.

Scheduling Problems

When you're a personal trainer, you have days like this: You have a 6:45 A.M. workout at Client A's home and a 10:30 A.M. workout at Client B's house, which is 10 minutes from Client A's. The only problem is that you have a 9:00 A.M. workout at Client C's club, which is 30 minutes away from Client A's and Client B's! Argh!

Unfortunately, despite your efforts to make sure that you schedule appointments close to each other to avoid nonstop road running, sometimes it will be unavoidable. Also, clients sometimes need to change their regular appointments because of conflicts in their schedules. You must try to accommodate them but also try to structure your regular schedule so that such deviations are the exception and not the rule. The juggling act isn't easy, but it does get easier after you've established your clientele. In the beginning, it's really tempting to take any client you think you can help, no matter how far away.

An important word to the wise: Resist the desire to fill every waking moment with client sessions. You must include time for planning, preparing workouts, and doing administrative work. I suggest that you plan one hour of office work for every client session you schedule. In addition, be sure to schedule free time into your week. Burnout is a real risk for personal trainers! If you don't recharge your batteries on a regular basis, you will find yourself going through the motions, conducting workouts like a robot and losing your edge. Avoid this danger by planning ahead.

Travel Isn't Always Fun

Many personal trainers work in some combination of clubs and homes and therefore spend a fairly large portion of the day traveling. (Yes, you need a reliable car.) Although travel is inevitable under these circumstances, do anything you can to avoid excessive travel. Not only does it wear you out, but it also limits the number of hours you can work with clients. If you can't stand the idea of traveling a lot, consider a personal training job in a club.

Not Enough Hours in the Day

Speaking of hours, they won't be 9 to 5 in this gig. The reasons should be obvious. Most of the people you will be working with have jobs or other commitments and can't work out in the middle of the day. You will probably work what is effectively a split shift—three or four sessions in the morning and another three or four in the evening.

Many Jobs Rolled Into One

When you work for yourself, you have to wear many hats—manager, bookkeeper, and secretary as well as service provider. You need to decide whether you want to assume the responsibility of your own business. If you enjoy working with clients but would prefer not to deal with administrative responsibilities, consider strongly whether you should be in business for yourself. You may be better suited to working as an employee in a club.

Lugging the Equipment

It's not only enduring those long and irregular hours that will leave you feeling as if you've been pulled through a keyhole at the end of some days. Between carrying a heavy bag full of equipment from house to house and demonstrating exercises, you will learn what seems obvious: Personal training is a physical job!

The Good Part

Although some personal trainers work in a health club setting as employees, this book is written for those of you who are more entrepreneurial. If you currently work in a club and are frustrated by some

If You're Having Trouble Deciding . . .

. . .whether to become a personal trainer, think about this: If you decide to take the plunge and your business is successful, I guarantee there will be a beautiful, clear day when you are cruising along in your car, clad in brightly colored spandex, liberated from the business attire that binds so many of your friends, listening to tunes in the middle of the day rather than the annoying babble of office gossip, bathed in sunshine rather than complexion-sallowing fluorescent light, wondering what took you so long to decide to become a personal trainer.

of the limitations imposed by the need to see a minimum number of clients in a day or by management restrictions on how you design your programs, you should consider striking out on your own. Having your own business has tremendous rewards that make all the hard work worth it for many. You will be able to provide better, more personalized service, and you will be able to use your knowledge and skill to design innovative programs for your clients.

Flexible Hours

Irregular hours are also flexible hours—time in the middle of the day for other things like grocery shopping, buying stamps, doing your own workout. All of these things can be done at times when most other people are working—a definite advantage.

Creative and Expressive Freedom

One of the most rewarding things about doing personal training is the opportunity to help clients set goals and reach them. Each client is a new opportunity for you to apply your knowledge and skill to reach a desired result.

Fulfilling Professional Relationships

My clients are the greatest people who have ever walked the face of the earth (and I'm not just saying that because I know many of them are reading this). They think I've changed their lives, but it's really the other way around: They've changed my life. I draw inspiration from their determination. I look forward to hearing about all the interesting things they're doing. I feel fortunate to run ideas by them and get their advice. It's a mutual admiration society, which shouldn't be surprising. When you help someone achieve something as significant and life-changing as becoming fit, watching her transform not only her body but her attitude, you become a part of that transformation. And the really amazing thing is that it transforms you, too.

Threshold Question 2: What Do I Need to Get Started?

After you've figured out whether personal training is right for you, the next questions you need to ask yourself are about your own readiness. You may need more training, and that might affect your decision to go ahead with starting your own personal training business.

Do I Need a Degree?

A degree is like a computer. No, you don't *need* one, in the sense that you can get by in life and in business without it; however, you'll get a lot farther with it. Suppose a potential client wants to hire Joe Muscleman to train him. Joe barely made it through high school and will never be mistaken for Albert Einstein's long-lost twin brother. What's wrong with this picture? From a legal and regulatory standpoint, nothing. At least for the present time, personal training is a self-regulated industry. Consumers are free to hire anyone they want, and service providers don't need any credentials.

That's theory; here's reality: Both individual clients and managers at quality clubs who hire personal trainers tend to be well educated, and many of them understand what qualifications and educational background they should demand in a personal trainer. Surveys have shown that fewer than half (in some surveys, fewer than 25%) of personal trainers surveyed have earned a degree in a fitness field. But because most clients looking for a personal trainer have degrees, they will choose a degreed trainer almost every time, even if it costs them more money.

I suggest that you acquire at least a bachelor's degree in exercise physiology, exercise science, physical education, or some related field. If you don't have a degree yet, begin taking classes. Some colleges and universities have special programs for fitness enthusiasts looking at careers in personal

5

training. Courses in anatomy and physiology, nutrition, exercise physiology, and related subjects will be invaluable to you; and potential clients are much more likely to become actual clients if you have taken such classes. You will be able to pursue your career as a personal trainer and get clients while you're in school, provided that you get certified by a reputable organization.

Do I Need Certification?

Unlike a degree, which is still at least officially an optional requirement, certification is essential. For one thing, the overwhelming majority of personal trainers are certified. If you aren't, you'll come up way short by comparison. Second, you'll find it impossible to get liability insurance without certification.

Flip to the back of any bodybuilding magazine, past the photographs of the massive, tanned hulks with the bikini-clad admirers draped across their impressive chests, and page through the ads. No doubt you'll see several advertisements for certification programs, some of which require nothing more than writing a check and completing a home study program. You might be tempted to write said check and get started tomorrow. That seems like a

Reasons to Get Certified by One of the Top Programs

- Your professional credibility will be enhanced.
- You will learn something while preparing for the exam.
- You will be able to get liability insurance through the organization.
- You will be able to get referrals from physicians and other health professionals.

lot less hassle than one of these highfalutin programs that make you get a degree and take a written (and maybe even a practical) exam. So you might reasonably ask, "Does it matter which certification I get?" The short answer: Yes.

I recall a conversation I had once with an extremely inarticulate muscle-bound gym rat who told me that he was very confident about his ability to work with clients because he's "certified by four organizations." I didn't have the heart to tell him that certifications are sort of like situation comedies: There are a lot of them, but only a few are any

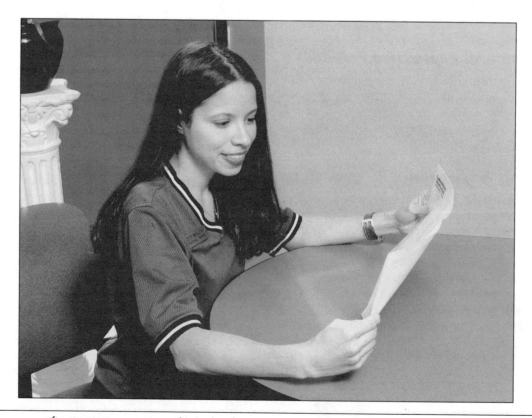

Getting your certification is a reason to smile. It identifies you as a professional.

good. Approximately 300 organizations certify trainers, or purport to certify trainers, and new ones are created every day. But only about a dozen are in the top echelon. Some personal trainers, or some people who want to be personal trainers, seem to think that just saying they are "certified" ends all questions about their qualifications. Well, I can tell you that I'm a "singer," and I might be the next Celine Dion or I might just enjoy singing in the shower. It's the same thing with the word "certification." Call me crazy, but to me, just because somebody has $400 for a weekend workshop and can fog a mirror, that doesn't make him a qualified personal trainer.

Certifying organizations range from those that require you to pass a written and practical exam (such as the American College of Sports Medicine, or ACSM) to those that require only that you pay a fee (usually hefty) and attend a weekend seminar. I know of at least one program founded for the sole reason that existing certification programs like ACSM's set such high standards and have such "extremely clinical" education materials. They make no bones about the fact that they want to set the bar low enough so that anyone with a detectable pulse and a valid credit card can make it over! These substandard programs are tempting because some of them permit a great deal of flexibility not only in their requirements but also the dates and times you can take their tests. As previously mentioned, some even permit home study and testing.

Before you write your check, though, consider this: Fitness consumers are beginning to understand the differences among the various certification programs, so you should aim high and get the best certification you can. Your decision about certification will affect whether you will get referrals from other health professionals and whether you can get access to clubs and gyms. If anyone can just pay the fee and get the organization's certificate, is it really worth anything? What sort of reputation does this certification have? Does it have high standards? How long has the program been in business? Will you be able to get liability insurance with this certification?

Recommended Certifying Bodies

Aerobics and Fitness Association of America (AFAA)

15250 Ventura Blvd., Ste. 200
Sherman Oaks, CA 91403
818-905-0040 or 800-446-2322

American College of Sports Medicine (ACSM)

P.O. Box 1440
Indianapolis, IN 46206-1440
317-637-9200

American Council on Exercise (ACE—formerly IDEA)

5820 Oberlin Dr., Ste. 102
San Diego, CA 92121
800-825-3636

National Dance-Exercise Instructors Training Association (NDEITA)

1503 South Washington Ave., Ste. 208
Minneapolis, MN 55454-1037
612-340-1306

National Strength and Conditioning Association (NSCA)

P.O. Box 38909
Colorado Springs, CO 80937
719-632-6722 or 402-476-6669

The ACSM certification is the gold standard in the field. I highly recommend it. The American Council on Exercise (ACE, the most widely held certification), the Aerobics and Fitness Association of America (AFAA), the National Dance-Exercise Instructors Training Association (NDEITA), and the National Strength and Conditioning Association (NSCA) certifications are also highly regarded. Don't waste as much as several hundred dollars on a substandard certification. Make the effort and go the extra mile. Get certified by ACSM, ACE, AFAA, NDEITA, or NSCA. You will be glad you did, and so will your clients.

Do I Need a License?

Sometimes it seems as if anyone can claim to be a personal trainer—the muscular bag boy who helps out at a friend's gym in his spare time, the veteran of countless aerobics classes. The reason it seems that way is that, theoretically at least, it's true: Anyone can! Personal training is a self-regulated industry, and any individual, qualified or not, can claim to be a personal trainer.

Though several states have considered requiring licenses for fitness instructors and personal trainers, none have enacted such regulations. (However, Louisiana recently enacted a license requirement for clinical exercise physiologists, those who work in cardiac rehabilitation programs under the supervision of physicians.)

Although you may be relieved that you don't need a license, you should know that many potential clients have serious concerns about the competence of personal trainers, and they will be looking for evidence that you are more than a friendly personality and a hard body. They are likely to look to your academic background, experience, and certification.

Do I Need CPR Training?

CPR is like your local fire department or the Maytag repairman—you hope you never have to call them, but you're awfully glad they're there if you do. Speaking of your local fire department, they sometimes offer CPR classes. You can also get your CPR card by attending a class and passing a test at your local YMCA or American Red Cross chapter. Be sure to do so well in advance of the deadline for sending in your certification exam registration. You will need to send a copy of your CPR card along with your exam registration form.

It is absolutely necessary that you obtain and maintain current CPR certification. Aside from the remote possibility that you will actually have to use your lifesaving skills, most certification programs require that you have a current, valid CPR certification in order to register for the exam. The legal standard in most U.S. communities dictates that a reasonable and prudent personal trainer will have a current CPR certification, and your liability insurance carrier may ask for proof of your compliance with this requirement. Unquestionably, if you ever find yourself in a position where your legal status matters, it will be significantly weaker if you don't maintain current CPR certification.

Threshold Question 3: *Do I Have What It Takes?*

You've got a degree, and you're certified by ACSM. Your knowledge of anatomy, physiology, biomechanics, and nutrition is first-rate. Is this enough? Unfortunately, it isn't. To move into the upper echelon of professional personal trainers, you also need superior communication skills and a personal commitment to fitness.

Superior Communication Skills

A personal trainer must be able to explain and clarify, simplify the complex, and focus the client's attention on making that all-important mind-muscle connection. It's more than just breaking down biomechanical technicalities.

Contrary to popular belief and practice, listening is the biggest part of communication. Your function is not to demonstrate how much you know by controlling and dominating the session, filling it with a nonstop lecture. You are there to help your client reach his goals, and you need to adapt to his needs and wants. Listen and be flexible to create the most effective and enjoyable personal training experience possible.

Words mean things—usually different things to different people. Choose them carefully and tailor them to your client. Your goal is to make yourself understood. Using anatomical and scientific words may be appropriate in some contexts. I have clients who are physicians, nurses, and chiropractors. With these clients, it is not only appropriate, it is more understandable to say "iliac crest" rather than "hipbone." On the other hand, a novice exerciser who has no background in anatomy is likely to think the iliac crest is something you encountered on your last ski vacation. One of your goals should be to educate your client about her body. Eventually your client's anatomical vocabulary should improve enough to include some of the most commonly used body landmarks. During your first few months together, she will have more than enough to remember. Keep this in mind when deciding which words to use and when.

"God gave us two ears and one mouth for a reason."

Ancient proverb

Don't forget the role of nonverbal communication. Do you arrive at your session round-shouldered and head hanging, looking like you've lost three nights of sleep, your wallet, and your last friend? What message does your posture convey? Tired, low energy, zero enthusiasm? Ask yourself—would you want to work out coached by you?

Personal Commitment to Fitness

A friend of mine recently attended a workshop on parenting. As she listened to the lecturer sharing her insights about how to get children to behave, a thought occurred to her. She raised her hand and asked, "How many children do you have?" The young woman seemed a little flustered, and said hesitatingly, "Well, none." Needless to say, that revelation affected her credibility like a needle affects a helium balloon. The audience's attention drifted from the speaker's words to football standings, TV sitcoms, and similar topics of greater seriousness. Like most intelligent adults today, they had little patience listening to someone who has never done something tell other people how to do it.

"Do as I say, not as I do" may work for some parents (not many, I suspect), but without genuine passion and commitment, you will not be an effective fitness coach. A successful personal trainer must have a personal commitment to fitness. He must feel passionate about what exercise can do for the body, the mind, and the spirit. He must infect his client with this passion so that the client feels it, too. Going through the motions won't cut it for you or your clients. You will lose your tolerance for the challenges inherent in a personal trainer's day. Soon you will lose your clients, too.

"The difference between the right word and the almost right word is the difference between the lightning and the lightning bug."

Mark Twain

Approach personal training with alacrity and commitment, and watch your satisfied client base grow!

Threshold Question 4: Do I Want to Start My Own Business or Work for Someone Else?

Like attorneys, architects, accountants, and other professionals, personal trainers can work for themselves or as employees for someone else. The decision to start your own business is like the decision to get married—that is, very serious and not to be entered into without some sober deliberation. Owning and operating a business, even if it has only one employee (you) is not for everyone. Here are some reasons that people who start their own businesses often give to explain why they did so, and some things to consider about each one.

Dope Avoidance

Perhaps you think back on a job you had, or even about the job you have now. Your boss was (is) a dope. Maybe, you think, *My next boss could be a dope, too, even a worse dope if that's possible. That's for the birds! I'll work for myself. Then I'll be the boss!* That sounds good, until you consider that when you run a service business, you have not one boss, but many—your clients. The reality is that we all have a boss; even your boss, the dope, works for his superiors, or, if he's the head honcho, for the customers or the clients of the business. Of course, we hope that none of your clients will be dopes, but whether they are or not, you may have to work with them to keep the business running, at least until you can replace the income that they bring in. If you are motivated by a desire to avoid dealing with an idiot boss who wastes your time and tries to break your spirit, be clear about this point. As an entrepreneur, you will have some choice about whom you work for, but as any entrepreneur will tell you, the only dope-free zone is the Betty Ford Center.

Freedom, Independence, and Control

You don't want someone, almost certainly someone who doesn't know one-tenth of what you know (i.e., the dope), telling you what to do and when and how to do it. You want to design the workouts that clients do. You want to decide when you work and where. You want to tell them what kind of spandex to wear. OK, I'm kidding about that last one, but the point is that you want to be in charge. You don't want to have to get your programs approved by some higher authority or answer to anyone other than yourself and your clients. You want to take time off when you want. You are not only the boss, but also the expert, right?

Yes, but even a boss/expert must work within situational limitations. You want to work "when you want," but your schedule will necessarily revolve around the times when the paying customers are available to work out, which is usually early in the morning (often *very* early) or in the evening after work. In addition to actually performing the service for clients, you will also be responsible for sales and marketing, billing and other accounting matters, and every other aspect of the business. With all these demands, you will soon discover that "flextime" means that you get to set your own hours, which are usually 24/7. So much for all that free time you thought you'd have by becoming the boss.

But even if you have to work long and weird hours, when it comes to the actual workouts, at least you can do whatever you want. You've got that going for you, right? Not exactly. Though in one sense it's true that you will have complete freedom to design the programs and instruct your clients in how to perform them, this freedom brings with it a mountain of responsibility. Most obviously, you have the responsibility to avoid hurting anyone, which attorneys call the legal duty to avoid negligence (i.e., to conduct yourself and your programs as a reasonable, prudent professional personal trainer would under similar circumstances). If a client sues you for negligence, your conduct will be judged against recognized industry standards, such as the American College of Sports Medicine's Guidelines for Exercise Testing and Prescription.

In other words, your freedom is constrained by the limits of what is considered acceptable in the field. Your program design, choice of equipment, instruction, and any other aspect of conduct with respect to the client will be scrutinized against these standards if anyone gets hurt. That's when what once appeared to be an innovative, cutting-edge exercise regimen becomes, in hindsight and with the assistance of a skilled personal injury attorney, an obviously dangerous, negligent, injury-producing scheme that even you, in your pathetic impersonation of a fitness professional, should have known better than to ever attempt with this client. In addition, you will have to operate within the confines of laws against nutritional counseling by nonprofessionals, and similar laws and regulations.

Most important, even if your clients are all the warm, wonderful people that I suspect they will be, remember that they are still your ultimate bosses. Repeat after me: "*You* are working for *them*." (Or should that be "*I* am working for *them*"? Whatever—you get the idea!) This is a mantra for all successful service professionals who recognize that the people who write the checks are the ones in charge. These people pay professionals to use their knowledge and expertise to solve problems for them. In your case, they pay you to help them reach specific fitness goals. If you consider the opportunity to yell, boss people around, and otherwise boost your ego by being "in charge" as a perk of owning your own business, perhaps you should consider looking for a gig as a crossing guard.

Creative Expression

You know that you would really enjoy creating innovative, safe, effective programs for a variety of different types of clients, and you want to be able to do that without an employer breathing down your neck and asking you to explain everything you do. Personal training does offer the opportunity to use your knowledge and experience creatively to design something "perfect" for every client. It's challenging and fun to try to come up with new ways to do the same old exercises, and, provided that you stay within the confines of accepted industry standards, you are limited only by your imagination. The chance to be creative is a win-win: You will get enormous personal satisfaction when your clients appreciate the time and effort you put into designing safe and effective workouts while keeping the boredom beast at bay. Your clients will reward you not only by becoming devoted to you, but also by singing your praises to their friends and acquaintances, which is the very best form of marketing.

Although it's not necessarily a bad thing, the freedom to be creative carries with it the responsibility to take the time to genuinely think about every aspect of the client's program. You need to be able to explain why this exercise is appropriate for this client. Of course, if you are ever asked for that explanation, chances are the question will not be asked in the context of an interview with a network news show or for *People* magazine. Best-case scenario: You have a curious client who is eager to learn. Worst-case: It is asked as part of an adversary proceeding (lawsuit), and the person asking it will have the benefit of perfect hindsight. In that light, it's easy to see how much more carefree you can be when someone else tells you what's contraindicated and what's OK.

Big Bucks

If you're going to work hard and be the best you can be, why not reap most of the financial reward? As an employee, you will probably be paid 40% to 60% of the per-session rate that clients pay. For example, in many large health clubs, clients pay $30 to $60 per session, and trainers are paid $15 to $35. Although this may seem unfair to employee trainers, to remain profitable, service businesses typically pay 30% to 45% of gross revenue to their employees. If they exceed this guideline, they won't make it (Justice 1996).

Given this apparent disparity, the answer to the question "Should I start my own personal training business?" might seem to be a no-brainer. If you don't open your own business and make twice as much, you're either a dilettante or a fool. Like many things that appear obvious at first, though, this choice isn't. The flaw in that analysis is that it's not about what you make. It's about what you keep. Consider the following:

• **Taxes.** Most people have heard of the supposed tax advantages of opening their own businesses, and it is true that business owners may have the opportunity to take certain deductions unavailable to employees. The value of a tax deduction depends on factors such as marital status, home ownership, and the myriad of other variables that make up an individual's tax status. So in the end, those "great" deductions might not be enough to buy a newspaper and cup of coffee. In addition, it comes as a shock to many new entrepreneurs to learn to what extent the hydra-headed monster of government—federal, state, county, and city—has invaded the private sector. When you see all the papers that you have to file, you'll be amazed that anyone can stay in business and still make a living!

• **Administrative expenses.** Filing all of those papers requires a lot of time and effort. Unless you're an accountant, you'll need to hire one if you own a business. Come to think of it, even if you are trained as an accountant, you won't have time to do your own accounting. If you work as an employee, your employer takes care of tax filings and all the other required paperwork to keep a business running and out of trouble. Employees get their paychecks prepared by a bookkeeper or payroll service. If you are the boss, you will have to write the checks to pay your suppliers or prepare the invoices that you need to send to clients to make sure that you get paid.

• **Facilities and equipment.** Most employers provide the equipment that you use to train clients. In a club setting, they spend thousands of dollars on the building and equipment, dollars that you don't have to spend when you show up to train a client. If you work for yourself, you will have to buy some equipment.

• **Marketing.** Business owners invest in advertising and other promotional activities that highlight the features and benefits that the business has to offer. These expenditures inspire prospective clients to call. As an employee, you don't have to find clients yourself; they come to you. Granted, often they come to you because of your personal reputation, but that takes time to establish. In the beginning, before any word-of-mouth promotion, it costs money to let the world know how great you are. If you own the business, that money will come out of your pocket.

Business owners must pay for innumerable other expenses, such as office supplies, membership dues for professional organizations, postage, supplies, and the ever-popular "miscellaneous expenses." After all these expenses are paid, a well-run service business will earn a profit of 5% to 15%. Any less than that and it's time to pull the plug.

The Bottom Line

Ultimately, the decision to start your own business turns on one very important question: Why do you want to run your own business?

The decision about whether to be your own boss or someone else's employee depends on your personality and your personal situation. Although most of us have formed our basic personalities by the time we hit preschool, our life situations are always changing. Even if you were the kid who always had a lemonade stand, a paper route, or some other way to separate your schoolmates from their allowance money, what works today may not work tomorrow. At the beginning of your personal training career, you may decide that you would benefit from working under the supervision of a more experienced trainer. Your family situation may not allow you to spend the extra time you'd need to run a business and be a professional personal trainer. For these reasons, and any one of a gazillion others that are unique to every personal trainer, it would make sense to work for someone else. After a while, your circumstances may change and you might want to try striking out on your own.

If You Do Decide to Start Your Own Business, Start Here

If you do decide to start your own business, do yourself a favor and write a simple business plan. Most people get a knot in their stomachs at the mere mention of the words "business plan." They fear that it will be too difficult, too time consuming, and too confusing. If you are one of those people who would rather have dental work without anesthesia than even think about writing a business plan, here's a suggestion: Don't think of it as a business plan. Think of it as a way to organize your thoughts and plans and decide how you can best invest your time and money. Isn't it better to find out that you live in an area that can't support the high-end, luxury personal training business you have in mind? Of course it is! Otherwise, you will end up wasting your time (and probably a considerable amount of money) trying to make an unworkable idea work. You will end up frustrated, exhausted, and broke. Now that you are convinced, consult chapter 2 for a sample business plan, how such a plan can help you get off to a successful start, and instructions on how to write one of your own.

Threshold Question 5: Do I Want to Work in a Club or in People's Homes?

Personal trainers work in many environments. Commercial health clubs need personal trainers. So do community wellness centers, hospital fitness facilities, and bodybuilding gyms. Many of the most successful personal trainers work in people's homes.

These clients appreciate the privacy and personal service this type of arrangement brings. Here are some factors to consider as you think about the place you want to fill with your knowledge, enthusiasm, and positive energy.

- **Income.** Clients are willing to pay more for the privacy and convenience of having a professional personal trainer work with them in their homes. This sort of personal attention is the ultimate in service, and they know it. They also know that personal trainers who travel between locations must charge more to compensate them for the opportunity cost associated with traveling to different locations.

- **Opportunity cost.** "Opportunity cost" is just a fancy term economists use to describe a simple fact: You can't be in two places at once. When you're traveling between client locations, you can't be working with (and billing) a client. That unbillable travel time can destroy the profitability of your business if you aren't careful.

- **Equipment.** Do you want to put your client on a stepper for 10 minutes, then a treadmill for 10, then an elliptical trainer for 10? How about having him do a squat using a Smith machine, then a seated leg curl, followed by a Hack squat? This type of workout is generally possible only in a health club (although high-powered, wealthy clients will often buy whatever you suggest they need for their in-home gyms). What if your in-home client doesn't have any equipment? Get used to schlepping those 15-pound dumbbells in and out of the house.

- **Isolation.** When you work in a club, you have people around you all the time. If you have a question, there's usually someone you can ask. When you work for yourself, you spend a lot of time alone. That's not necessarily a bad thing. Some people enjoy solitude. Others find the silence deafening. Only you can decide.

Don't Stress Out

Remember that **you always have the option of a do-over.** Although important, the decisions about starting your own business and working in a club or in clients' homes are never etched in stone. Genuine professionals know that their first-rate skills and impeccable reputations let them write their own tickets.

Advantages of Working for Yourself

- Greater income potential
- Freedom to decide when, where, and with whom to work
- Freedom to design and execute workouts as you see fit
- Freedom to decide what to wear
- Higher status
- Potential tax advantages

Advantages of Working for Someone Else

- No investment in equipment, marketing, or business organization costs
- Responsibility limited to showing up on time and doing the one job for which you were hired
- No need to sell or look for clients
- No responsibility for administrative activities required to run a business (tax filings, zoning and other regulations, payroll)
- Shared responsibility for avoiding negligence
- Employer-provided benefits such as medical insurance, liability insurance, continuing education

Advantages of Working in a Club

- No need to purchase equipment
- No need to lug equipment between clients' homes
- Large variety of available equipment
- No pets, children, ringing phones, or other distractions for you or your client
- No unbillable travel time
- Ability to interact with other trainers and benefit from their knowledge

Advantages of Working As an In-Home Trainer

- Higher dollar revenues and income
- Less monotony, less potential boredom
- No annoying loud music
- No need to share equipment or "work in" (i.e., asking another gym member to let your client do a set while the gym member is resting between sets)
- Friendlier atmosphere
- More privacy

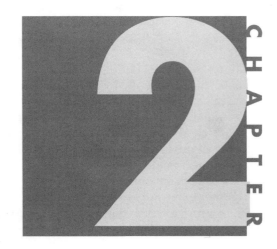

CHAPTER 2

Business and Legal Matters

Questions we'll answer in this chapter:

- How should I structure my business?

- What are the pros and cons of incorporating my business?

- How much should I charge my clients?

- How do I know if I'm making money?

- What taxes affect my business?

- What specific actions can I take to reduce the chance of being sued?

- Will a waiver protect me from a lawsuit?

- What are the ethics of personal training?

The following text is provided for general informational purposes only. Every person's situation is different, and your personal situation might require the attention of an attorney licensed to practice in your state. This information is no substitute for the personal advice of knowledgeable advisors (a licensed attorney, a good accountant) who have reviewed your circumstances. When you're deciding whether to incorporate, what to do about your tax situation, or a similar important matter, do yourself a favor—get a good lawyer and an honest accountant!

How Should I Set Up My Business?

Let's take a look at some general information about the various ways that you can structure a business. As stated previously, this information is a starting point, designed to give you a framework for organizing your thoughts so that when you meet with your attorney and your accountant, you will be able to decide on the best type of business structure for you.

The three basic types of business organizations are sole proprietorships, partnerships, and corporations. There are some other, more specialized ways to set up a business, such as limited liability companies, but those need not concern us here. Your business will probably be one of the basic three types. Let's look at each of them.

Sole Proprietorship

For many entrepreneurs, who tend to be rugged individualists by nature, the sole proprietorship is the way to go. It is formed by a person who decides one day, "I want to start my own business," and hangs out a shingle (literally or figuratively, by selling a product or providing a service for a fee). Most personal trainers who start their own businesses do just that and are therefore sole proprietorships.

The advantages of the sole proprietorship structure are

- ease and affordability of formation, and
- total control over business operations and financial decisions.

The disadvantages of the sole proprietorship are

- unlimited legal and financial liability,
- no additional and complementary skills of others, and

- no opportunity to raise capital for the business by selling shares to investors.

Limited and General Partnerships

The two types of partnerships are limited and general.

In a limited partnership, one partner, called the general partner, is responsible for day-to-day business operations and decisions. The other partners, called limited partners, are simply investors who share profits and losses but don't get involved in running the business and have very little say in how it is run. This form of business organization is often chosen by entrepreneurs who need investors but don't need any additional expertise or manpower to manage day-to-day operations.

The other type of partnership, called a general partnership, is like a marriage in many ways. The decision to form one is every bit as serious as with marriage, and the termination of one can be every bit as acrimonious and painful. In a general partnership, partners share the profits coming into the business and are equally liable for the business's expenses, including debts incurred and expenditures for business-related goods and services made by any partner, even if these purchases are made without the knowledge or consent of the other partner(s).

Let's say you and a friend decide to open XYZ Partners Personal Training in a small studio. Without your knowing about it, he goes out and signs on the dotted line for thousands of dollars' worth of exercise equipment. If he then changes his mind and skips town, you are stuck. The equipment seller doesn't know or care that this rotten bum who used to be your best friend is now somewhere in South America. Why should he? His deal is with XYZ Partners, and he's still got one partner—you—on the hook for the dough. He kindly reminds you that he does take most major credit cards.

This unfortunate example illustrates an important point about general partnerships. As in a marriage, each partner has an equal right to manage the daily affairs of the business. (I know, I know, the man is the king of the castle. My husband says that stuff too, but who listens?) To stay with the marriage analogy, let's say one spouse wants to use the family nest egg to buy a new car and the other wants to spend it on a dream vacation. What happens? At best, some long discussions, some whining, and maybe even some raised voices. At worst, slammed doors, thrown lamps, and nights spent in separate rooms. Eventually, most spouses are able to compromise about important issues and come to some understanding. The thought of angry marital quarrels reminds us that most partnerships, like marriages, start out all lovey-dovey, but when they break up badly, it can get very ugly.

Of course, in one important respect, marriage is different from a general partnership. With rare exceptions, unless you take some simple, voluntary actions like signing a couple of papers and saying the words "I do," you will not end up married without realizing you've taken this big step. It is possible, though, to be deemed the business partner of someone without deliberately intending to be. This inadvertent partnership can result if an innocent third party provides a benefit to the business because you "consented" to the appearance of being partners with someone else. Let's say you and your rich uncle go to a friend to borrow money for your new business. The two of you meet with this friend and discuss your new business. Your uncle appears to be involved in every aspect of the business. Reasonably assuming that you and your uncle are partners and relying on your uncle's substantial assets in making his decision, your friend loans you the money. You go broke. Your friend could argue that at least as far as he was concerned, your uncle, who still has plenty of money, was your business partner and therefore should be held liable for the debt.

The take-home message here is that you need to pick partners very carefully, and you need to be sure that you don't let anyone assume you are another person's business partner if that isn't your intention. If you really feel the need to go into business with someone else, you should consider forming either a limited partnership or a corporation. If you decide to form a general partnership, have your attorney prepare a partnership agreement providing for your respective contributions to the business, both financial and service related, and setting forth a procedure for dissolution. This sort of business "prenup" will make it possible for your former partner to stay your current friend.

The advantages of a general partnership are

- shared responsibility to complete tasks,
- complementary skill sets (you're a great personal trainer, he's a great salesman, for example), and
- ability to cover business responsibilities during personal emergencies or vacations.

The disadvantages of a general partnership are

- joint liability for your partner's actions,

- all partners share profits equally regardless of their contribution (unless their partnership agreement provides otherwise),
- analysis-paralysis from shared decision making, and
- potential personality conflicts.

Corporations

When I formed my corporation, I joked with my attorney, a longtime friend of the opposite gender, that this occasion was the only time that he and I could go into a room together and create a new person without having a lot of 'splaining to do to our spouses. This was true because a corporation is in fact a separate legal "person."

There are two principal advantages to incorporating. The first is the ability to sell shares in the business to raise working capital. If you need $10,000 and you can convince someone to pay you $10 a share for 1,000 shares, you're there. The second advantage is that the liability of a corporation is limited to that corporation's assets. People doing business with a corporation must look to it for payment of debts and bills. In general, if the corporation is sued, only its assets can be used to satisfy a judgment. For example, suppose that a personal trainer employed by XYZ Personal Training, Inc. fails to properly instruct a client, resulting in the client's injury. The client sues XYZ for $2 million. XYZ's assets total $1 million. Although it's true that XYZ will probably go out of business if the client wins his case, his recovery will be limited to $1 million. He cannot look to the shareholders of XYZ to pay any additional damages, even if they are more than able to pay. The exception to this rule is what attorneys call "piercing the corporate veil." This occurs when the corporation is so closely identified with the shareholders (or, typically, an individual shareholder) that a court will agree that the shield of the corporate identity should be disregarded. Since that is often the case with small personal-service businesses, it may not make sense for you to incorporate.

The protection of this separate corporate identity is not without a price. The rules governing the creation of a corporation vary by state, but in every case, you must file articles of incorporation with the secretary of state and pay a fee to establish your corporation. In addition, there are annual fees and filings to keep your corporation viable and in legal compliance. If you don't need to raise money, it may not be worth the hassle, time, effort, and extra expense, especially when you're first starting out in your business.

If you do decide to incorporate, be sure to discuss the option of choosing a special type of corporation called an S corp. S corps are creatures of the Internal Revenue Code, specifically subchapter S. They were created to help small businesses avoid the double taxation that traditional corporations face. Remember that corporations are separate legal persons; therefore, they pay separate taxes—most importantly, income taxes. For example, if a corporation earns $10,000 in income, it must pay income tax on this income before any of it is distributed to shareholders as dividends. Once the shareholders receive all or part of the $10,000, they must pay taxes on these dividends as well. An S corp doesn't pay separate income taxes. Instead, the income passes through to the shareholders, who pay income tax on it once. In addition, any losses the corporation sustains can be used to offset other income earned by an S corp shareholder, which can be very helpful in reducing a family's total tax liability.

The Internal Revenue Code imposes restrictions on the creation of S corps, such as limitations on the number of shareholders and time limits on filing for the S corp election. When you consult your attorney and accountant to discuss the best way to organize your business, you should also consider whether an S corp is the right choice for you.

The advantages of a corporation are

- the possible protection of personal assets and
- the ability to sell shares to raise capital.

The disadvantages of a corporation are

- the cost of formation and
- the administrative costs of required annual filings.

In my opinion, most personal trainers beginning a new business do not need to be concerned about incorporating. The main reason to incorporate is to attempt to shield yourself from personal liability. I suspect that this is less of a concern for you than for some businesses because

- you are doing everything you can to avoid potential liability;
- you have not worked with any clients before making sure that your liability insurance is in force; and
- since you are the entire business, if you do injure someone, you'll likely be called to account regardless of your corporation status, since lawyers like to pierce the corporate veil.

If your business expands and you hire one or more employees, you should discuss incorporating with your attorney and accountant.

How Much Should I Charge?

A recent issue of Club Industry magazine contained a letter to the editor that in many ways epitomizes the sad state of our public education system. The author was an AFAA-certified fitness instructor working at a YMCA who said that she "always felt

Why Consult an Attorney?

Think I'm a nag for telling you to consult an attorney? This guy wishes he did.

Here's a plan: remodel your basement and spend $60,000 on professional equipment. Then the clients can come to you. You'll have the comfort and privacy of in-home training without the hassle of transporting equipment or the expense of nonbillable travel time. That's probably what one personal trainer thought when he did just that. His in-home gym was located in a residential subdivision. He saw 20 to 25 clients a week there. All was well until someone complained that both the subdivision's restrictions and the municipal zoning prohibited the carrying on of any industry, business, trade, occupation, profession, or commercial activity of any kind within any residential premises. The city sued the personal trainer and won. The take-home messages:

- Before you invest the time and effort to start a business in your home, make sure that there are no private or legal restrictions against doing so.
- The time to hire a lawyer is before you need one (City of Madeira v. Furtner, 1994).

I will also remind you that since most cases like this begin with a complaint from a neighbor, if you do decide to operate a business in your home, be a considerate member of your community. Don't allow your clients to obstruct parking, and avoid any obtrusive signage that might make your neighbors think their homes have been magically transported to the Vegas strip.

cheated out of decent pay by the various clubs and gyms [she] had worked for." She continued her lament by citing that her main concern was the clients who attended her classes, who "deserve qualified, competent, and skilled instructors to teach their classes. The only way they're going to get (and keep) this type of fitness professional is if the industry standards change" (Letters, Club Industry 2002). Her solution to changing industry standards was to suggest that fitness instructors in her area unionize!

It's probably not her fault that she doesn't understand the first thing about capitalism or free enterprise. Education in that area is pathetic in our society. If it weren't, instead of writing letters to the editor complaining about making $7.50 to $8.25 an hour or looking for ways to further distort the market, such as unionization, this instructor would realize the reason that she is paid this paltry sum. It's not because of industry standards. It's because that's what the customers are willing to pay. Just as consumers who shop at Wal-Mart are not willing to pay $300 for a pair of shoes so that the people making them can be paid $30 an hour, those who belong to the YMCA are not going to pay $1,000-plus annually to come to group exercise classes. If I were counseling this unfortunate and confused fitness professional, I would tell her what I'm about to tell you: Setting rates for services in a free-market economy is a function of many factors. The take-home message from this tale is that if you want to maximize your income, you must create perceived value in the mind of the consumer of your services.

Some Important Questions

The first step in setting your rates is to gather some information so that you can answer these questions:

- **Who do you want to train?** Extremely affluent consumers actually prefer to pay more for services, thinking that low-cost service providers must provide inferior service. The CEOs and celebrities of your town will probably be receptive to a fee of $250 to $300 a session. On the other hand, if you want to train senior citizens on fixed incomes, you are going to meet with enormous resistance at anything over $30 a session. I'm certainly not suggesting that you avoid working with low-income or price-sensitive populations. Money isn't everything, and it's not the only reason to pursue a career in fitness. I'm only suggesting that you be aware that there are differences in how people perceive cost and value, and take that into account when setting your rates.

- **What is your service area?** It's simple: Personal trainers who work in large cities can charge more than those working in rural areas or small towns. Find out what other personal trainers within a 10-mile radius of where you want to work are charging, and set your rates accordingly.

- **What competitive options are available to your customers?** Pretend that you are a prospective client of your services. You are looking to solve a problem. That problem might be the need to lose weight. It might be the desire to improve performance in a recreational sport. Consider every other possible option a customer could consider to solve that problem other than you and your services. There are not only other personal trainers, but also clubs and gyms with group exercise programs as well as videos, books, and similar self-directed plans. The latter operate as a ceiling on what all personal trainers and health clubs can charge. After all, if the customers perceive personal training or health clubs as too expensive, they will resort to trying to solve the problem on their own. Investigate how much other personal trainers in your service area charge, then ask yourself how your service is different and, we hope, better than theirs. The only way you'll be able to justify charging a higher fee is if the consumer can justify paying it. When considering two possible alternatives, prospective clients will ask themselves, What's the difference? If the higher-priced alternative doesn't seem superior, there's no reason to shell out the extra dough. As of this writing, personal trainers charge a broad range of fees, anywhere from $30 to $250 a session.

- **What do other trainers with similar qualifications charge for their services?** The key to this question is "similar qualifications." Some "trainers" may have no educational background, certification, or experience working in clubs, but if you have a master's degree in exercise physiology, ACSM certification, and years of practical experience, you're in a different league. Let's face it: You didn't spend all that time and effort getting your degree to earn less than the typical street musician. Unless you're independently wealthy and you want to do personal training for your own enjoyment, you need to get paid what you're worth. The converse is also true: If you've been lifting weights for 10 years but have no educational background, no degree, and no certification, it's not realistic to expect to get paid top dollar. A trainer with an impressive background can certainly make the case for charging a higher rate than one without these credentials, but note that you do need to make the case. It's not enough to say, "I have a master's degree." That's going to provoke a big "So what?" in many members of the public, which is why our friend from the YMCA is wrong about the solution to low pay among fitness professionals. The average person doesn't know the difference between someone who got their "certification" by sending in $400 to a P.O. box on a matchbook cover and someone with a master's degree in exercise physiology from a top university. If you want to get the big bucks, you've got to explain the difference. It's true for every good or service in the marketplace. The unique, the distinctive, and the special command the most dollars from the consumer. The fungible (interchangeable), the run-of-the-mill, and the mediocre do not. To maximize your income, you must convince your prospects that you are one of a kind. (For more on the issue of maximizing your income by creating a unique identity and positioning, see chapter 3.)

Factors to Consider When Setting Your Rates

- Your education
- Your experience
- Your geographic location
- Rates charged by other personal trainers in your area
- The length of your sessions
- The location of your sessions
- Your cost of doing business
- Anything that makes you unique versus fungible

Other Factors to Consider When Setting Your Rates

Once you have completed your initial market analysis, you will have a ballpark idea of how much to charge, but your work isn't done quite yet. You need to address a few other issues before you settle on that final number.

Don't Set Your Rates Too Low

It's tempting to set your rates lower than the competition's, but it's crucial to avoid this common pitfall. Of course, you'll get lots of new clients, especially if you are very good at what you do. Imagine how many clients you could get if you

worked for free! You get the point. If you set your rates too low, you will end up frustrated, exhausted, and resentful. Sooner or later, you will either quit in a fit of burnout-induced disgust, or you will have to impose a rate increase. When you do, it may be difficult to explain to clients why they should pay more today for the same thing that they were getting for less yesterday. Many of them will leave, and you'll be back to square one, having to build up your client book again.

Length of Sessions

Most trainers' sessions last approximately 1 hour, and the suggestions about billing I'm making here are based on the assumption that your sessions will last that long. Once you determine your hourly fee, you'll have a basis for deciding how much to charge for shorter sessions, if you decide you want to do them. For example, you might decide to offer half-hour sessions to address individual client needs, such as learning sport-specific exercises or for "checkups" with clients to whom you've taught a routine and who have been working out on their own for a while.

Travel Time

Another factor to consider is travel time. Sometimes you will decide to work with a client outside your usual geographical service area. If you do, you should consider billing at least some part of your hourly fee as travel time. Let's face it: In your business, your time is your stock-in-trade. One way to ensure that you end up exhausted and underpaid is to accept clients over a huge service area. To avoid wasting a lot of time traveling, limit your service area to appointments within 30 minutes of your home or office. Don't be afraid to turn down clients who call you from outside your service area. Instead, establish mutual referral relationships with other personal trainers who work in these areas. This type of networking is a classic win-win!

Most Important Factor

You might find doing volunteer work very rewarding, but unless you don't need to make a living, you need to make sure that your business makes money; therefore, to effectively decide how much to charge, you need to know how much it costs you to keep the business running. See the sample business/marketing plan (pp. 23-25) for more information about figuring out the cost of doing business.

Whatever You Decide, Decide Something!

Decide carefully your rates and methods of billing. Think about whether you're going to bill your clients monthly, per session, or in some other way. Will your charge per session be the same no matter how many sessions a client signs up for, or will you offer package deals? Will you bill clients for canceled sessions? If so, under what circumstances? Whatever you decide, decide now!

You need to have a policy so you can respond to potential clients. Imagine this: You're sitting around one day waiting for the phone to ring, hoping it's a potential client, when it actually does! You and the person have a very pleasant conversation, during which you explain all your wonderful qualifications and all the miraculous things you can do for her, and she seems very interested in hiring you. Before it's a done deal, she just needs to know the answer to one question: "How much is this going to cost me?" You've got to be able to answer that, and fast; otherwise your prospect will be an ex-prospect before you can say "Body by Jake."

A Recommendation About Billing Your Clients

I, like you, can probably think of at least one type of professional who shows up at somebody's house for a private, shall we say, "consultation," and then leaves with a wad of cash, but I don't think that those folks would be characterized as health professionals, nor do I think that you should collect your fees the way they do. So why do so many personal trainers seem to think it's a great way to do business? Not only is this billing system, if you can call it that, unprofessional, but it also has the potential to cause a tremendous loss of income for a lot of trainers, and even increase the chances of their being sued. Let me explain.

Like all professionals, personal trainers need to have a professional billing system. Otherwise, I see four potential problems:

1. **Unprofessional impression.** Accepting money at the beginning of a session not only adds time to the length of your visit, but it is also very distracting to what you are there to do. Even worse, it diminishes the impression your client has of you as a health professional. Your doctor doesn't ask you for money when you're sitting there in the examining room, does he? No, someone else handles that, so that your relationship remains, for lack of a better word, pure. Collecting money during your sessions reinforces the belief that your client should treat you as a manicurist or a hairdresser. What happens if you drive 20 miles to a client's house for your session and he tells you he doesn't have any checks in his checkbook, and can he pay you next time? What impact will that have on your focus during the session?

2. **Lost income.** Second, there's the issue of lost income. If you don't get paid until you go to a client's home, how are you going to be compensated for your time if somebody cancels at the last minute? Some of you may think you'll be able to collect for scheduled sessions from clients who cancel at the last minute, but you've got a better chance of sprouting wings and flying than you do of getting clients to pay you under those circumstances. On the other hand, if you've billed a client at the beginning of the month for all the sessions that month and you have a firm written 24-hour cancellation policy, then it will be easy—or at least easier—for you to be compensated for this lost time. And remember, a personal trainer's time and knowledge are his stock-in-trade. That's why it's very important that you be compensated for late cancellations. When you block out time for clients, you can't commit that time to someone else. It's gone forever. If you don't get paid, so is the income that you would have earned for that session. If this happens often enough, your business will suffer dramatically. Monthly billings in advance eliminate this problem automatically.

3. **A hammer for clients to use on you.** Sometimes, as much as I try to keep her locked up, my inner lawyer gets out, so bear with me. The overwhelming majority of your clients are going to be wonderful, honest people who would not dream of taking advantage of you. Your relationships with all your clients should be based on commitment, integrity, and trust, and I'm sure that they will be. Once in a while, though, you might run into a bad apple, so it's important that I tell you this because it may not be immediately obvious: Clients who owe you money have a built-in incentive to find reasons to sue you. Here's an example illustrating how it could happen. A client owes you several hundred dollars for previous training sessions. When you press her for it, she suddenly discovers this horrible pain in her back that she never had until she started working out with you. She doesn't want to talk to her lawyer, she explains, but money being as tight as it is, she might have to—medical bills are so expensive, and she also owes you that several hundred dollars. Oh, didn't you know she'd seen the doctor? Oh, yes, and the doctor said that without a doubt, you are the cause

of her pain. Of course, if you're willing to forget what she owes you, she's willing to forget the whole thing. She just doesn't see that she has any choice, she explains pitifully. Of course, you lose this deadbeat as a client—maybe you could refer her to your "favorite" competitor—but in the meantime you're out that income. If you bill clients monthly and do not allow them to fall behind in their payments, you eliminate the temptation for someone to stiff you, using the threat of a lawsuit as a hammer.

4. **Absence of a cancellation policy.** I alluded earlier to a late cancellation policy and I urge you to have one. What do I mean by that? I mean if clients do not give you at least 24 hours' notice of a cancellation, they will be billed for the session. Some trainers have a specific cancellation fee; that is, they don't bill clients for the entire missed session if cancellation is given within a certain time frame. You could consider something along those lines if you think it is fair. But whatever you do, have a firm written policy on cancellation as part of your billing system, and make sure every client understands it from the beginning. There's nothing more detrimental and souring to a relationship between you and a client than arguing about cancellations and whether the client is going to pay you for them.

Writing Your Business Plan

Most people find the prospect of preparing a business plan about as appealing as preparing their tax returns, and even when they are excited about a business idea, they avoid the important planning process. People who are seeking funding from banks or venture capitalists, however, have no choice. These third parties require a business plan before disbursing any funds. The business plans they require are much more comprehensive and detailed than the one presented here (figure 2.1), which is intended to give you an idea of the type of analysis you need to do for yourself.

Even if you are not looking to impersonal suits to loan you the scratch to get started, putting everything down on paper is a good idea. It makes the business seem real and gets you thinking as a businessperson. You will start to realize how important it is to control expenses if you're going to make it. You will think analytically about whom you are going to serve and how you are going to reach them. Ultimately, the purpose of doing a business plan is to gather information that will answer the question, "Can I make a living running this business?"

When you prepare a business plan, you investigate every aspect of the business you want to create.

In addition to visualizing exactly what the business is going to look like, who its customers will be, and what you will do to distinguish yourself and your business from your competition, you will do a projection of earnings and expenses. The business plan will enable you to explain your uniqueness very effectively because you will have analyzed your competitors thoroughly. That's the easy part. The tricky part is coming up with the numbers: how much revenue you will generate and how soon you will be able to break even. Though it may seem that you're just pulling numbers out of the air, do your best to make these estimates as realistic as possible. Otherwise, your business plan will be nothing more than an optimistic fairy tale, and you'll waste a lot of time trying to create a business that has no chance of succeeding. For example, unless you know that all of your clients will be generous gazillionaires, you wouldn't want to project your earnings based on a rate of $500 a session. You also don't want to allow your exuberance to cause you to overlook mundane but inevitable expenses like taxes and insurance.

As you can see from the sample business plan we've provided, this project doesn't have to consist of volumes of pages. A short, simple plan will do the job, so don't become overwhelmed at the prospect of writing one. View this exercise as an opportunity not only to refine your ideas about your business and clarify your vision about how to make it special, but also to avoid making a lot of mistakes.

Most business plans, including the one provided here, are divided into several sections, each of which looks at a different factor that will determine how feasible your business idea is. Let's take a look at each one:

• **Market analysis.** This section looks at how many potential buyers you have for your product or service. For example, if you want to sell those red-clown noses, you need to know how many practicing clowns live within driving distance of your store, and how many people are considering entering the field. (Let's hope that it's not too many.) If you discover there are no clowns in your community, your business idea is probably not a good one. (At least you live in a clown-free zone, though, so you've got that going for you.)

• **Competition.** If your idea is a good one, that is, if you discover that there are many potential buyers for what you have to offer, chances are you will have some competition. If no competitors are in place, that will mean one of two things: either you are so visionary that you are the very first one in your area to think of this great idea, or no market exists for what you want to sell. With personal training, unless you move to an extremely remote area, chances are the competition will be in place. How can you make yourself distinct from them? What services can you offer differently or better? You need to answer these questions to show how you will get your share of the market pie.

- **Services and operations.** The services and operations sections are the place to sketch out the practical details of the business by explaining specifically what it is you do, including the hours.

- **Feasibility.** Conclude your plan by constructing a reasonable estimate of expenses and revenues. Don't let your enthusiasm lead you to an analysis that is the triumph of hope over experience. Be honest and realistic. Better to underestimate how much you can earn than to dream of pie-in-the-sky projections that never materialize.

Sample Business/Marketing Plan for Fit to Be Tried Personal Training, Inc.

This plan presents the results of our analysis of the feasibility of profitably operating Fit to Be Tried Personal Training, (FBT) a one-on-one personal training business specializing in the needs of attorneys, paralegals, legal secretaries, and judges in downtown Springfield, USA, an area of approximately 2 square miles (5.18 sq km) consisting of high-rise office buildings and a courthouse/judicial center.

Our analysis shows that it will require an initial investment of $10,000 to establish the business. Most of these funds will be used to lease equipment and build out the studio. In addition, the owner will use her existing car and computer in running the business.

MARKET ANALYSIS

Springfield's metropolitan area consists of approximately 600,000 adults. Of these, 3,842 are licensed to practice law, and 2,000 of these practice within a five-mile radius of downtown and the courthouse. They are supported by approximately 1,500 paralegals and legal secretaries. This population is the market that FBT will serve.

As an industry, personal training has experienced explosive growth in the last 10 years. The International Health, Racquet & Sportsclub Association (IHRSA)/ American Sports Data Health Club Trend Report shows that from 1999 to 2000, the number of Americans who used a personal fitness trainer grew by approximately 32% to just over five million. FBT hopes to capitalize on this trend in Springfield.

COMPETITION

- Springfield YMCA—A large YMCA with a swimming pool and fitness center serves downtown Springfield. It costs approximately $650 annually for membership in this facility. Current membership is approximately 1,200.

- Labby's Total Fitness—This national chain of health clubs has a full-service club three miles from the courthouse. It has a lap pool and a free weight room and offers aerobics classes in the morning and evening. After paying the $200 initiation fee, members pay $480 annually to be a member of this club. Labby's offers personal training services at approximately $40 per session.

- Fitness for Women Only—This new chain recently opened a 6,000-square-foot facility in the Springfield Mall, four miles from downtown. They offer only group classes and do not have showers.

While these competitors offer similar services to that planned by FBT, FBT will occupy a unique and specialized subset of the market for fitness/wellness services.

- Unlike the YMCA, FBT will not market to families or seniors as a primary client base.

- Unlike Labby's, FBT will target a professional clientele that tends to be older, more highly educated, and more affluent. The pricing for Labby's personal training reflects this fact. FBT's clients are those who don't object to paying more for higher quality as compared to mass-market consumers.

- Unlike Fitness for Women, which specializes in group classes and whose primary consumer benefit is privacy and a "non-judgmental" atmosphere, FBT will pitch professionalism, time-efficiency, and effectiveness.

(continued)

Figure 2.1 Sample business plan.

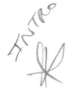

(continued)

SERVICES AND OPERATIONS

Services to Be Offered by FBT

Our primary service will be one-on-one personal training for time-challenged adults, particularly those working in and supporting the legal profession. We will specialize in our 30-minute "power sessions," designed to be the fastest way to reduce body fat and improve overall cardiorespiratory fitness. This power workout will be our primary product. We will also offer traditional one-hour personal sessions.

Management

FBT is being founded by Dana Carter, MS. Dana has been a personal trainer for two years, working in a variety of club settings in Springfield. She is certified by the American College of Sports Medicine as well as several other organizations. In addition, Dana is a former paralegal, which makes her uniquely qualified to speak to the target market.

Initially Dana will operate the business and be the only one-on-one trainer. Initially, she will have one part-time additional employee, a bookkeeper/receptionist.

Operations Plan

Operating Hours

Initially, FBT will offer sessions the following days and hours:

5:30 A.M.–10:00 A.M., Monday, Wednesday, Thursday, Friday

11:30 A.M.–1:00 P.M., Monday through Friday

4:00 P.M.–7:00 P.M., Monday, Wednesday

We anticipate adding additional hours as market demand increases, probably adding the early-morning hours to Tuesdays, and possibly adding Saturday mornings.

Facility

FBT will operate out of a 6,000-square-foot studio on the ground floor of an office building. To design the studio, FBT will use the services of a space planner specializing in efficient exercise facilities. The planner is experienced in equipment selection and will assist with outfitting the studio with the best equipment for FBT's needs.

Prices

FBT plans to price its services as follows:

- Power workout—$75 per session for a12-session program, $70/16 sessions, $55/24 sessions
- One-hour sessions—$95/12, $75/16, $70/24

Although there are no personal training businesses charging these rates in downtown Springfield, these rates are comparable to those charged by premium service providers in metropolitan Springfield, such as Prestige Personal Training, 20 miles (32.18 km) north of downtown, which happens to be the area where many Springfield professionals live.

Marketing Plan

Dana has an established reputation in the community and hopes to use this goodwill to generate interest in FBT, resulting in many new clients. Her strategy is to use the following marketing methods, all of which rely more on investments of time and energy than on substantial outlay of funds:

- Quarterly ads in the *Legal Times,* a free weekly tabloid that blankets the downtown area and that surveys show 87% of the legal community reads every week
- Small phone book ad, necessary because competitors appear there
- Postcard direct mailing to all law firms in downtown Springfield

In addition, Dana has enrolled in the Speakers' Bureaus of the Springfield Rotary Club, the Springfield Bar Association, and the Springfield Women's Bar Association. She plans several presentations to these groups as part of her marketing efforts.

FBT's target market is educated, affluent, and time challenged and will therefore be moved to action by appeals to effectiveness and efficiency; therefore, all of FBT's marketing and advertising efforts will emphasize the following consumer benefits:

- The professionalism and credentials of staff
- The effectiveness of FBT's programs
- The time efficiency of FBT's programs

Eventually, word of mouth will be FBT's primary method of advertising.

FEASIBILITY

At these rates, and given the number of sessions anticipated a week, FBT anticipates first-year revenue at approximately $50,000 and second-year revenue at $72,000. After the first year's operating loss, the business will generate approximately $20,000 in profit and is therefore feasible.

Statement of Estimated Monthly Revenues and Expenses—1st Year

Revenue

Personal training services	$4,200
Newsletter subscriptions	80
Total	**$4,280**

Operating Expenses

Salaries	$3,000
Payroll taxes	600
Other taxes	400
Insurance	45
Rent	3,000
Telephone	60
Web page/Internet	25
Advertising	25
Office supplies	10
Certifications	30
Continuing education/seminars	15
Dues and subscriptions	10
Professional services	
Attorney	15
Accountant	15
Depreciation	10
Total	**$7,260**

Statement of Estimated Monthly Revenues and Expenses—2nd Year

Revenue

Personal training services	$9,000
Newsletter subscriptions	200
Total	**$9,200**

Operating Expenses

Salaries	$3,000
Payroll taxes	600
Other taxes	400
Insurance	45
Rent	3,000
Telephone	60
Web page/Internet	25
Advertising	25
Office supplies	10
Certifications	30
Continuing education/seminars	15
Dues and subscriptions	10
Professional services	
Attorney	15
Accountant	15
Depreciation	10
Total	**$7,260**

Bookkeeping and Financial Records

I cannot overemphasize the importance of keeping accurate records of dollars in and dollars out. I could call this section of this book "Follow the Money," because that's what establishing your record-keeping and bookkeeping system is about. There are two reasons to do it: the basic reason and the scary reason.

1. **The Basic Reason.** If you're going to bill your clients monthly in advance and impose some sort of a cancellation policy, you need to keep track of how many sessions they paid for; how many they actually had; how many of those were credited cancellations; and how many were late, and therefore no-credit, cancellations.

2. **The Scary Reason,** or **Whose Hand Is in My Pocket?** You need to keep track of money coming in and going out not only to see if you are achieving that first goal of running a profitable personal training business, but also to address the second goal, avoiding tax problems. It's not enough to just collect money haphazardly and deposit it in your personal checking account along with the Christmas gift from Aunt Tillie and the money you got from another job.

It's very important to be able to isolate the proceeds that you receive from personal training. Why? Because of the government, specifically, the ever-popular guilty-until-proven-innocent branch of our government, the Internal Revenue Service. The IRS, as you know, requires you to pay income tax and to file an income tax return every year. As your accountant will tell you, though, every dollar that you receive is not necessarily taxable income. For example, the expenses you incur in conducting your business will reduce your taxable income. You'll have to print business cards, maybe brochures. You may buy some equipment. You may place ads to market your business. All of these things are expenses that can offset the revenue that comes into your business, and this will reduce your tax liability. Now, if you've been just taking all the money that you get from your clients and plunking it into your personal checking account that contains money from God-knows-where in addition to that from personal training, how are you going to know how much income to charge those expenses against? You're really going to have a hard time separating income from personal training from other income, on which taxes may have already been withheld, and from gifts. And if you can't prove it's not income, the IRS will say it is. Picture yourself sitting at the kitchen table surrounded by piles of papers and adding machine tapes and probably a really, really big bottle of aspirin, wondering why you didn't just set up a separate checking account and create a separate bookkeeping system.

Getting Financially Organized

So as soon as you have established your business (ordered your business cards, gotten your liability insurance in place), and before you accept a single client, open a separate checking account for the business and set up your bookkeeping system. You should do this even if you aren't incorporated and even if you have only one or two clients.

How Do I Find a Lawyer and an Accountant?

In my experience, the best way to select a lawyer or an accountant is to ask trusted friends, especially other small-business owners, for a referral. Get two or three names of possible service providers. Make a list of what you want these professionals to do for you, and call each candidate. Explain your situation as a new small-business owner, tell her what you need (prepare my tax returns annually, review my waiver form—whatever the specifics are), and ask lots of questions. Here are a few to get you started:

- Do you handle many small-business clients?
- How do you bill for your services, by the hour or by the job? (If you can negotiate a flat fee for some services like preparing your annual tax returns, you will be able to save some money.)
- How can I reach you in an emergency? (You want to make sure that the person you hire is responsive and that if you really need help in a short time frame, you can get in touch with her fast.)

If you like the answers you get, schedule a face-to-face meeting. It's never a good idea to hire a professional sight unseen. You'll get better service if he and his staff have met you, have seen your sunny smile, and can put a face with a name when you call.

Incidentally, the worst way is to pull a name out of the phone book.

Your bookkeeping system doesn't have to be elaborate. Nobody's asking you to put on a green eyeshade and sit there all day without ever seeing the sun 'til you develop the pasty, fluorescent-light complexion of an accountant. That's what you have your accountant for. He or she will help you set up a bookkeeping system, and the good news is that, just as we live in a time of e-mail and miraculous medical treatments, today we're fortunate enough to have many wonderful computer bookkeeping programs. So there's no reason to avoid setting up good bookkeeping and record-keeping systems for your business. And if you don't, you will definitely regret it—if not today, then on April 15th.

Most small-business owners keep their books on a cash basis as opposed to using the accrual method of accounting. With cash basis, you record income when you receive it and expenses when you pay them. Your business is small enough that once you get some help from your accountant in setting up your books, you should be able to keep them yourself. You can set up your books either manually or on a computer. I highly recommend the latter. Using a computer simplifies the process of figuring out income and expenses for tax purposes at the end of the year.

Here's the method I've used, which worked quite well for me. At the beginning of the month, bill your clients for the month's sessions in advance. Prepare the invoices on your computer, using either your bookkeeping program or a separate database program. Keep track of each client's sessions in your appointment book, and at the end of the month, before sending out the next month's invoices, figure out whether any credits for missed or canceled sessions are due. Compute the amount due for the upcoming month. This is the amount for next month's invoice.

What About Taxes?

Each individual's income tax liability is dictated by that individual's specific situation. (Married? Single? Children? Homeowner? Renter? The considerations are endless.) The important thing is, as mentioned previously, you don't want the IRS breathing down your neck! You should consult an accountant or other professional tax advisor about your specific tax situation. A few things to think about:

• **If you earn income and you are not an employee who has taxes withheld,** you will need to pay estimated quarterly taxes, estimates of the amount of the taxes you will owe when you file your annual return.

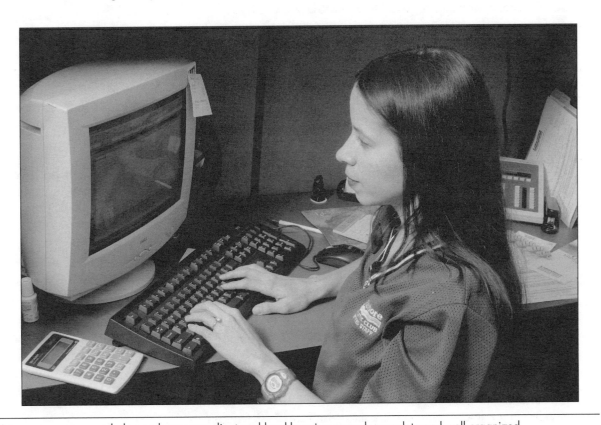

Using a computer can help you keep your client and bookkeeping records complete and well organized.

- **If you do personal training as a second job,** or if you do personal training part-time as an employee of a club and the rest of the time as an entrepreneur, do not assume that because you have taxes withheld at your job, you don't have to pay estimated quarterly taxes. The amount of your withholding at your job covers the wages that you earn at that job. It does not take into account additional amounts you might earn moonlighting. If you should pay estimated taxes but don't, you may owe penalties and interest in amounts that will make you seriously regret ignoring this little detail.

- **If you have decided to incorporate your business as a C corporation** (as opposed to a subchapter S corporation—remember, you're going to discuss this issue with your lawyer and accountant), your corporation may owe corporate taxes separate from individual income taxes.

- **As a service business with only one employee (you), you probably won't have to pay sales taxes,** since most localities don't tax services. (I say "probably," but I don't know your state and local laws. If you aren't absolutely positive about your local laws

and regulations, find someone who is, and ask!) You will, however, need to pay payroll taxes on the salary that the business pays you. Your tax advisor can help you through the mechanics of computing the amount of the payroll tax and making the payroll tax deposit.

Licensing and Other Burdensome Governmental Requirements

In addition to taxes, your state, county, or municipality might impose additional obligations on you and your business, such as business franchise taxes, or, if you sell products, sales taxes. In addition, some jurisdictions require that businesses file a fictitious name certificate, a document stating that, for example, Hard as a Rock Personal Training is owned by Sally Jones, an individual, or, if the business is incorporated, by SJ, Inc., a corporation doing business as Hard as a Rock Personal Training. If you don't understand these things backward and forward yourself (and most of us don't), do yourself a favor—consult a competent advisor.

What About Licensure?

Some personal trainers and other fitness professionals believe that many of the problems in the industry could be solved, or at least ameliorated, if personal trainers were licensed. They cite the fact that many states require other professionals to be licensed, even though their professions appear to require less knowledge and expertise. "Is it right that hairdressers and manicurists need to be licensed, but any bonehead can claim to be a personal trainer?" they whine. They also believe that having the state's seal of approval would open the door to insurance reimbursement along the lines of physical therapists and other allied professionals. Not only that, but a state license would give consumers a uniform standard of professionalism to look to in evaluating personal trainers. Let's face it: Most members of the public don't know a quality certification from a credential advertised on a matchbook cover.

All of that may sound pretty convincing, but consider the following:

- **Insurance reimbursement may not be the panacea that many think it is.** Think about it. What's happening to physicians' incomes in this age of managed care and third-party payment? They are declining because insurance companies set their reimbursement rates below many doctors' fees for services. Would you really be that much better off having a lot of clients whose insurance companies pay you $30 a session, especially if you had to fill out a gazillion forms to get it?

- **A license may or may not equal professionalism and high standards.** It depends on who writes the exam and how it is administered. Suppose that the owners of large health club chains, who are not known for their high standards in hiring personal trainers, decide to pay a visit to the state legislature and lobby aggressively for the exam to be the one that they are currently using for their personal trainers, an exam that consists of showing they can fog a mirror and fit into the spandex outfit. Suddenly, the personal trainer with a PhD in exercise physiology and the Jake Jr. who doesn't know a rotator cuff from a pant cuff are equal in the eyes of the public. So licensure wouldn't eliminate the incompetent or unqualified. It would just make it harder to sort them out.

Some states have debated licensure, but currently only one state—Louisiana—requires that fitness professionals be licensed, and its license requirement applies only to clinical exercise physiologists working in cardiac rehab under the supervision of physicians.

Avoiding Lawsuits

We all know that there has been an explosion in medical malpractice cases over the last 25 years. I have a theory about that, which has nothing to do with greedy personal-injury lawyers, whom I'll revisit later. First I want to tell you about a conversation I had with a client back in my personal training days, someone who happens to be a physician. He has managed to get himself into the unfortunate position of being in charge of cost containment, and no, he doesn't hold it against me that I call him an "HMO Nazi." He was lamenting the fact that he was constantly having to plead with his colleagues to stop giving patients so many—as put he it—"unnecessary tests." He said that whenever he asked why a doctor felt the need to give someone so many tests, the doctor would reply, "I don't want to get sued." I told him that he should say this: "Since anyone can sue anyone anytime, we can't let that affect our medical judgment. After all, I could sue you for divorce"—and he would be saying this to a male colleague—"and until you went in to court and got it dismissed, you'd be 'sued.' It's stupid to base our patient care decisions on that." And it's true.

A couple of years ago the Wall Street Journal ran a story about a guy who found a great way to make a living. He was an ex-stockbroker who had figured out that by threatening to sue major corporations, he could extort $2,000 to $3,000 out of them for the price of a stamp. Here's how it worked: He sent each company a letter, alleging that the board of directors' decisions financially damaged him, a shareholder of the company, and threatened a shareholder lawsuit. The company realized that hiring a lawyer to get this thing dismissed would cost more than the $2,000 to $3,000 he was asking for, so they just paid him off. It didn't matter that in most cases, he never even owned the stock. They didn't even check. It also didn't matter that he made only about $30,000 a year doing this. He didn't need much money, since he was in prison! There's a guy who gives new meaning to the term "jailhouse lawyer"! But it's a perfect illustration of how even major corporations can be so freaked out at the possibility of being sued that they lose the ability to think straight. Don't let it happen to you!

Many personal trainers have never stopped to think about the fact that a lawsuit could be filed against them and are downright terrified when they discover this. It's an unfortunate fact that we live in an extremely litigious society, and anyone can sue anyone. We all heard about the woman who spilled hot coffee in her lap and then sued McDonald's. The courts are filled with other outrageous examples of careless, silly people trying to avoid responsibility for their own actions and achieve victim status and the dollar payoff that goes with it. Is it inevitable that you will face a lawsuit? No, I don't think the picture for personal trainers is that bleak. Though it's true that exercise is not without risk, and injuries do happen sometimes no matter how careful we are, you shouldn't lie awake at night worrying about getting sued.

The best protection against lawsuits is to avoid problems by screening your clients; designing safe, effective programs; and exercising care while working with your clients. If you are sued despite doing

Torts, Liability, and Other Scary Legal Words

Tort is one of those words that you probably can't define unless you attended law school. The study of torts is part of the core curriculum in every law school in the common law world. That notwithstanding, it has been said that a really satisfactory definition of the word has never been found. Leave it to the law professors and legal theoreticians to worry about semantic abstractions. Here is a workable definition of tort: A tort is an act or a failure to act that violates a legally created right and allows the injured party to sue for damages or injunctive relief; that is, it gives rise to liability. For the personal trainer, a tort means causing an injury to your client, which is usually physical but could be emotional.

Liability—what is it, and why should you care? Being liable means being legally responsible for the consequences of one's actions or omissions. If your actions result in injury or loss to someone, have you committed a tort and subjected yourself to liability? You have if the following elements are met:

- Duty: You have an obligation to do or refrain from doing something.
- Breach: You do not live up to this obligation.
- Proximate cause: Your act or omission causes the injury.
- Damages: Someone is injured as a result of your act or omission.

> ## Three Legal Basics to Remember That Will Make You Feel Better
>
> - **Legal basic 1**—Anyone can sue anyone for anything at any time. Once you realize this, it's a lot less scary, isn't it?
> - **Legal basic 2**—Waivers will protect you, if handled properly. For some reason, most people believe that waivers aren't worth the paper they're written on, but that's not true if you do it right.
> - **Legal basic 3**—A lawsuit without damages is not a hammer, it's a squirt gun. No harm, no foul.

these things, you will be way ahead of the game if you have a degree and are certified by one of the nationally recognized organizations (see chapter 1). You can also strengthen your credentials by taking continuing education classes, something most of the certifying bodies require for you to maintain your certification. If you consistently follow good safety procedures for handling equipment, you minimize the risk of making a mistake. Finally, remember that the personal trainer–client relationship is first and foremost just that: a personal relationship. If you show genuine concern for your clients' needs, desires, and well-being and you really do relate to clients as individuals, your chances of being sued are greatly diminished. Concern for your clients is more than showing genuine warm feelings. It is also performing your job as a professional and exercising care to avoid any potential harm to your clients. Read on.

Taking Care: Ensuring Your Clients' Safety

As a personal trainer, what does this mean to you? When you work with your clients, you have an obligation to use ordinary care to refrain from causing injury. Ordinary care means that your actions are consistent with those of a reasonable, prudent personal trainer. This is a way of referring to the legal concept of the "standard of care." If you are ever hauled into court to answer for allegedly injuring a client, and your state does not require trainers to be licensed, you will probably be judged by a standard of care based on

- the standards set by the leading national certifying organizations, and
- expert witness testimony about what a careful personal trainer would have done in the same situation.

The following are specifics of how to ensure your clients' safety.

Instruction and Supervision

As a one-on-one trainer, you are responsible for providing proper instruction and supervision. So what exactly does that mean? Glad you asked. It means the following:

- **Individualized and continuous instruction.** To achieve this properly, you must stay in physical proximity to your client with all of your attention focused on her.
- **Accurate instruction.** This means ensuring correct form and technique for every exercise and paying attention to proper body mechanics for every exercise. The Resistance Workout Guide (part III of this book) is an invaluable resource in this respect. Once you have written the exercise prescription for your client, review the material in the guide for each exercise you will ask him to do, and be sure it's in your head as well as in the book!
- **Supervision.** This means executing proper spotting technique and giving attention to things that could cause an unsafe situation in the workout area or with your client herself, such as not wearing a belt during squats. Again, the Resistance Workout Guide contains essential tips on proper supervision.

Handling Equipment

A big part of your job as a personal trainer will involve handling equipment: machines, free weights, and similar items. For clients who have never set foot in a gym or lifted a weight, your expertise with equipment will be one of the main reasons they retain you. Sometimes those of us who spend most of our time with these tools of the trade can get a bit complacent about them, not consciously aware of how powerful and, if misused, how dangerous they can be. Rest assured that if your client gets injured, such lapses in concentration can be very costly. Always remember to ask yourself, "What's the worst thing that can happen if I do this?" (or don't do this, as the case may be). The answer is the risk that you are assuming. Is it an acceptable one for you and your client? Following are several precautions you must consistently follow.

Check and Double-Check

You'd be amazed at how easy it is to pick up two dumbbells of different weights and not notice the difference, especially between 15s (6.8 kg) and 20s (9 kg). This is not a disaster unless you hand them to your client. He is depending on you for guidance, instruction, and support—how's it going to look if you hand him the wrong dumbbells?

Dumbbells

As you know, dumbbells come in many varieties, shapes, and sizes. You've got the premolded, one-piece type, sometimes covered in colorful thick plastic, with a distinct hue for each different weight. There are also the adjustable ones, basically a short bar and a pair of collars that you use to anchor plates to it. The number and size of the plates determine the weight of the dumbbell—for that set, anyway. Many gyms have a hybrid variety that started out as adjustable units but have been welded or held together with screws so that they remain a designated weight. Each of these variations has its advantages and disadvantages. The adjustable type costs less, of course, than a complete set of individual, premolded dumbbells, especially the fancy, shiny chrome ones. You buy one bar and a couple of collars, and as few or as many plates as you need. They also take up less space and can be more portable. After all, it's easier to carry the bars and collars in the trunk of your car than it is to haul pairs of dumbbells from 3s (1.36 kg) to 20s (9 kg).

One major downside of the adjustable dumbbells is the hassle of reconfiguring them every time you want to do a set. It's nearly impossible to do a drop set (in which you have your client do a designated number of repetitions with one weight, then, immediately after completing them, continue the exercise with slightly lighter weights). Thoughts of the difficulty and time spent in dumbbell reconstruction will definitely put a damper on your creative program design. They are also not as safe as premolded dumbbells. If the collar loosens on one side in the middle of a set, the plates can suddenly crash to the floor or, even worse, onto your client's stunned face. For this reason, I suggest that if you are working with an in-home client, you recommend that she purchase premolded dumbbells in the sizes you need. That makes your workout time much better spent, gives you the flexibility to do more intense

protocols like drop sets, and avoids the potential danger of breakaway adjustables.

Whatever type you are using, before you suggest that a client pick up a dumbbell (you should not hand your client the dumbbells, since handoffs can be tricky), make sure you have the right dumbbell, or dumbbells. If you are using two, make sure that they are both the same size. If you are using adjustable dumbbells, especially the hybrid type, be sure to check that the dumbbell hasn't been so loosened by repeated dropping that it's about to fall apart. This problem is unlikely with in-home clients, who don't tend to appreciate the melodious sound of heavy metal objects slamming against their floors. In gyms, even without the irritating propensity of many gym rats to conclude their sets celebrating with a triumphant cry and a dumbbell drop from 5 or 6 feet (why *must* they do that?), dumbbells get loose from constant use, so be sure to check them.

Machines

Make a notation in the client's workout record form (see appendix A) of the position she uses on a particular machine. If you have to adjust a seat on a bike or machine, make sure the pin is in place by sitting on it yourself before you allow the client to sit on it. Also, pay attention to the position and condition of cables on machines. Do they look frayed? Are they off the track? Check the hooks connecting the cables to pull-down and pushdown bars. Sometimes these hooks bend due to the amount of force they have to handle in a typical gym or club. I don't hesitate to suggest that a client refrain from using a particular bar if it appears the item is nearly worn through. Make sure equipment is clean. (Some clients are more comfortable placing a towel on a bench before they lie on it, which I encourage.) In short, check everything: the equipment, its condition, and any adjustments you make before you let your client use it.

Don't Modify Equipment

Sometimes in gyms you see people using equipment in, shall we say, innovative and creative ways. There may be no problem with this sort of thing if you are not responsible for anyone else's well-being. As a professional, however, you must realize that a lawsuit can turn on the issue of design for a particular purpose, as in a lawn mower isn't designed to be handheld and used as a hedge clipper. For example, the gym where I work out has a seated horizontal bench press machine. It's clear that this machine was designed with one exercise in mind. The subject places her hands on short handles that are directly in front of her shoulders. The handles are not adjustable. Seeing this inflexibility as a design defect, some people attempt to correct it by placing a straight bar between the two handles so they can do a close-grip variation of the exercise. I see people do this almost every day. It should be apparent to you that this procedure might not be safe, especially with a beginner. Remember the question: What's the worst thing that could happen? The bar could slip, fly up, and whack the client in the face. When this or any workout accident is reviewed in hindsight, what seemed like a reasonable and creative way to work a particular muscle group will usually be transformed into a clear example of trainer negligence and stupidity. In fact, it will probably seem that this was the dumbest thing that any trainer ever did. How could you do such a thing? You couldn't, you wouldn't, and you won't if you follow this simple rule: Don't modify equipment.

Free-Weight Smarts

As you no doubt know, working with free weights is different than working with machines. Here are a few rules you need to follow:

1. Always use collars on bars.

2. Do not hand weights to your client. Have him pick them up himself to avoid potential hand-off problems.

3. Always be aware of other objects and people in the workout area.

4. If you approach a loaded Olympic bar on a cage-style rack, get some help stripping the plates. Don't try to pull them all off one side and then the other, because if you do, the weight remaining on the bar after you've pulled it all off one side may cause the bar to flip up in the air and crash to the ground. The best thing that will happen is a very loud, embarrassing crash. I don't think you want to imagine the worst thing. This won't happen on a safety squat rack where the bar rests on an angled support.

5. You might have noticed that gyms are minefields: There are usually dumbbells, handles, barbells, and other paraphernalia on the floor and heavy objects moving through the air, sometimes seemingly without guidance. Watch out! Pay strict attention to things on and off the floor. Never move in a direction without looking first. Warn your client of these hazards, too.

Proper Spotting Technique

One of your jobs during the workout is to properly spot the client. Proper spotting requires that you understand the exercise well enough to select the biomechanically efficient place to spot and have your complete attention focused on your client while he is doing the exercise. Follow these rules:

1. **Preview.** Before you begin the exercise, explain to your client that you will be spotting him on the exercise just to make sure he can complete his final repetition safely. Tell him that your assistance may be in the form of applying a little help by touching the bar or dumbbells or by stabilizing a body part by applying a little direct pressure to it (the elbows, for example, during a dumbbell press). This is a good time to explain to clients, novice weightlifters especially, that you will be placing your hands on their bodies, in a purely professional way, of course. You don't want to startle someone hoisting a weight by touching him unexpectedly.

2. **Communicate.** Baseball outfielders can attest to the importance of always communicating with your partner in a common enterprise. "I've got it, I've got it" is important in the gym as well as in the field. Imagine this unfortunate scenario: Your client is using a pec deck. You think, *She's doing just fine controlling this weight. I don't need to keep my hands on the pads.* She thinks, *I can try to force out a couple more reps. She's spotting me.* The client loses control of the pads and is seriously injured. All of this could have been avoided if you both were on the same page. I like to tell my clients in advance where I will be spotting them (elbows on a flat dumbbell press, waist on a squat, for example) and how we will proceed. ("You should pick up the right dumbbell first, and when we have finished this set, please lower the dumbbells and bring them down to your side. Then I'll take the left.") Be sure that you apply equal assistance to both arms in a dumbbell exercise. Otherwise, you can throw the client off balance.

3. **Focus.** A distracted spotter is worse than no spotter because he gives the lifter a false sense of security, which, if relied on, can lead to disaster.

Remote Control

One other area that raises legal issues for personal trainers over and above the general liability matters previously discussed is that of "remote" workouts. You might think it's a great idea to take your client out on a power walk in a remote area (and by remote, I don't mean some secluded hideaway, I mean a place other than the one in which you typically conduct workouts). What if an emergency arises in that place, where there might be no phone and no way to get help if you need to? For example, how about taking your client out for a bike ride or in-line skating? These situations raise the issue of premises liability. If you recommend an unusual location for a workout, you have a duty to warn your client about dangers that might be present.

If you decide to do this (although it's hard to know why you would), I have four suggestions:

1. Visit the area ahead of time and investigate it for obvious dangers that you definitely want to avoid and potential problems that you want to be aware of, work around, and warn your client about.

2. Check with your insurance carrier to make sure your liability policy covers outdoor workouts.

3. Have your attorney prepare a specialized waiver or informed consent for this type of workout.

4. Finally, if I were to take a client on this sort of workout, I would take a cellular phone along just in case of an emergency. Make sure the area is served by 911, or if not, find out the emergency number. Write it on a card and take it with you. Better yet, tape it to the phone.

The subject of remote workouts may raise in your mind the question, "Hmm . . . do I need to check any equipment my client will be using in his aerobic workouts?" The answer is no, *no*, a thousand times NO! Don't go down that road by taking responsibility for equipment for which you do not have custody and over which you have little or no control. If you assume this responsibility, you could be held liable over things that are rendered unsafe due to factors completely beyond your control. HUGE MISTAKE! Other than your own equipment, making sure that the things the client uses are safe and well maintained is your client's problem. The very most any personal trainer should do—and then, only if specifically asked—is to recommend that clients comply with the suggestions in manufacturer-provided owners' manuals.

Recommending Equipment

You'll get a lot of questions from your clients about what type of equipment to buy. The rule here is not to recommend anything without knowing the reason for your recommendation and being able to document it. If you aren't sure about a piece of equipment, say so, but try to help your client by recommending a good fitness equipment retailer where he can go to discuss the right product for him. Notice I said a *good* fitness equipment retailer. I don't mean some cavernous 100,000-square-foot sports superstore where customers can be seen wandering aimlessly through the aisles and a knowledgeable employee is rarer than a snowstorm on Maui. Once you've decided to do personal training, build a relationship with a quality retailer. Go into the retailer's establishment. Introduce yourself. Ask whether you can leave some of your cards. When you get an equipment inquiry, suggest that your client go to this retailer, and be sure he mentions your name.

Handling Emergencies

If you provide proper instruction and supervision, you probably won't have to deal with injuries or other emergencies, but remember that proper instruction and supervision include proper response to emergency situations. Suppose your client drops a dumbbell on her foot. Did you make sure that your client had control of the dumbbell when she picked it up? That is, did you say, "Do you have it?" Did you recommend that your client wear gloves when lifting weights? Were her hands sweaty from her warm-up, making them more likely to be slippery? Were you standing close by and spotting your client properly? Did you take the dumbbell when it looked like she was failing? These are the questions that are relevant to the issue of proper instruction and supervision. The time to think about emergencies is before they happen. Failure to have an emergency plan is negligent and irresponsible.

If despite your best efforts an accident should happen, you should follow standard first-aid procedures. In this example, you should make sure that your client sits down and gets off her foot. You might need to call an ambulance, depending on how serious the accident is. Do not attempt to treat injuries that are beyond your knowledge or ability. The other extremely important thing you need to do is to document exactly what happened. Immediately after you have seen to first-aid matters, sit down and write a summary of the accident. Be specific and answer the following questions:

- Where does the client feel pain or discomfort, if anywhere? (Describe the specific body part affected.)
- Was the injury caused by direct contact with an object, including the ground?
- What specific action was the client doing when the injury occurred?

Emergency Plans Summary

When it comes to safety and injury prevention, fitness professionals should adopt what I like to call a PDQ strategy: prevent, document, and status quo. You need to take every precaution to prevent injury, including close supervision, proper instruction, and attention to details. If an unfortunate event occurs, you need to be sure to accurately and completely document what happens. Finally, if an injury happens, you need to preserve the status quo, as in don't let it get any worse! Do whatever you can to achieve this objective until help arrives. Here are a few points to remember.

1. Always remember that actions taken during the event of an emergency will be evaluated in hindsight. Take-home message: Be prepared *before* something bad happens.

2. Require all participants (and parents of minors) to sign a valid, legally binding (reviewed by an attorney licensed in your state) waiver/assumption of risk form before participation.

3. Educate clients about potential risks of participation and the policies of your facility designed to minimize them. Before participation, athletes should understand and appreciate all the risks associated with various exercises.

4. If you have employee trainers, be sure to educate them about their responsibility to prevent injuries.

5. Maintain your equipment, and do not ignore reports of defective equipment.

6. Spend some time educating your clients about exercise safety, especially beginners who are inexperienced with exercise and equipment.

7. Be prepared for emergencies. Make sure that you

- know the location of the nearest phone and proper emergency numbers (this means you'd better be sure that if you're relying on your cell phone, your battery is charged and you're not running out of minutes or about to be cut off because of not paying your bills!),

- have emergency information for each client always available when you are with that client, and

- maintain current CPR certification.

8. If an accident happens, be sure to document immediately the details of what happened. Memories fade. Be as specific as possible. Imagine that you will not be able to explain in person but that this written explanation will have to speak for you. Don't use pencil, which can smear. Make sure to include the names and phone numbers of any witnesses. Don't admit fault or apologize, because these sorts of statements can be used against you later. Remember that your relationship with your client is your number-one protection against getting sued, so show concern, but don't admit blame.

- Were there any warning signs that something might be wrong, as in complaints about pain or discomfort shortly or immediately before the injury occurred?

- Was there a pop, crack, or any other body-generated noise when the injury occurred?

- Has this client had a similar injury before?

- Were there any obvious outward physical signs of injury such as bleeding, skin discoloration, or swelling?

- Who was present when the injury occurred?

- What was the date and time of the injury?

- What action did you take?

- Was 911 called?

This information could be important to your client's physician. Be especially careful to address the questions in this paragraph. If you did everything right, you'll want to have it on record. See appendix A for a sample injury report form.

One other note about emergencies: Never make any statements that suggest that the accident was your fault. Even an innocent apology can be used against you later. Focus on accurately documented facts, not opinions about whose fault it was.

This is probably a good place to mention that these days, cell phones have become so inexpensive that even kids operating lemonade stands use them to call their moms and ask for more ice. I recommend that if you don't have one already, you get a cell phone that you can use not only for emergencies, but also to accept client and prospect calls.

Insurance

Liability insurance is like your spare tire: You hope you never have to use it, but you certainly are glad it's there when you need it. I don't have a lot to say about liability insurance, except this: Get it, and don't talk to a single client or potential client until you have it. Not that liability insurance will protect you from getting sued. It will protect you if you are sued, though, and that's the important thing. In addition, most potential clients are going to ask you if you have liability insurance. The reason they will is not because they don't have confidence in you, but because everyone realizes that no matter how smart or how careful people are, accidents happen. That's what insurance is for. If and when an accident happens, your insurance is there to protect you and to compensate anyone who may have been injured as a result of the accident. Let's face it: Exercise can be dangerous, and with all those heavy objects swinging through free space and things on the floor, gyms are minefields. So given that fact, only a real beanbag would avoid having liability insurance. Think about it: You're a safe driver, but you still have auto insurance, right? Of course you do.

Some other people also might be interested in whether you have liability insurance. If you are lucky enough to be allowed to come into a gym or health club as an outside trainer, the owners will at a minimum insist that you provide them with evidence of liability insurance.

You should direct any specific insurance questions or requests from third parties to your agent. All you need to worry about is making sure that you satisfy yourself that you have adequate and current coverage, and of course, that your premiums are paid.

Insurance is another advantage of certification, because you can often get affordable liability insurance through your certifying organization. ACE, NSCA, and ACSM offer liability insurance, as do several other certifying organizations. However you get it, just get it! It is extremely important that you have liability insurance in force before you do any personal training. Pay close attention to the date and time that your policy becomes effective and expires.

Waivers and Informed Consents

Before you start working with a new client, you should require her, in addition to filling out a health history questionnaire, to sign a waiver and informed consent form. As we previously mentioned, exercise is a powerful therapy, and as such has risks as well as benefits. The waiver and informed consent advises your client of the risks and benefits of the program and may give you some protection if a lawsuit is filed against you. Although the legal concepts of "waiver" (surrendering a legal right or benefit) and "informed consent" (the process of a legally competent adult's acknowledging the risks he's assuming and knowingly agreeing to assume them) are distinct, they are related and so are often combined in one form as we've done on our sample form in appendix A. For convenience, we'll refer to this form as the waiver, even though it includes both separate legal acts by your client.

Enforceable Waivers

I can see some of you now with shocked expressions on your faces, saying, "But, Ter, I didn't think those things were worth the paper that they're printed on!" Wrong-o, my friend. Courts enforce properly drafted waivers every day of the week. The key phrase is "properly drafted," which is why it's extremely important to have your waiver form reviewed before you use it by an attorney licensed to practice in your state.

In general, here are the kinds of waivers that courts uphold:

- **Clear and unambiguous.** This is no time to pussyfoot around. Remember the question that should always be in the back of your mind when it comes to working with clients (this is only the first time that you'll hear this phrase when we discuss the subject of getting sued; it definitely won't be the last): "What's the worst thing that could happen?" Whatever the answer is, you need to say that explicitly in your waiver. My waiver form specifically mentions the risk of death during exercise. Have any of my clients ever died during a workout? No, but we all know that astounding and unexpected things can happen during exercise. One day an employee of mine, a personal trainer, and I decided to try a spinning class at our club. Her husband, a lean, fit, nonsmoking 35-year-old, decided to join us. We had a great time and all was well. About three weeks later, while running at the track, he collapsed in cardiac arrest. It was only then that doctors diagnosed a congenital heart defect. So bad things can happen when you least expect them to, and your waiver needs to mention them.

- **Explicit.** You need to be explicit in describing not only the risks but also what activities you intend to cover with the waiver. If you're going to be doing fitness testing in addition to workouts, be sure to cover that. If you're working out in the client's home, make sure you provide for the risks inherent in using equipment that you don't maintain or control. If you think of it, just say it!

• **Consistent with state law.** The law in this area is constantly changing. Not only that, but it varies state by state. Some state courts have defined "magic words" that you need to use to protect yourself. It's not your job to know those words. That's your attorney's job. Have your waiver form prepared by a qualified lawyer who knows your state's law, and things should be just fine.

• **Knowing.** In addition to being clear, explicit, and consistent with state law, a waiver is more likely to protect you if it is what lawyers call a "knowing" waiver; that is, you don't want anyone to be able to say that it was signed without having first been read and understood, or that there was any pressure to sign it.

A sample waiver and informed consent form is given in appendix A. Although these forms are not intended to substitute for the judgment and skill of an attorney licensed to practice in your state, you can give them to your attorney to use as a template. This is likely to save you money because in many cases the attorney will simply have to review the forms and make minor revisions.

Proper Waiver Administration

It's not enough to have a waiver form, though. You've got to know how to use it. After your attorney has assured you that your waiver form is valid, there is one more step you need to take to make sure it is legally enforceable: You must learn how to administer the waiver properly. This step is just as important as the content of the waiver itself because if you don't administer it correctly, you can invalidate the whole darn thing. Here are suggestions for proper waiver administration:

• **Explain what the waiver is and the reason you're asking the client to sign it.** This is because exercise, even when done appropriately and under proper supervision, has inherent risks that the client is willingly assuming as a condition of your working with him.

• **Don't minimize the significance of the waiver.** When explaining the waiver, never say any of the following:

- "Oh, it's just a formality."

- "It doesn't mean anything, but my lawyer makes me do it."

- "It's just for insurance purposes."

Statements like these can invalidate the waiver because courts can find that the client didn't really understand the full legal effect of his signature on the document. You aren't trying to trick anybody. You want it out front and above board: If you do what you're supposed to do, but he or she gets hurt anyway, you don't want to be sued.

• **Don't hover over the client waiting for him or her to sign it.** I recommend that once you have agreed to work with a new client, you send the waiver to him or her in advance of your first session. You can say, "I'll be sending you my new-client packet, which contains my policies and some other information that will help us get a good start. It also includes my waiver form that I want you to read carefully, and have your attorney read if you'd like. If you have any questions about that, please give me a call." The point is that you don't want there to be any suggestion of coercion or pressure on the client to sign. These things are the opposite of voluntary assumption of risk and are therefore the opposite of what you want here. Either enclose a self-addressed stamped envelope or have the client fax the forms back to you in advance of that first meeting so you don't waste time going to a client's home only to find out he or she hasn't signed the waiver.

• **Keep all waivers in a safe place for the appropriate length of time.** A signed, appropriately administered waiver won't do you much good if you can't find it, so preserve these important documents in a safe place. Your attorney will tell you how long to hang onto them. The statute of limitations differs from state to state.

• **When in doubt, card 'em.** A minor cannot enter into a legal contract, which a waiver is; therefore, if you work with minors, or have any doubt about the age of your client, ask him or her to produce some ID. When working with minors, you might consider an "agreement to participate," which is not a contract but might provide some protection. Consult with your attorney to see whether this form would be a good adjunct to your personal training practice (Eickhoff-Shemek and Forbes 1999).

• **Keep one thing in mind:** The best waiver is one that you never have to refer to again because of your strict attention to proper safety procedures.

Health Forms

Appendix A contains a sample health history questionnaire as well as a sample physician's consent form. As in the case of the waiver, these forms are provided for informational purposes only and are not intended to substitute for the judgment of an attorney licensed to practice in your state.

Here are the forms you'll find in appendix A:

- **Letter of agreement.** The letter of agreement summarizes all the terms and conditions of your business relationship with your client, including the rate per session, how your client will be billed, and that all-important cancellation policy. Specifics are included in the "Policies" section of exhibit A.

- **Health history questionnaire.** As discussed in more detail in chapter 4, you will need to screen your clients to determine their risk of cardiovascular and metabolic disease as well as pre-existing orthopedic problems that you will need to work around. This form gives you the information that you need to do so.

- **Medical clearance and physician's consent to participate.** Some clients will have pre-existing medical conditions that require that they see their doctors before you work with them. This form is a short, easy way for busy docs to let you know what's OK and what to avoid.

- **Goal inventory and lifestyle questionnaire.** These forms address the changes that will take place inside your clients' heads. The information requested gives you a heads-up about your clients' attitudes toward exercise and food so that you can customize your motivational strategies for maximum effectiveness.

- **Workout record form.** This form will help you keep track of your clients' progress and keeps the information in an organized format.

Statutes That Might Affect You

Most states have laws against practicing medicine without a license, but what is meant by "practicing medicine"? Every state defines this phrase differently, through either statute or case law. Penalties can be severe. (In Illinois, for example, the unauthorized practice of medicine is a felony. Unauthorized practice of medicine includes not only diagnosing and treating illnesses, but also attaching the title "Doctor" to your name to represent yourself as authorized to treat illnesses.) Clearly, no personal trainer should attempt to treat diseases or other medical problems with supplements, special diets, or similar modalities.

Your clients might ask your advice on the treatment of injuries. You should always preface any response to questions about treating injuries with the statement "Of course, I'm not a doctor, and I can't diagnose your injury," or something similar. Limit your advice to general statements about RICE (rest, ice, compression, and elevation) and recommend that your clients see their physicians for diagnosis and treatment of injuries. Continue to monitor reported injuries by asking your client to keep a written diary about them and report on their progress regularly so that you can make necessary modifications in their workouts.

Some states regulate activities that personal trainers sometimes engage in. For example, in Illinois, there is a statute that regulates the giving of advice on nutrition. Your state may have similar laws or regulations. Consult with a licensed attorney to find out which restrictions affect you.

The Best Protection Against Lawsuits

The very best protection against lawsuits is not certification, insurance, or even a well-written waiver form. The very best insurance against lawsuits is a good professional relationship with your client for whom you have designed safe, effective, well-thought-out programs. There is no greater protection because the personal trainer-client relationship is just that—a personal relationship. If you show genuine concern for your client, your chances of his suing you are greatly, greatly diminished.

Some experts who have analyzed the explosion in medical malpractice lawsuits over the last 20 to 25 years found they had less to do with a decline in the quality of medical care and more with a decline in the quality of personal relationships between physicians and their patients. They noted how the physician-patient relationship had changed from the days of the avuncular Marcus Welby–type coming to the house to look after a sick child, to the time-pressured HMO doctor who is cognizant of every second ticking away as he hurriedly deals with each patient's problems. The same thing applies to you. If you have a good relationship with your client, even if an accident happens, you'll be less likely to see a lawsuit resulting from the accident.

The Ethics of Personal Training

Is personal training a "learned profession"? It should be, in the ordinary sense of the words, since it requires knowledge, expertise, and skill to do it right. Traditionally, though, the learned professions were law, medicine, and the priesthood. This "learned profession" thing goes back to the Middle Ages, when those were the only professions. Today, other professions that also require knowledge, education, and advanced expertise—from accountant to zoo horticulturist—(see www.azh.org for the mission and bylaws of the Association of Zoo Horticulturists) have codes of ethics, mission statements, by-laws, or similar documents setting out their goals and what it means to be a professional. In the opinion of many, including yours truly, personal trainers will never be regarded as genuine professionals until they all accept a uniform code of ethics. I think it is more important and will have more beneficial impact on the industry than any licensure law ever could. The reason is that a piece of paper is only as good as the people governed by it. I recognized that and attempted to address it when I wrote the eight core beliefs in the introduction to this book. The ACSM has thought of this issue, too. They adopted a comprehensive code of ethics to address these concerns. Their code requires that members

- strive to continuously improve knowledge and skill,
- maintain high professional and scientific standards,
- safeguard the public against members who are incompetent and unethical, and
- strive to improve the health and well-being of not only individuals but the whole community as well (ACSM Code of Ethics).

In her excellent article on ethical behavior in the fitness industry, Kathryn Hilgenkamp lays out the following 15 specific areas that fitness professionals need to consider to make sure that they are behaving ethically:

1. Competency. Formal education and certification are to being a professional what getting a driver's license is to being a good driver. It takes continuing education to stay competent.

2. Certification. Beware of certifications without a practical component from fly-by-night organizations.

3. Scope of practice. We know that practicing outside one's area of expertise and competence is not only unethical; it can be illegal.

4. Conflict of interest. It would be highly unethical to work for competing employers and potentially share trade secrets. It is also a potential conflict of interest to sell products like supplements to clients, since you may be influenced by your own financial concerns to sell them things they don't need.

5. Client autonomy. The client is always in charge, and genuine professionals never forget that. They don't try to create dependency or take advantage of their clients' trust in them.

6. Communication. Professionals are always completely honest and explain the terms and conditions of everything to their clients.

7. Harassment and discrimination. In some contexts, harassment and discrimination may be illegal. They are always unpleasant to be around and are the mark of a genuine oaf.

8. Dual relationships. Personal relationships with clients are a bad idea. If you must get personal with a client, refer him or her to another personal trainer.

9. Screening and risk stratification. Clients hire professionals to solve problems, but you can't solve a problem without first identifying it. A personal trainer is often the first one to detect a potentially serious medical condition because it's not possible to design safe and effective programs without screening.

10. Use of testing information. It's not appropriate to give a standardized series of assessments. Although everyone will need to be screened for cardiovascular and metabolic problems, medications, and musculoskeletal conditions, not every client needs a body composition test. Use professional judgment in test selection.

11. Informed consent and informed refusal. Once again, clients are in charge and have full veto power over the tests they choose to allow you to administer after being told of the risks, benefits, and uses for the information obtained.

12. Confidentiality. The confidences and secrets of a client must be held strictly confidential.

13. Test accuracy. Make your tests meaningful by making them as accurate as possible.

14. Exercise program efficacy. You must design a safe, effective program to meet your client's goals, and to keep him or her motivated to reach those goals. Cookie-cutter programs won't do it.

15. Copyright infringements. It is not ethical to violate the copyright laws by using workout music, videos, or software without the consent of the copyright holder. Ethical professionals do not knowingly break the law (Hilgenkamp 1998).

Most of these things are just common sense, but thinking about them in this organized, specific way will help you decide whether you should or shouldn't take a particular action. Ms. Hilgenkamp's article also contains a self-assessment test that you can use to test your ethical score.

Being an ethical professional enhances your reputation, your self-esteem, and your income. Those who pay premium rates want to hire the very best and only the very best.

Meet Your Fitness Goals or Die Trying

Early on the morning of October 1, 1998, 37-year-old Anne Marie Capati, a mother of two and a knitwear designer for a large national company, arrived at Manhattan's Crunch gym to work out before she went to the office. Her personal trainer, August Casseus, whose Crunch brochure read, "Meet your fitness goals, or die trying," met her. Anne Marie told her trainer that her head had been hurting for several days, but she proceeded to warm up by doing some light squats. She felt nauseated and weak. She stopped exercising, threw up, and passed out. At 9:45 P.M. that same day, she died as the result of a massive cerebral hemorrhage.

After Anne Marie's death, some interesting facts came to light. Her husband found a handwritten list of instructions in her gym bag. The instructions were written in the same hand as a diet plan that her trainer had given her, and listed several recommended supplements that Anne Marie should take to help her lose weight. He also read an entry in her diary indicating that August Casseus had accompanied Anne Marie to a vitamin store around the corner from the gym to purchase supplements (Brownlee 2000). The recommended supplements included products that contained ephedra, an herbal product that is strictly contraindicated for anyone with cardiovascular disease. Anne Marie was such a person. She had hypertension for which she took the drug Normodyne (Chase 1999). In June 1999, Anne Marie's husband filed a $40 million lawsuit against Crunch Fitness, August Casseus, and several supplement manufacturers (Brownlee 2000).

What lessons can we learn from this tragic story? First and most obvious, personal trainers have no business recommending supplements to their clients. Going to the store to help the client purchase them is beyond stupid. Unless you are a licensed physician, the most you should do in this regard is recommend reference resources for clients to read. Second, a personal trainer should be familiar with a client's current medical condition. Although many people get headaches, in a person with hypertension, a headache can precede a serious cerebral vascular event. When in doubt, err on the side of safety and have the client skip the workout and go see the doctor. Third, although many fitness professionals are tempted to add a supplement profit center to their businesses, this course of action presents a major ethical dilemma. The income potential of selling these pills and powders is enormous, and therefore so is their siren song for personal trainers. You are only one person, and you can see only so many clients a week, but you can sell thousands of bottles of capsules to thousands of people every single day. If you sell them online, you can even sell them while you're asleep. Given this enormous potential payoff, do you really think you will be able to avoid recommending them to every single one of your clients? Clients—what am I saying? Before long, you'll probably be buttonholing people on the street and saying, "Do you want to buy some fat burners?" The point is that it's impossible to devote yourself 100% to what's good for your clients when the thought of the potential for augmenting your own bottom line is always in the back of your mind.

I've got nothing against supplements. I take them myself. If you decide to make your living selling them, more power to you, provided that that's all you do. In my opinion, personal trainers who sell supplements put themselves in a potential conflict-of-interest situation every single day.

Marketing Your Business

Questions we'll answer in this chapter:

- How do I attract potential clients?

- How do I market my services by stressing my unique features and benefits?

- How do I write an effective ad?

- What items do I need to have in place before I meet with a potential client?

- What items does a prospect need to have in place before my first meeting with her?

- What "powerful questions" can I use to understand my client's "heart's desire?"

- How do I overcome a prospect's objections to becoming a client?

You may think that your goal is simply to "get clients." If you are laboring under this mistaken impression, let me suggest a more profitable alternative. Instead, your goal should be to develop a book of long-standing clients whom see you week after week, month after month, and year after year.

You want your business to be characterized by the following:

- **Minimal client turnover.** Each standing client represents, at least at the crass financial level we're discussing here, a stream of several hundreds, or even thousands, of dollars in income. To the extent that you don't have to continue replacing lost clients, that income stream continues in an uninterrupted way.

- **Minimal marketing expenditures.** The very best marketing, hands down, is word of mouth. One very satisfied client is worth thousands of dollars in advertising and marketing expenditures. If you have lots of clients singing your praises, you won't have to spend much, if anything, on marketing.

- **Efficient use of time.** Recognize that as a personal trainer your product is your expertise, your knowledge, and, most of all, your time. You need to try to avoid wasting it.

- **Effective programs.** Effective programs equal not only satisfied clients but also job satisfaction for you.

Knowing how to achieve these characteristics in your business is what this chapter is all about.

Marketing

Marketing is simply promoting your business and attracting clients. It's getting the word out in a general way. Marketing is to sales what a radio broadcast is to a telephone call. The former is general, directed to a large number of people. The latter is personal, a one-on-one conversation. Marketing is what makes the phone ring by piquing the interest of potential clients, what salespeople call prospects. Marketing is to sales what love is to marriage. It comes first and if things go well, it leads to a happy conclusion. Since your relationship with your client begins with marketing, let's start there.

You should approach marketing your business just as you approach any important project, by setting objectives and mapping out the steps to reach them. Think of it this way: Somewhere out there are scads of people who will benefit from working with you. They're just waiting for you to reach out, tap them on the shoulder, and tell them how you can enrich their lives. That's where marketing comes in.

Appealing to Your Customer

There are three steps to successfully marketing your business:

1. Identifying your potential customers
2. Establishing your positioning in the market-place
3. Spreading the word

Who Is Your Customer?

Identifying your target market—answering the questions "Who do I want to work with?" and "How do I reach them?"—is your first step in getting clients. You might be thinking, *I'll work with anyone! I just want to do personal training!* What's wrong with that? Simply this: You can't do everything, and do everything well. Remember, your goal is to be the best in your field, and to be your best, you need to concentrate on what you do best. You shouldn't decide that you want to train bodybuilders preparing for competition if your background is primarily in teaching aerobics. If you spent several years in competitive swimming, you'd be uniquely qualified to work with swimmers, designing programs to help them improve their performance. A woman in my master's program, a student who returned to school after raising her family, decided that she wanted to work with physically active people over age 50 who live or work near her home. This is her target market. Here are a few exercises to help you get started finding yours.

List Your Qualifications and Profile Your Ideal Customers

The first things you must think (and write!) about are the qualities that make you unique as a personal trainer and the kinds of customers you are especially qualified to work with. So here are your first two tasks:

- **List your special qualifications.** What benefits can you offer people that someone else with similar education cannot? Have you participated in a sport in addition to weight training? For example, are you a golfer, tennis player, or swimmer who can coach these sports as well as provide advice on general conditioning?

- **Write a profile of your ideal customer.** Be as specific as possible. How old is she? Where does she live? What sports does she do? What does she do for a living? What is her annual income? It's important to get a clear picture of this client, so spend some time and effort doing it. After you have come up with a specific, detailed picture of your customer, you will be able to find her.

Think About the Problem You Will Solve for the Customer

Studies have shown that people hire personal trainers for three main reasons:

1. To improve their muscle tone or body shape
2. To control their weight
3. To improve their exercise adherence

With that information, plus your detailed description of your target client, you should be able to come up with a dynamite ad that will really push the buttons of your target audience.

The following examples can help you begin to think just how to appeal to the ideal customer you've identified.

- **You've decided that your ideal client is a married woman between 30 and 60 years old** who has gained the typical 15 to 25 pounds that is unfortunately average for this population. She wants to get rid of this extra weight and return her now flabby arms and legs to their pre-childbirth firmness. Your ad needs to stress your ability to raise her metabolism, burn fat, and sculpt shapely contours in a minimum of time. Your ad should say something like, "It's a scientific fact: Studies have shown that people who do resistance training lose three times as much fat as those who do cardiovascular exercise alone." Make this provocative statement the headline, then follow with some copy, such as, "If you would like to reshape your hips and thighs, flatten your tummy, and regain the strength that you had before life (kids, husbands, jobs) showed up, give me a call. I can show you how to achieve these benefits safely and with a minimal investment of time. You won't even need to leave your house because I come to you and bring all my expertise and motivation along. No gym, no travel time, just a new you. Call today!"
- **Your ideal client is a business executive whose passion is golf.** "Would you like to add 20 yards to your drive?" is your headline, with appropriate golf graphics that you or your newspaper's designer can supply. The copy states, "Research has

shown that golfers who do resistance and flexibility training can do just that. Not just any 'exercise' will do the job, though. To achieve these benefits, you need a program designed to strengthen certain muscles and stretch others. You need to build endurance and power by engaging all the muscles in your 'power core.' It doesn't have to take lots of time from your busy life, if you know how to do it right. I do, and I can show you. Please call me today. Mention this ad and I'll send you a free copy of the study I mentioned."

You get the idea. You and your programs offer certain features (education and expertise, great customer service) that mean nothing to the customer unless you stress benefits (weight loss, reshaping body contours, improved sports performance) that he craves like an ice cream cone on a hot summer evening.

Envision Where Your Customer Can Be Reached

You wouldn't reach middle-aged executives who like to play golf by advertising in a decorating magazine, would you? Of course not. Since you've clearly defined your customer, you shouldn't have any problem figuring out where he likes to go and what he likes to do. Answer these questions about your ideal client:

1. Where does your ideal customer go on a regular basis?
2. What publications does your ideal customer read?
3. What activities does your ideal customer like to participate in?

Returning to our examples, to reach the weight- and appearance-conscious females in your target market, consider some cross-marketing with a tanning or hair salon in which you leave some coupons at these establishments offering a "free consultation" for their customers. Women who worry about having a good tan are probably very looks-conscious, and so your pitch about losing fat and firming up will speak to them at a deep and emotional level. For the golf-crazed execs, look into placing an ad in a golf publication in your area. I don't mean national magazines, whose fees can run to several thousand dollars. Even if you could afford these rates, you'd be telling thousands of people thousands of miles away about a service that is literally out of their reach. Instead, look into local publications. Many small local newspapers

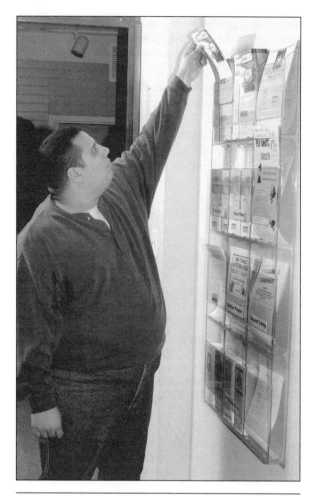

To reach your ideal customer you should identify his interests—where he goes, what he reads, and what activities he likes.

periodically run special sections featuring topics like golf to appeal to potential advertisers. Some locales have local golf publications, magazines, or tabloid newspapers that would be ideal ways to reach your target customer. Do some research and see what is available in your area.

Establish Your Positioning in the Marketplace

The key to being successful in personal training, in terms of both your income and your impact, is to specialize and to make yourself unique. Whatever you do, you do not want to be perceived as "fungible," or interchangeable with a dozen others. What is fungible is devalued. The number-one criterion for deciding where to purchase a fungible commodity is price. Here's an obvious example: Books are fungible. If you want the latest best-seller by your favorite author, the copy you get will be the same

whether you get it at a discount store, online, or at a small specialty bookstore; therefore, your decision about where to purchase the book will most likely be based on where you can get it for the fewest dollars.

On the other hand, what is unique is prized. To be one of a kind, you need to be able to state the following, in a 30-second "elevator speech":

1. What you do
2. Who benefits from what you do
3. How you are unique from everyone else in your profession

For example, Tom Trainer is a personal trainer who works with time-challenged professionals. He is the only personal trainer in Anytown who offers clients the option of a massage after their workouts. Kerry Koach is an optimum-performance coach who teaches tennis players how to get to and stay at the top of their games. Unlike other tennis coaches, she has a master's degree in exercise science and is a former tennis champion.

What can you do that will make you different from everyone else? Here are some questions to help you define your uniqueness.

• **What is your educational background?** If you have an MBA as well as bachelor's degree in kinesiology, you could stress your ability to deal with your clients' issues as with a business turnaround, something that would appeal to the denizens of corporate offices.

• **What unusual experiences have you had that might help you bring a unique point of view to the personal training process?** If you are a cancer survivor, you bring a unique and inspirational perspective to everything you do. If you are a mother of six who somehow has managed to fit exercise into your life, you've got some secrets to share.

• **What additional skills and/or training do you have?** In our Tom Trainer example earlier, we mentioned that in addition to being a personal trainer, he is a massage therapist. Can you take clients through a directed meditation at the end of the workout because you spent 10 years sitting on a Tibetan mountaintop under the tutelage of a Zen master? If so, that makes you unique! (I know: Duh.)

• **What personal training experiences make you special?** Have you worked with celebrities? Appeared on local television as an expert in residence? Do you write a health and fitness column for a newspaper? Any of these experiences make you special because out of all the personal trainers in your area, you have been selected as the most qualified expert to give advice to either large, general audiences or people who theoretically could choose anyone. If you work with Mr. Big Celebrity for whom money is no object, you must be good! The very fact that you are Mr. B.C.'s trainer will make many others want to hire you just so that they can attend cocktail parties and tell their friends, "My trainer Sally? Oh yes, she's Mr. B.C.'s trainer, too."

Give this a lot of thought because it will drive all your marketing. Your business cards, brochures, direct mail letters, Rotary Club speeches, and any other vehicle you use to get the word out about your services should emphasize your positioning in the marketplace. If you've decided to specialize as we discussed in "List Your Special Qualifications" earlier, all of your marketing materials should trumpet the fact that you are uniquely qualified to coach these specific clients. Say, "the last word in optimum performance for the serious golfer," or whatever your specialty is, and say it loud, big, and often.

Outline a Strategy

With a clear understanding of your ideal client and of what is unique about the services you will offer, start planning your marketing strategy. For example, after doing a little snooping around, you determine that most of the people in your target market shop regularly at a small sporting goods store downtown. You also learn that most of the people in your target market read the afternoon paper. You should approach the store's owners about putting some of your business cards by the register, and place an attractive display ad in the afternoon paper. Then wait for your phone to ring!

Advertising

Many personal trainers have begun their businesses with one well-designed, well-placed ad. Once you have identified your target market, you should be able to figure out where and when to run this special ad and what it should say.

Print Ads

Sometimes newspapers or magazines offer small businesses substantially discounted rates if they agree to advertise every week, or at some other regular interval for an extended period. This seems like a bargain, but it will be one only if the ad pulls in customers. Otherwise, it will be a millstone around your neck, taking dollars away from what would otherwise be an effective marketing program. Try a single ad in the paper and see how that works for you. If you get enough calls, consider asking the ad representative about discounted rates.

Every time you create a print ad, include each of the following elements, and make sure you've paid close attention to the material describing what makes each of these elements effective.

- **Headline.** Begin with a provocative, attention-getting statement that will get potential clients to read the rest of the copy.

- **Subheading and explanation of the benefits you are stressing.** Here's where you explain what you have to do with the provocative statement or question in the headline.

- **Visual focal point.** Most print ads have a photo or graphic because these elements attract the eye. Consider putting something eye-catching in your ad. If you can't think of an appropriate visual, ask the designers at the publication you are using to help. Often they are very experienced at this process and very good at coming up with something terrific.

- **Call to action.** It does no good to interest prospects in your services if you don't lead them by the hand to the next step, so say, "Call today and let's talk about how you can go into the new year fitting into those jeans in the back of your closet. Mention this ad and receive a free gift. Offer good through January 15." The reason you say a "free gift," instead of specify what that gift is, is that you may want to run this ad several times and you don't want to limit yourself to a particular item that you may have in limited quantities. You might also want to change the freebie based on the time of year to create a holiday tie-in. Asking callers to mention the ad lets you track which publications are drawing a lot of interest (advertise in these again) and those that don't stimulate a single call (lose the phone number of their ad department). Including an expiration date not only inspires a sense of urgency to deter procrastination but also protects you from having someone show up a year later asking for a free gift when you no longer have anything to give.

- **Contact information.** Include not only your phone number but also your e-mail address because these days many people prefer to communicate through e-mail. If you have a Web site, say, "For more information, call 555-5555, or visit our Web site [include the Web address here] for more information." You could put a list of FAQs (frequently asked questions) there and conclude the FAQ page with your e-mail address.

Referrals

Some of the best methods of marketing won't cost you anything! Without a doubt, word of mouth is the very best source of new clients. The fact that your current client recommends you sells you as a competent, professional personal trainer. Being recommended by a client is one of the highest forms of praise you can get!

Referrals from other professionals also cost you nothing. One advantage of getting at least a bachelor's degree in exercise physiology, exercise science, or a related field is that you will have a much easier time marketing your services to physicians, chiropractors, physical therapists, and other health professionals. It's not that only people with degrees know anything. I know some competent, excellent personal trainers who are self-educated. It might seem unfair, but health professionals, wary of liability and degreed themselves, tend to be extremely reluctant to recommend anyone without formal credentials. If you have a degree and are certified by a reputable organization, you can confidently approach health professionals and offer your services to help them get their patients started on safe, effective fitness programs.

Marketing Materials

Sometimes people ask me how to come up with a business name. Everyone wants something clever but not cutesy, something people will remember. Unfortunately, there's no easy way to find these little gems. In my experience, the best ones are often the result of serendipity. They seem to sprout from that special precious spot in the brain, pass through the heart, and spring to our consciousness ("Aha!"). Failing an "aha," you could do some brainstorming, either alone or with friends. Write down without hesitation everything that occurs to you and see if anything inspired pops out. If not, don't despair. There's nothing wrong with using your name, and there's at least one advantage: You don't have to do any costly name searches to see if anyone is already using your perfect name. If you do decide to use a catchy name for your business, your attorney can advise you on how to do a search to see if it is taken. In most cases, this process will not be difficult or costly.

Your Business Card

The most important marketing piece you have is your business card (see figure 3.1). It is the item that most people will keep and remember you by, so get the best-quality card you can. Do everything possible to make it look professional. Use high-quality card stock. Strongly consider hiring a graphic designer to come up with a logo for your company.

A word about titles: If you don't have a master's degree, should you put any initials after your name? I suggest simply the title "Personal Trainer" under your name. Sometime when I wasn't looking, some trainers started using the initials "CPT," which I now realize means "Certified Personal Trainer," after their names. I've seen this title a lot lately, especially in health clubs. (The first time I saw this CPT business, I thought the card's presenter was a physical therapist!) Perhaps it's my legal background, but I'm not sure I can recommend that approach. It seems like a misrepresentation. It always appears to me that the person is trying to overstate his credentials, as if he's saying, "No, I don't have a degree, so I can't use the initials MS, MD, or PhD, so I'll use some other initials. Maybe if I'm lucky they'll get confused and think I'm a physical therapist or something." Most people are not fooled by this, at least not those who can afford to pay your fee, and it only calls attention to the fact that you don't have a master's degree. List your phone number and a catchy tag line if you've been able to think of one.

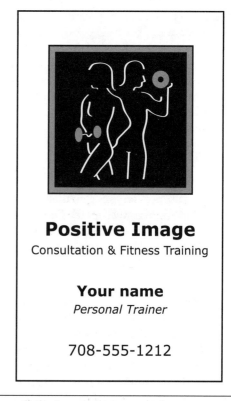

Positive Image
Consultation & Fitness Training

Your name
Personal Trainer

708-555-1212

Figure 3.1 Sample business card.

Brochures and Leaflets

A business card is really the only essential marketing piece that you need. If you desire, and if you have invested the time and effort in creating a logo, have some brochures printed to help promote your business. Describe the benefits of your service and any special features you offer. Not only do you not have to spend an arm and a leg on these, I suggest you don't. I'm not saying you should create some cheesy-looking thing that could be mistaken for a ransom note, but it's the content that counts most. As with your business card, use quality paper and spend some time considering the design of the piece, but remember that the most important aspect of the brochure is substance, not style. By this stage, you will have given serious thought to what makes you special and sets your service apart; that information will be the strongest "selling point" in your brochure, so be sure you highlight it.

Some Questions to Ask Yourself When Designing Your Brochure

- What benefits will clients get from hiring you? List them and use them in your brochure.
- What business are you in? Be specific—not just "personal training," but "training people over 50 in Anytown, USA."
- How will this piece be distributed? Eye-catching design is more important if you plan to leave your brochure on store counters than if you plan to mail it. And speaking of mailing, consider whether you want to design your brochure to be a self-mailer, that is, one that requires no envelope because one panel has room for the mailing address on it.

Sales: Your First Contact

All good salespeople understand that selling is not simply about getting people to hand over money. The best salespeople view themselves as professional consultants who serve their customers by selling solutions.

The First Rule: Listen!

Many personal trainers make the mistake of thinking that people hire them because of how much they know. As a result, they spend about twice as much time talking as they do listening. This is the exact reverse of what they should be doing. The key to getting hired is effective listening. Yes, a prospective client wants to hire a knowledgeable, well-educated professional personal trainer, but his initial concern is not whether he is speaking to the smartest person in the room. He is focused on himself and whether the trainer can help him achieve a goal.

The first time you talk to your prospective new client, you will have a limited amount of time to impress him with your professionalism, knowledge, and infectious enthusiasm. The best way you can do this is by asking intelligent questions, listening carefully to your prospective client's answers, and by sharing with him just enough relevant knowledge to let him know that you are equipped to handle his concerns. The information about why most people hire personal trainers discussed earlier is just the beginning of your understanding of how to help *this* client. Don't assume that every person who calls you is looking to get "buns of steel." Every client is unique. So use this limited time to find out what this client wants and how you are in a unique position to answer his perceived needs. This is such an important aspect of being an effective (and successful!) personal trainer that we'll talk in greater detail about how to listen in chapter 9.

Typically, your first contact will be over the phone. Begin by asking how she heard about you. This information sets the tone for the rest of the conversation. If she heard about you from one of your current customers, you don't have to spend as much time giving her your entire educational and professional biography, although you should still give basic information. If she is responding to an ad, encourage her to tell you about her current fitness situation and what she hopes you can do for her.

What comes next depends on how serious you perceive this prospect to be. Let's face it: You'd like to work with everyone, but there is only one of you and you have to ration your precious time carefully, if not ruthlessly. Everyone wants to know how much things cost, of course, but if a prospect seems concerned about cost to the exclusion of everything else, I suggest that you send her a rate card describing your services and the prices for each. If price, not quality, is a prospect's primary concern, why spend a lot of time describing all of your qualifications? If you are a well-educated

Check Off These Items Before Your First Prospective Client Contact

- Do you have current knowledge of anatomy, physiology, and biomechanics? In short, do you know what you're doing?
- Are you certified by a reputable organization?
- Do you have liability insurance?
- Do you have the following forms?
  - Health history questionnaire
  - Waivers
  - Goal inventory
- Has your waiver form been reviewed by an attorney licensed to practice in your state?
- Do you have written policies in place regarding payment, cancellation, and credits for canceled workouts?
- Do you have current CPR certification?
- Do you have a separate business checking account?
- Do you have a bookkeeping system in place?
- Do you have all required business licenses and/or other permits required by your city or state?
- Do you have a separate phone line (probably your cell phone) for your business, or at least have you made arrangements to have your business calls handled professionally?

professional, you will never be able to compete on price, because, as we have discussed, the world is full of less-than-qualified people who are willing to work for slightly above minimum wage. Let your rate card speak for you. On the other hand, if after a few minutes of conversation it is apparent that this prospect really wants to work with you, and she hasn't asked you yet about price, you should tell her your rates. If she isn't scared off by that, arrange a meeting at a mutually convenient time and place.

Items Your New Client Should Have on or Before Your First Meeting

- Brochure
- Business card
- Letter of agreement
- Waivers
- Health history questionnaire
- Goal inventory
- Self-addressed, stamped envelope (if you plan on having the forms mailed back to you)

Ask the Powerful Questions When You Meet

This meeting is for the benefit of both you and your potential client. I strongly believe that before either of you enters into any sort of trainer-client relationship, you should meet, talk briefly, and make sure you're comfortable with each other. If you're planning to work out in the client's home, meet there. That will give you the opportunity to inventory the available equipment, see the available space, and otherwise prepare for any special needs dictated by the workout area. If you'll be working out in a club or gym, the meeting gives the client a chance to see the facility, find out about memberships, and get comfortable there. Bring your packet of new-client forms with you to this meeting.

The following are powerful and open-ended questions designed to get prospective clients to talk and reveal important clues about what they are looking for. Don't interrupt them. Instead, pay attention and take notes. Then use this information to address their specific needs, concerns, and goals.

- **Question:** Tell me about your exercise history. Have you exercised much in the last year? In the last five years?

  Reveals: whether compliance is an issue for this person

- **Question:** How did you hear about me?

  Reveals: how effective your marketing is, what his or her initial impression was of you and your services

- **Question:** Have you worked with a personal trainer before? If so, why did you stop?

  Reveals: what's important to this person in a personal trainer, and how a personal trainer can disappoint

- **Question:** Have you ever gotten injured during exercise? If so, what happened?

  Reveals: information about specific problems to be aware of; gives you an opportunity to talk about your expertise; probing can reveal if this person has ever sued a personal trainer

- **Question:** Have you given any thought to the type of exercise program that you think would be fun for you?

  Reveals: the type of program you should design to please this client

- **Question:** How often do you think you might want to work together? What time of day would work for you?

  Reveals: how committed this person is and where he or she might fit into your existing client base and current schedule

- **Question:** If we were to work together, how would you evaluate my performance as your trainer?

  Reveals: what you really need to focus on

If all goes well, congratulations—you have a client!

Handling Common Prospect Objections

Even though usually your first contact with a potential client will come when he calls you, that doesn't mean that he's ready to write you a big check. If you've done it right, your effective marketing will have him so intrigued that he's got to find out what this personal training thing is all about. Still, prospects typically exhibit some resistance to signing up and handing over the cash.

Reasons for Objections

The three most common reasons for prospects' objections are inertia, failure to appreciate the benefits,

and having had a prior bad experience with a similar service.

- **Inertia.** As the old saying goes, the only person who likes change is a wet baby. It seems to be human nature to resist change. The prospect may be thinking, *Sure, I'm a little overweight and I need to start exercising, but I can just get a tape or a book and get started on my own. What if I bite off more than I can chew here?*

- **Failure to appreciate the benefits.** You've got to give the prospect a good reason to become your client, one that answers the question, "What's in it for me?" Every single human being in the Western world (and probably a large percentage of the rest of the planet as well) knows that it's good to exercise, and we know that most adults in America don't do it. Your prospect needs to have the vague "good to exercise" message translated to "Once you sign up with me, Mr. Prospect, your life will be different and better from that day forward because I can show you how to get what you really want, what you crave, what you lust after." It's got to be that compelling. That's the reason that producers of commercial products don't just say, "Buy our soap. It will get you clean so you don't have BO, and it's not expensive." Instead they show images of incredibly attractive people using the product and experiencing an outpouring of affection from their fellow human beings, giving the subliminal message that you, too, Ms. and Mr. Viewer, can be popular and attractive by using this soap.

- **Prior bad experience with a similar service.** If your prospect has had a bad experience at a health club with one of these uneducated, dangerous fitness enthusiasts masquerading as a personal trainer, she might be a little skittish. She wanted the benefits of personal training and got burned. Now, it's once bitten, twice shy. She's thinking, *Will this trainer be a jerk like that last loser?* Find out the details of the earlier disaster and be prepared to show how that sort of thing could never happen if she goes with you. Help her understand that you and your service are different, wonderful, and exactly what she's hoping for!

Some Typical Objections and How to Handle Them

Absorb the following objections and the responses to them so you'll be prepared to counter your prospect's inertia and fears.

- **Objection:** "I need to discuss this with my spouse (partner, mother, dog)."

This one reminds me that whenever my husband wants a new golf club, regardless of the price, he never feels the need to discuss the purchase with me. Why should he? He knows what this club can do for him and he "needs" it. So, this objection indicates that the prospect doesn't have a firm, tangible, and—most important—*personal* appreciation of the benefits of your service.

Response: "I can appreciate that, but I think we both know that you are the one who wants to flatten your tummy and increase your energy level. This is something you're going to do for yourself, not anyone else, so you are the ultimate decision maker."

■ **Objection:** "My friend hired a personal trainer who was always late and even didn't show up a couple of times."

Response: "That's terrible! Customer service is a serious priority for me, and I'd be happy to give you the names of several clients who can vouch for my punctuality and dependability. Last week I was five minutes late to one client's house because of a serious auto accident that blocked traffic, and when I got there, she said, 'Oh, I'm so glad that you're here! I was so worried because you're never late. I can set my watch by you.'"

■ **Objection:** "What can you tell me that I can't learn from reading a book or watching a video?"

Response: "For one thing, a book or a video isn't going to be able to assess your current biomechanics and determine which exercises are safe for you to do, and how to correct your posture so that eventually you can do every exercise and activity you want. Perhaps you're the rare exception, but most adults have some muscular imbalances in their backs and shoulders that make some common exercises downright dangerous. Also, you should ask yourself whether a book or video is going to pop itself into your hands or into the VCR and make you stop putting off your workout. It can't. I will."

The Number-One Objection: Price

Of course, the number-one objection will be to price. In chapter 2, I warned you about what a mistake it is to underprice your services. The simple fact is that if a prospect's number-one concern is price, that person is not a desirable potential client. If that's where your relationship starts, that's probably where it's going to end; that is, this client is going to nickel and dime you by counting the minutes of every session, arguing about paying for every canceled session, and expecting even better service than your other clients who may pay more. In short, this person will be a troublemaker. And you don't need the headache because, remember, your goal isn't to try to get as many clients as you can. You need only enough to fill your working hours, an automatic scarcity situation. What is scarce is valuable, which puts you in the driver's seat when it comes to price objections.

The first step to handling price objections is to have confidence in the value of your service. If you don't think you're worth $100 a session, it will be impossible for you to convince others that you are. In addition, here are some suggestions to help you handle price objections:

• **Deal with price objections immediately and with confidence.** For example, I used to say something like this: "Yes, I did say that my rate is $80 per session, and yes, I know that the personal trainers at the YMCA charge half that much. If price is your number-one consideration for hiring a trainer, I'm probably not the best choice for you. You can drive a Lexus, or you can drive a Yugo, after all. Although I can't recommend any of these economy personal trainers, I do know where you can find some."

• **When you state your price, always couple it with a statement of value.** Don't say, "My rate is $80 per session." Instead, say, "My rate is $80 per session and that includes periodic fitness assessments and designing your cardiovascular program."

• **Don't invite comparisons among different packages or options.** If you give a prospect too many choices and ask him to compare too many options, it takes the focus off the value of your service and puts it on price.

Remember that your goal is to get a steady stream of clients who are delighted to pay your fee because you've done so much for them. If you keep that thought in mind, you will find price objections an insult, and you'll be able to dispense with them easily.

A Sample Script

This is an example of what a personal trainer might say after listening to the prospect's answers to the Powerful Questions.

"Ms. Prospect, based on what you've told me, here are my thoughts on how we should proceed.

"You mentioned that you've been exercising on your own, but you haven't gotten the results that you want, especially with upper-body strength and reducing your body fat. I'm sure that together we can achieve some improvement in these areas.

"You mentioned that you'd like to do some strength training, and I agree that that would be one key to achieving your goals. I'm excited about designing a safe and effective resistance-training program for you. We need to make sure that we address that left shoulder that bothers you when you try to lift boxes or put things up on shelves. That's another reason that you are going to love lifting weights! It will make you stronger and less likely to get these annoying aches and pains.

"You mentioned that you would be available three times a week at 5 P.M. Why don't we get started next Monday and plan to work together for two months, and see how much we can accomplish? After that, we can reevaluate where we are. You may decide that you want to continue working with me three times a week, or you may want to work out on your own once a week and see me once or twice a week. We'll have to be flexible about that and see what works best for you. The important thing now is to get started so that you can get where you want to be!"

Keeping Track of the Results

After you've been at this for a while, you will discover which methods of reaching potential customers are most successful. Of course, the sooner you obtain this information, the less time and money you'll waste building your client base. You could spend months sitting around twiddling your thumbs because you select the wrong advertising vehicle, only to switch and find yourself working nonstop. At this point, you'll be thinking, *Where were you (successful ad vehicle) several hundred (or, God forbid, thousand) dollars ago?* You can avoid asking this question by asking prospects who call how they heard about you. Chart this information and cut your losses.

Working With
Your Client

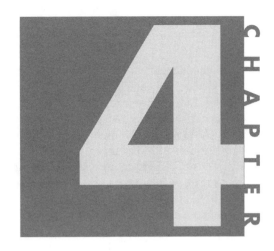

The Art of Exercise Program Design

Questions we'll answer in this chapter:

- What are the general principles that underlie effective program design?

- What are the components of a well-designed fitness program?

- What are the steps of individualized program design?

Your client hired you for a number of reasons. He might want someone to provide motivation and encourage him as he reaches his fitness goals and makes the sometimes-tricky transition from junk-food junkie to healthful eater. He might want to have a regular appointment to force him to be consistent with exercise. In many cases, though, the number-one reason clients hire us is to have someone show them what to do and how to do it correctly. You probably know that a lot of confusion exists about which exercises to do to achieve particular results. When you throw in the variables of age, medical history, and previous injuries, many people will simply throw up their hands and decide they'd be better off just sitting on the couch. That's where you come in.

General Principles of Program Design

Before we get to the specifics of program design, let's review some general principles that apply to every client's program.

To design safe, effective, and personalized programs for your clients, it's essential to understand the basics of exercise physiology. Just as good auto mechanics must understand the workings of engines, carburetors, and the other components under the hood, professional personal trainers must know how the human body functions. Among the questions they must be able to answer are the following:

- Where does the body get the energy it needs?
- How do muscles get stronger?
- Why does heart rate increase during exercise?
- How do I know if I'm getting in better shape?
- How do I burn fat?

These are the questions, along with many others, that clients will throw at you.

This brief review of exercise physiology basics is not intended to turn you into an expert. Given the complexity of the subject, that is beyond the scope of this book. Nor will it guarantee that you won't have to hit the books to answer a curious client or to pass a certification exam. It is intended as a simple summary of the exercise science behind the practical programs personal trainers design. With this knowledge, your programs will be more effective and your presentation more confident. That's the reason that every major certification exam contains a section that tests proficiency in this area.

Thus, the chapters on designing the specific components of the client's program include general overviews of the science behind the art of exercise prescription for each component. If you've taken a college course in exercise physiology, this material will be a review. If you haven't, it will provide a good introduction to this essential information. The suggested readings section that begins on page 243 describes a number of excellent resources on the science behind the art.

Once you have the scientific foundation necessary to understand what you're doing, you must apply these general principles of program design to your work with every client:

- **A well-designed fitness program is complete.** A well-designed fitness program has four components:

  - Resistance training
  - Cardiovascular conditioning
  - Flexibility training
  - Proper nutrition

A program that does not include all four components is incomplete and will not accomplish the goal of a strong, healthy, and *functional* body.

- **A well-designed fitness program reflects an understanding of human movement and basic principles of biomechanics.** A safe, effective strength and conditioning program depends on developing balance between the joints on both sides of the body. Muscular imbalance is a primary cause of injury, especially to the vulnerable back and shoulders.

- **A well-designed fitness program is based on clearly defined goals and objectives.** You should ask, "What is the objective?" about every exercise. The term "objective" in this book has a dual meaning. First, it is the rationale for everything in your client's program. Why do you want your client to do leg extensions? Why are you using a free-weight exercise rather than a machine to work a particular muscle group? Why did you suggest a treadmill and not a bike? Your objectives will provide sound answers to these questions. Second, the objective is the guide and goal for your client. Once you've decided to include a particular exercise in the routine, explain what you want your client to do. In the case of leg extensions, for example, you'll see much better form if you say, "Your objective is to straighten your legs at the knee joints while keeping your hips relaxed."

- **A well-designed fitness program is planned around each client's unique constellation of goals and objectives.** When I talk to groups, I am often asked, "What should I do to get in shape?" This is a lot like asking, "How do I get there?" without telling you where "there" is. You can't design an effective program for a person without understanding her specific goals and objectives. No two people are exactly the same. Your exercise prescription must reflect this fact. One-size-fits-all programs don't fit anyone properly.

Steps of Individualized Program Design

With these foundational principles in mind, you're ready to work your magic. Your knowledge and expertise about the body in general, and about this unique and special person you call your client in particular, makes it possible for you to create his or her unique program, the one that will change his or her life. When it comes to achieving optimum function and performance, one size definitely does not fit all!

Step 1: Evaluate and Screen Your Clients

A health history questionnaire will give you the information you need to screen your clients and determine which ones absolutely cannot begin your program without written permission from their physicians. (A sample health history questionnaire is included in appendix A.) You should recommend that all clients, even apparently healthy ones, see their doctors for checkups before beginning an exercise program. This is especially true of sedentary people over 40. I use American College of Sports Medicine guidelines to decide whether to require that a client obtain written consent from a physician before beginning an exercise program.

The ACSM guidelines divide clients into three categories:

1. Apparently healthy, with the subcategories "younger" and "over 40 (men)" or "over 50 (women)"

2. Individuals at higher risk

3. Patients with disease

I strongly suggest that you consult ACSM's *Guidelines for Exercise Testing and Prescription,* 6th edition (see suggested readings) for a more thorough understanding of these important screening criteria.

Occasionally, the answers you get on the health history questionnaire dictate that you decline to work with a particular client. Do not hesitate to refer a client with special needs to another trainer or other health professional (for example, a physical thera-

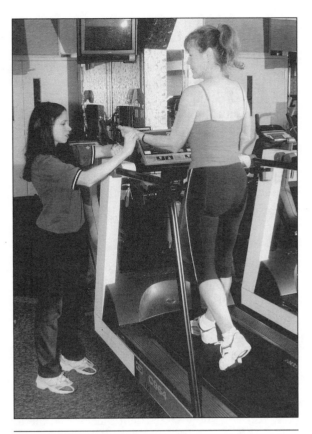

A treadmill can help you assess your client's current cardiovascular fitness accurately.

pist or kinesiotherapist) who might be better able to help her. You do no one, especially yourself, any favors by taking on clients whose needs and challenges are beyond your knowledge and ability.

Why Do a Fitness Assessment?

There are a number of vital reasons you must do a fitness assessment:

• **To gather information.** Many people never begin an exercise program because they don't have a clue about where to begin. The answer is, of course, to begin at the beginning, which is wherever you are now. The fitness assessment tells you where the client is now in terms of his cardiovascular fitness, strength, and flexibility. It gives you the information you need to design a program that will condition all the major muscle groups, promote balance in every joint, and condition the heart and lungs. It gives you a record you can look back at to see that you have accomplished your goals. It shows you where your client is and where you want to go together.

• **To focus on objectives.** Good program design requires a thoughtful, careful analysis of the

Challenging but Achievable

Most people find it difficult to continue anything that they find extremely uncomfortable or feel awkward doing. Many previously sedentary people fear beginning a program in the first place for just this reason. If you know your client's fitness level, you can design a program that will be challenging but achievable. Your client will experience success and positive reinforcement and be highly motivated to continue exercising.

methods, reasons, and manner of each exercise or protocol. The fitness assessment helps you answer these what's-the-point questions about your client's program. For example, if a client is in excellent cardiovascular condition but is too weak to carry in a medium-sized bag of groceries, you know that you need to focus on improving strength.

• **To motivate the client.** One of the strongest motivators to continue a program is seeing progress. How can you show your client that he has made progress if you don't have a record of where he started?

• **To detect special fitness needs.** In my experience, most adults have tightness in the neck, shoulders (especially the internal rotators), low back, and hamstrings. Your client might be the exception to this general rule. If she's not, though, you need to know about it. You also need to know if she stands with a swaybacked posture, if her toes point out excessively (think of Charlie Chaplin), or if one hip is higher than the other. Why? Back pain, twinges in the hip, and achy neck and shoulders can often be attributed to bad posture or structural asymmetry. You need to know which muscles need to be strengthened and stretched to correct these problems and help your client achieve optimal balance and function.

• **To design a realistic program.** It's difficult to say which has caused more human misery, good intentions or the unrealistic expectations they create. Compare these two clients, who both begin a 3-month program with you. The first expects to lose 40 pounds (18 kg) and 15% body fat. The second expects to lose 10 pounds and 5% body fat. Both lose 15 pounds (6.8 kg) and 7% body fat. Which client do you think will be happier? Which will be disappointed, perhaps so much so that she will conclude that she's been working for nothing?

The Body Composition Test

Clients tend to feel about body composition tests the way many of us feel about IQ tests: We have an almost irresistible impulse to know the result, an uneasiness about the possibility that the result might not be as good as we hope, and a terror of anyone else finding out. I can say without hesitation that every single client you work with will want to know what his or her body fat percentage is after you explain the concept of body composition, lean weight versus fat weight, and the insignificance of the number of pounds he or she weighs. I also guarantee that clients will fear the result. In fact, some clients approach these tests with sheer dread. You need to recognize that for these clients, seeing what they consider the "wrong" number in this test result is a crushing personal failure. Try to avoid this counterproductive reaction by explaining the real, rather than imagined, implications of the test, how what you're really measuring is a *range* within which her body fat falls, and how uncontrollable variables unrelated to body fat (water retention, for example) can affect the result. If your client understands that a few millimeters' difference in a skinfold measurement can show up as a 5% difference on a body composition test, it's less likely that she will spend any time crying over the result. (Yes, I've had clients cry over the results of their body fat tests!)

I suggest that you measure subcutaneous body fat (the body fat directly under the skin, as opposed to

Suggested Tests to Perform During Your Clients' Fitness Assessments

- Height
- Weight
- Blood pressure
- Resting pulse
- Body composition
- Anthropometric measurements
- Sit-and-reach test
- Finger-touch test
- Curl-up test
- Push-up test
- Posture evaluation

Advise your client that she should feel free to stop exercising any time she feels dizziness, light-headedness, chest pain, or nausea, or for any other reason.

intramuscular fat) with calipers and take measurements with a tape measure. Specific instructions on performing the body fat tests and tables for interpreting them are contained in the reference books in the suggested readings section. To compute body fat percentage, see appendix B, pages 230 and 231.

Flexibility Tests

As I mentioned previously, you should encourage your clients to work on their flexibility as well as other aspects of fitness. To find out where your clients are starting from, I suggest that you do two flexibility tests on all of them, the sit-and-reach test and the finger-touch test (pages 232 and 233, respectively, in appendix B). I selected these because they address the two areas that are problems for most adults: the hamstrings and the rotator cuffs. Remember that flexibility is joint specific. A person can be like Gumby when it comes to his hamstrings, yet have such tight rotator cuffs that he looks like the Hunchback of Notre Dame!

Cardiovascular Fitness Tests

Cardiovascular fitness can be measured in many ways, some more accurate than others. The most accurate tests are done in sports medicine labs or clinics and involve expensive, bulky equipment. These tests will give the most accurate results, but you can do the three-minute step test described in appendix B (p. 234) without costly equipment to measure your client's cardiovascular fitness.

Evaluating Posture and Muscular Imbalance

Good posture is functional posture. It is a natural body alignment that allows you to move in a pain-free, efficient way. Unfortunately, many of us develop bad posture early in life and spend the next several decades cementing our joints in these misshapen twists and warps. Overcoming bad posture requires identifying the problem and taking corrective action, stretching the shortened structures and strengthening the opposing muscle groups. In my experience, the overwhelming majority of adults suffer from some very common postural deficiencies. The typical new client that I see has rounded shoulders; a tight, almost spasmodic neck; and a hanging head. Often these conditions are accompanied by other dysfunctional conditions: locked knees; outward-pointing toes; and excessive lordosis, commonly known as swayback, which is an exaggerated forward curvature of the spine that causes the stomach to stick out and the low back to arch excessively. Others have kneecaps that turn in toward each other, usually due to tight hip rotators.

"A steady and pleasant posture produces mental equilibrium and prevents fickleness of mind."

B.K.S. Iyengar, noted yoga master

Visual Inspection

Many of us, confronted with our less-than-exemplary posture, react to this reminder as if we've been zapped with an unexpected bolt of electricity, hyperarching our backs into exaggerated military contortions that would embarrass a corps of West Point cadets. To avoid this reaction, evaluate your client's posture without comment and before telling her that you are doing any sort of evaluation. The posture evaluation should begin the minute your client walks through the door. Chances are this posture will be her real posture, as opposed to her "I'd-better-stand-up-straight-to-do-well-on-this-test" posture. Do the following posture check to see where she stands.

Do You Need To Do Every Test on Every Client?

The short answer is no, of course not! If, for example, you're working with a well-conditioned weightlifter who wants your help increasing the strength and flexibility of his rotator cuff, you might not do a cardiovascular fitness test or a body composition test. There are clients whose medical histories dictate that they avoid any cardiovascular testing outside of a medically supervised environment. This is a judgment call, but as always, err on the conservative side. If you have any doubts about whether to do a particular test on a client, don't do it without consulting the client's physician. Some clients with no medical limitations will specifically request that you not ask them to do a particular test, and since they are ultimately in control of this whole process, that's their choice. You should explain why you think it's advisable to do the testing, but if they decline, proceed cautiously, even more so than you normally would with someone of this age, gender, and medical and exercise history. Specifics on performing the fitness tests are contained in appendix B.

• **Hangdog head, or "computer buzzard."** We spend so much time looking down that we often fall into the habit of walking around looking down. Not only does this make you look like you lost your last friend, it causes enormous stress in the muscles of the neck and upper back as they struggle to hold up the weight of the head and keep the chin off the chest. These muscles were never intended to do this task, and like any workers forced to do jobs outside their job descriptions, they complain loudly and frequently until this condition is corrected. Hangdog head often goes in tandem with lordosis and excessively pointed toes. As the body tries to bring the head into alignment with the lower spine, which, when these conditions are present, is out of functional alignment, it puts the head in a contorted and inappropriate position.

• **Shoulder at 1 o'clock, not 12 o'clock.** Ask your client to visualize his shoulder from the side as the face of a clock. The top of this clock face (12 o'clock) should align with the end of the collarbone. It should not point forward (1 o'clock).

• **Four-finger space.** Is your client's rib cage lifted up and out from the pelvis with an identifiable space between her pelvis and rib cage, or is she slouching so that you can barely slide a sheet of paper in between them?

• **Winging scapula.** Is your client's scapula flat against his spine, or is there a palpable space, almost like a little vertical shelf, where his scapula sticks out? Winging scapula often occurs in conjunction with hangdog head. That's because the levator scapulae muscle, which originates at the base of the skull and inserts at the top of the scapula, becomes very tight when it tries to resist the weight of the hanging head. As a result, the scapula is pulled up and out of its proper alignment.

• **Swayback.** As mentioned before, this is known by the scary name lordosis, but by any name it's a major problem. It can cause low-back pain and sciatica (pain in the legs caused by pressure on nerves), not to mention making your belly stick out in front like you're carrying a sack of dirty sweat socks. The derriere sticks out in back like a shelf attached to your lower spine. This is caused by the pelvis tilting forward, out of its proper alignment.

• **Locked knees.** If a person stands with her knees locked, two things are happening—the knees are not serving the shock absorption function that they should under ideal circumstances, and the person is not using the powerful muscles in her legs to move. If knees are locked, walking is initiated at the hip and the quadriceps and hamstrings are not functioning as they should.

• **Toes excessively pointing out.** Often related to swayback, hangdog head, and round shoulders, walking with your feet out like Charlie Chaplin's Little Tramp character can cause pain in hips, knees, and ankles.

• **Sagging ankles.** Are the ankles straight and directly below the knees, or do they cave in?

After you've had the chance to casually observe your client and his natural, albeit less-than-perfect posture, you can confirm your suspicions by putting him next to a plumb line or grid to see if indeed structures are not aligned properly.

Compensation and Pain

Pain is a symptom of a problem. So is moving in an unnatural manner to avoid pain that you know will result if you move normally. Ask your clients about pain during their daily activities. You might discover things about their work habits, workstations, or other activities that are causing problems that you need to address, either directly or by referral to another appropriate health professional. It might be obvious to you which muscles need to be stretched and strengthened to correct the conditions you observe. If not, suggest that your client consult with a physician, physical therapist, or other qualified health professional. Don't try to treat conditions beyond your knowledge or ability.

Perfect Posture

Now that I've told you all about posture dysfunctions, how will you know perfect posture when you see it? Look for the following:

• Head erect, "floating" on the spinal column
• Four-finger space between rib cage and pelvis
• Shoulder joints in line with hip joints
• Shoulders level
• Shoulder blades depressed
• Hands at the sides, not with backs of the hands facing front
• Hips level
• Abdominals contracted to hold the pelvis in proper alignment
• Kneecaps directly over feet, not pointing inward
• Knees soft, not locked
• Feet pointing forward

Step 2: Consider Client Preferences and Limitations

Your client is much more likely to exercise consistently and effectively if she

- feels she has been a part of the process of program design,
- feels her particular special needs, if any, have been taken into account, and
- isn't required to do anything that she really despises.

Facilitate your client's workouts by making them as convenient as possible. For example, walking in her neighborhood after work might be more palatable to your client than driving to the club for a session on the treadmill. Another helpful suggestion: If she needs to do more CV exercise and lives in a cold climate, suggest that she invest in a piece of indoor equipment, pointing out how unlikely it is that she'll go out in the dark on a 10-below January day to do that power walk.

Step 3: Set Objectives That Are *TOPS*

What are TOPS objectives?

- **T**imed—Set a target date for reaching each goal.
- **O**bjective—A measurable goal is meaningful precisely because you can tell when you have reached it. Don't say, "Get leaner." Instead, say, "Reduce body fat by .5% each month."
- **P**ersonalized—In addition to general overall fitness goals that most clients have, such as reducing body fat percentages, your client probably has some specific things he'd like to work on. For example, he might be planning a spring ski trip and needs some specific attention to pre-ski conditioning. You need to include this in your goals.
- **S**pecific—Making the goals as specific as you can will encourage your client by giving him a clear objective. An example of a nonspecific goal is "I want to get in shape." What the heck does that mean? Compare "I want to exercise three times a week for 20 minutes per session." The latter statement is measurable. You know when you're there. There's no way to tell whether you've achieved the former "goal," because "being in shape" is a vague, undefined term.

Steps 4 through 8: Putting It All Together

There are a few other elements to incorporate into an effective fitness program.

- **Steps 4 and 5: Establish the cardiovascular and resistance components.** After considering your client's goals, you are ready to decide what her cardiovascular program will consist of and what she will do for muscular strength and endurance. Cardiovascular exercise can consist of indoor, machine-assisted activities (treadmill, stationary bike, rower) or outdoor exercise (walking, jogging). Consult chapter 5 for more specifics on designing the cardiovascular program. Your client can do resistance training by using free weights, machines, bands, or body weight. Usually it will be some combination of these varieties. You will learn more about designing this component in chapter 6.

- **Step 6: Write the program.** Include "homework" (any activities that you want your client to do between your sessions as described in chapter 6) and the flexibility training. In most cases, you will spend more time planning and writing the resistance portion of the program than the cardiovascular because you need to determine which muscles and muscle groups need to be strengthened and stretched to bring your client back to optimum posture and function. Consult the Resistance Workout Guide for information about which exercises target specific muscles and muscle groups. The cardiovascular portion of the program that you write will include the suggested modality, number of minutes, and intensity. Often the client will use these specifications to do the exercise on his own. It's useful to suggest that he keep a record of these workouts, noting the number of minutes and his perceived level of exertion during each. You will be able to use this information to adjust the intensity of his cardiovascular program.

- **Step 7: Set the time parameters.** Set realistic parameters for achieving specific goals in each area. When deciding what's realistic, you need to take several factors into account. First, you need to look at where the client is now and where he wants to go. If you've got a long road ahead, as in 50 or more pounds (23 kg) to lose, it's useful to break that goal down into baby steps that don't seem so daunting. It's realistic for most adults to lose 1 to 2 pounds (.50 to 1 kg) of fat a week in the beginning, assuming good compliance with exercise and avoidance of excessive calorie intake. Don't assume, though, that your client is like most. If her lifestyle consists of 60-hour workweeks,

Writing the Program: A Checklist

- Did you do a thorough fitness assessment? If not, why not?
- Has your client completed a health history questionnaire?
- If your client's condition dictates that you do so, have you obtained a signed medical clearance from your client's doctor?
- Has your client completed a goal inventory?
- Do you understand your client's goals and objectives?
- Have you discussed realistic goals?
- Have you considered this client's special needs and limitations, both physiological (diabetes, hypertension, or obesity, for example) and orthopedic (e.g., low-back, shoulder, or knee problems or arthritis)?
- Have you recommended that your client learn about nutrition, especially the benefits of a low-fat, low-sugar diet?
- Have you taken into account the available time and equipment?
- Is the workout one that your client can complete in a reasonable amount of time (less than 1 hour)?
- Have you examined your client's attitudes toward exercise in general and toward specific activities?
- Have you discussed the general benefits of exercise with your client?
- Have you explained the objectives of the program to your client?
- Have you included two to three resistance training workouts per week for every major muscle group, in the 8- to 12-repetition range, unless otherwise dictated by this client's needs?
- Is your resistance routine balanced, that is, does it work opposing muscle groups for balance around each joint?
- Have you included three to five cardiovascular workouts of 20 to 60 minutes' duration at 55% to 80% of the client's maximal heart rate in each week's routine?
- Have you included flexibility exercises and taught your client how to do them?
- Have you included stretching and muscle balance exercises for the low back and rotator cuffs?
- Have you established timed, objective, personalized, specific goals in the areas of body composition, cardiovascular fitness, muscular strength, and flexibility?
- Have you set a date for retesting?
- Have you discussed "homework" with your client—that is, the activity, time, and intensity of the workouts he should do between sessions with you?
- Have you kept the client's overall life in mind, making sure that the workout is realistic and doable for him?
- Have you designed a workout that your client will actually do on a regular basis, one that is challenging enough to improve his energy, fitness, and overall well-being but isn't so difficult that he will dread doing it and eventually stop doing it altogether?

lots of travel, and a family on top of it, progress, though still achievable, may take more time.

Step 8: Determine progress. Progress toward goals should be measured daily, weekly, and monthly. Assessing client progress is important for both you and your client. For her, it lets her know how far her hard work has taken her. The knowledge that all that perspiration has not been for nothing will be a powerful motivator. For you, it gives you vital information about how effective your program has been

so far, information that you can use to make important, progress-producing adjustments.

Now you're ready to put it all together: the ultimate, top-of-the-mountain goal, and all the plateaus along the way. Chapters 5 and 6 detail how to design the cardiovascular, flexibility, and resistance-training portions of the program as well as how to approach the nutritional component. Chapter 8 contains a sample goal map that sets out these short-, intermediate-, and long-term goals.

Designing the Cardiovascular, Flexibility, and Nutritional Components

Questions we'll answer in this chapter:

- What is metabolism?

- How does the body get the energy it needs for movement?

- What are the different energy systems available to the body, and when is each used?

- What adaptations occur in the body in response to training?

- What factors do I need to consider when designing my clients' cardiovascular programs?

- What advice about nutrition should I give my client?

All personal trainers should have a thorough knowledge of how the exercising human body works, which is why many readers of this book will have taken a college course in exercise physiology or studied it independently while preparing for a certification exam. This chapter is not to substitute for either of those activities, both of which I encourage. Think of this chapter as your Cliffs Notes on exercise physiology, either a refresher course for things that you already know or an outline of things that you want to learn more about. To do that, check out some of the references in the suggested readings section.

Please don't assume that because I've placed the cardiovascular, flexibility, and nutritional components all in the same chapter that they are less important than the resistance component, which has its own whole chapter. All of these components are essential to a complete, effective wellness program. The components sharing this chapter, though, are typically ones that your client will attend to on her own after some initial guidance from you. Let's face it: Most clients either don't want to or can't afford to pay $75 and up for someone to talk to them while they are on the treadmill. On the other hand, to do resistance training, clients need both evaluation of their current musculoskeletal and biomechanical condition to make sure that they don't do any exercises that are unsafe for them, and instruction on proper form. Most people already know how to walk, but very few, even among those who have lifted weights for years, know how to do a lat pull-down correctly.

Metabolism and Basic Energy Systems

Metabolism is the sum of all chemical reactions in living cells that provide energy for all essential physiological activities. Where does energy for physical activity come from? The laws of thermodynamics dictate that energy is never lost or created, and that all forms of energy are interchangeable. The energy living creatures on Earth use originates from the sun as light and is converted by chemical reactions in plants that store chemical energy. Animals consume this stored energy in the form of fruits and vegetables. We consume these plant products, as well as the protein that animals make from them, when we sit down to our meals.

We know that we get the energy for human activity from the foods we eat, but we don't get that energy directly. Our cells cannot grab an apple as it passes by in the bloodstream. (And even if they could, that would hurt!) Food must be processed into a form that's accessible by the body. The body's digestive system extracts energy by breaking down food into its basic building blocks, the macronutrients. The circulatory system carries these macronutrients to the cells, where they are used for growth, repair, and production of the body's energy currency, adenosine triphosphate (ATP). The respiratory system provides the oxygen necessary for metabolism and helps maintain the body's proper pH (acid-base balance).

The Macronutrients, Summarized

Carbohydrate (CHO)
- Body's preferred energy source
- Required by CNS
- Yields 4 calories per gram
- The only macronutrient that can generate ATP anaerobically (without oxygen)

Fat
- Body's primary energy storage
- Yields 9 calories per gram

Protein
- Last resort energy source (gluconeogenesis)
- Yields 4 calories per gram

ATP, the Body's Basic Energy Store

Adenosine triphosphate is a high-energy compound that stores energy in the body. Our bodies require a constant supply of ATP, but they store only a small amount (approximately 3.5 oz or 105 ml). Fortunately, we have the ability to manufacture ATP in several ways. The method used depends on the intensity, type, and duration of energy-demanding activity.

How Do Cells Make ATP?

ATP is produced by three energy systems: (1) the ATP-PCr system, (2) the glycolytic system, and (3) the oxidative system. It is useful to think of energy production in the body as falling into one of two broad categories, anaerobic (without oxygen) and aerobic (in the presence of oxygen).

The ATP-PCr System

The ATP-PCr anaerobic system of energy production is also called the phosphagen system or the immediate energy system. Using stored ATP and another high-energy compound, phosphocreatine (the "PCr" in the system's title), it supplies enough energy for 5 to 10 seconds of high-intensity activity. If activity continues, the body must find another energy source.

The Glycolytic System: Anaerobic Glycolysis

After the ATP-PCr system, the body will look to the process of enzymatic breakdown of glucose known as glycolysis. (The stored form of glucose, glycogen, which the body keeps tucked away in the liver and skeletal muscles, breaks down in a similar process called glycogenolysis.) Glycolysis occurs in the cell's cytoplasm. Anaerobic glycolysis consists of a series of 10 steps, during each of which enzymes act on the glucose molecule and produce a series of by-products. At the end of step 10, the ultimate by-product of glycolysis is pyruvate. If oxygen is present, pyruvate can convert to acetyl-CoA and enter the Krebs, or citric acid, cycle, and energy production can continue. Otherwise, lactic acid forms from pyruvate, and pain and fatigue will result in a cessation of activity. That's the reason that anaerobic glycolysis provides energy for only approximately 2 minutes of intense activity. It's also the reason that we can continue high-intensity exercise for only a short time. One mole of glucose yields 2 mol of ATP. If glycogen is the initial substrate, 3 mol of ATP result.

The Oxidative System: Aerobic Glycolysis

In the presence of oxygen, the pyruvate formed in anaerobic glycolysis enters stage two of glycolysis, the Krebs cycle, as acetyl-CoA. The Krebs cycle's primary function is to produce electrons for the respiratory chain or electron transport chain (ETC). This process of creating ATP from other chemical sources is called phosphorylation. In oxidative phosphorylation hydrogen atoms released from glycolysis and the Krebs cycle are carried by two coenzymes, NAD (nicotinamide and adenine dinucleotide) and FAD (flavin adenine dinucleotide), to the ETC. Here a series of reactions produces more ATP. At the end of the ETC, hydrogen combines with oxygen to form water. Oxidative phosphorylation takes place inside the mitochondria, organelles that are the cells' energy factories. Oxidative phosphorylation provides the overwhelming majority of the body's energy needs, approximately 90%.

At the end of glycolysis and oxidative phosphorylation, the catabolism of one molecule of glucose yields 38 ATP molecules.

Oxidation of Fat

Muscle and liver glycogen stores constitute only 1,200 to 2,000 kilocalories of energy. Contrast that with stored adipose tissue, or fat, which can supply 70,000 to 100,000! Fat is stored in the body's fat cells, or adipocytes, in the form of triglyceride. Triglyceride consists of glycerol and three molecules of free fatty acids (FFAs).

To be used as energy by the body, triglyceride is broken down to these components. This breakdown process is called lipolysis.

Glycerol and FFA Breakdown

The glycerol part of the triglyceride molecule is metabolized in anaerobic glycolysis. FFAs experience beta oxidation, the process that transforms the FFAs to acetyl-CoA, the compound that enters the Krebs cycle for continued energy production.

It's important to remember that the body cannot make glucose from FFAs, which means that they are not good energy sources for the central nervous system, which uses glucose as its primary fuel. This is one reason that low-carbohydrate diets are a bad idea; they can make you stupid.

Fat Burns in a Carbohydrate Flame

Another reason to avoid low-carbohydrate fad diets is that without adequate carbohydrate, the body cannot completely metabolize fat. Remember that acetyl-CoA that enters the Krebs cycle for continued energy production? In order to do that, acetyl-CoA must first combine with oxaloacetate (OAA). When carbohydrate level is too low, OAA level may become inadequate, which means that the acetyl-CoA produced during beta oxidation cannot enter the Krebs cycle. If this happens, ketone bodies, by-products of incomplete fat metabolism, accumulate in the blood. The resulting decrease in pH can cause bone loss, as the body tries to reestablish proper acid-base balance by pulling water out of tissues and leaching minerals from bones in the process. This excretion of acidic by-products of ketosis can also cause kidney stress.

Fat Metabolism Produces Much More ATP

For example, 1 molecule of a typical fat, palmitic acid, can produce 129 molecules of ATP versus 38 molecules of ATP from glucose (39 from glycogen). The reason is that because fat has more carbon, more acetyl-CoA from beta oxidation enters the Krebs cycle, and more electrons go to the ETC, where oxidative phosphorylation can produce ATP.

Protein Metabolism

It is possible for the body to produce glucose from protein in a process called gluconeogenesis. To use protein as an energy substrate, the body must first break protein down to its building blocks, the amino acids and nitrogen. (Recall that protein is the only macronutrient containing nitrogen.) The nitrogen must be removed from the amino acid molecule (deanimation) and excreted from the body. Since some amino acids are more glucogeneic than others, it may also be necessary to shift the building blocks around, a process called transanimation. (Deanimation and transanimation occur primarily in the liver but can also occur in the muscles.)

Because of the need to eliminate the excess nitrogen produced during gluconeogenesis, the body needs more water when protein is being used as an energy substrate, another reason that people lose a lot of "weight" (read: water) when they go on low-carbohydrate diets.

Some amino acids can convert to pyruvate. Others can convert to acetyl-CoA. In either case, they end up in the Krebs cycle for energy production.

An Energy Continuum

It's tempting to think of each energy system separately, but they all work together to provide the energy the body needs. The determining factors are the intensity and duration of activity. During lower-intensity activity, the aerobic system provides most energy with fat as a primary substrate. As intensity increases, the body begins to switch to burning glucose, which transfers energy more rapidly than fat. The key concept to understand is that the body is almost never using one energy system exclusively. Think in terms of a sliding scale of energy production, going from low to high intensity, with a lot of overlap among the systems.

Conclusions

There are two take-home messages from these facts about the body's energy systems. One is that athletes must train the energy system that they want to use in competition. For example, sprinters need to sprint in training to improve the capacity of their

ATP-PCr systems. Marathoners need to run long distances in training (although if they want to go fast, they also need to do some sprint training). When they do, they improve their capability to use fat for fuel, even at higher intensities, which spares precious glucose and therefore allows them to run well longer.

The second point to take from our discussion of the energy systems is that it's important for you to explain to the average adult, who is often obsessed with "fat burning," that the key to fitness, leanness, and lifelong functionality is burning energy, as in calories, through activity (figure 5.1, a-b). The more active your clients are and the more calories they burn, the less fuel they'll store as fat. In addition, as they condition their bodies, they will burn more fat even during higher-intensity exercise. Fat burning should not be a goal, but rather a happy by-product of a well-designed exercise program and good nutrition.

The Role of the Cardiovascular System

The heart and blood vessels deliver oxygen and nutrients to the tissues. They also help maintain the proper body temperature by shunting blood to the skin.

The Heart

The heart is the body's pump. It is divided into right and left sides, and into atria (the upper chambers) and ventricles (the lower chambers). The right atrium receives deoxygenated blood and sends it to the right ventricle and then to the lungs to be replenished with oxygen. The left atrium receives oxygenated blood from the lungs. From there, it goes to the left ventricle to the aorta for transport to the body's tissues.

The Blood Vessels

The oxygenated blood travels to the tissues in a system of blood vessels, the arteries and smaller branches called arterioles. The arterioles play a vital role in shunting blood to working muscles during exercise. They contain layers of smooth muscle that allow them to constrict or relax and thereby regulate blood flow. During exercise, muscles can receive up to 80% of available blood in the body. From the arterioles the blood travels to the place where the rubber meets the road, the capillaries. These are the tiny blood vessels that are so small that blood cells

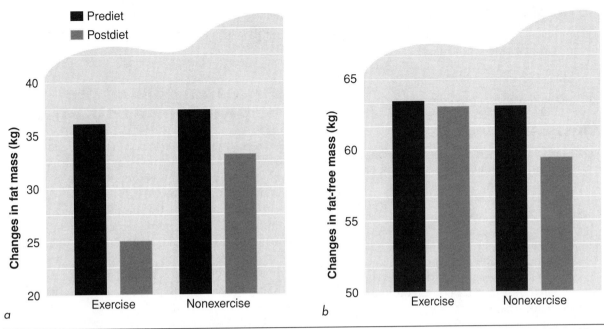

Figure 5.1 Changes in *(a)* fat mass and *(b)* fat-free mass resulting from a combined diet and exercise program and from dieting alone.

Reprinted, by permission, from J. Wilmore and D. Costill, 1999, *Physiology of Sport and Exercise*, 2nd ed. (Champaign, IL: Human Kinetics), 679.

must pass through them single file. Here, gases, waste products, and nutrients pass through the capillary walls to the tissues. The deoxygenated blood travels in a similar network of vessels. The capillaries feed their deoxygenated blood into the venules, which in turn pass the blood to larger vessels, the veins. Through the inferior and superior vena cava, the deoxygenated blood eventually returns to the right atrium and passes to the right ventricle for delivery to the lungs via the pulmonary artery. Muscular contraction assists in returning deoxygenated blood to the heart, which is why it's wise to cool down after exercise and reduce venous pooling, the tendency for blood to accumulate because of the force of gravity, in the extremities.

Other Important Cardiovascular Concepts

Of course, since we all have hearts and blood vessels, there must be more to it than that! The following concepts are key to understanding the workings of the cardiovascular system and the effect of exercise on it.

Stroke Volume

Stroke volume (SV), the amount of blood ejected from the left ventricle during systole, is the major determinant of cardiorespiratory endurance. This

fact makes sense when you consider that the body gets its oxygenated blood from the left ventricle.

SV is determined by the following:

- Volume of venous blood to the heart
- Ventricular distensibility (ventricle's capacity for enlargement)
- Ventricular contractility (ventricle's capacity for contraction)
- Aortic or pulmonary artery pressure

Another important cardiovascular concept is the ejection fraction, the percentage of blood entering the left ventricle that is actually ejected during contraction (systole). The average ejection fraction is 60%. Sometimes cardiologists will use this percentage to assess the degree of heart disease in a patient.

Cardiac Output

Cardiac output, often abbreviated Q, is the product of heart rate (HR) and SV. Even with training, SV does not change as much as heart rate, although it does increase with training. Cardiac output increases dramatically in response to the demands of exercise. For example, an average adult will have a resting Q of 5 liters per minute. This same person's Q will increase to as much as 40 liters per minute during exercise.

Maximal Heart Rate

Maximal heart rate (MHR) is the highest heart rate one can achieve during all-out effort. Because most of us don't have the use of a high-tech exercise physiology lab, we use the well-known "220 minus age" formula to estimate MHR.

Why Does SV Increase?

We've seen that Q increases because of an increase in heart rate, SV, or both. The increase in heart rate is obvious and dramatic. The increase in SV contributes less to increased Q but is still important. Why does it happen? Two reasons:

1. Frank-Starling mechanism. Ventricle contracts with greater force in response to greater filling; that is, the left ventricle stretches more while filling and experiences a boomerang-like effect during systole.

2. Increased contractility. As I'm sure you can see, even without increased end diastolic volume (the amount of blood in the left ventricle after filling but before systole), SV would increase if there was great contractility.

Both are involved. The Frank-Starling mechanism (ventricular distensibility) seems to be more involved at lower intensity.

Steady-State Heart Rate

When the workload is held constant at submax levels, heart rate rises rapidly and eventually plateaus and reaches what exercise physiologists call steady-state heart rate (HR). It's easy to understand why this happens. Think of pressing on a car's accelerator to reach cruising speed; steady state is the body's cruising speed, during which the heart has caught up with the body's increased oxygen demands.

As you would expect, the ability to achieve steady state improves dramatically with training. Trained individuals will usually reach it within 1 minute of increased cardiorespiratory demands, whereas the deconditioned take up to 3 minutes.

Cardiovascular Drift

With prolonged exercise, especially in a hot environment, at a constant rate of work, there is a gradual increase in HR and decrease in SV. Why does this happen? Two factors are usually cited. One is that cardiovascular drift is the result of progressive increases in the fraction of Q directed to the skin to attenuate rising body temperature.

The other is that there is a decrease in blood volume that results from the loss of fluid during exercise.

The Role of the Respiratory System

The respiratory system, consisting of the mouth, nose, trachea, bronchi, lungs, and alveoli, is responsible for providing the body with oxygen (O_2) and removing carbon dioxide (CO_2).

Inhaled air travels through the nose and is humidified and filtered before proceeding through the trachea to the bronchi. The bronchi provide the air a pathway to the lungs, which contain the alveoli, which is where actual gas exchange occurs.

Though technically ATP is the currency of energy production in the body, oxygen consumption is actually the true measure, because the greater an individual's ability to transport and use oxygen, the greater his or her ability to produce energy. (Recall that most energy is produced aerobically.) For this reason, the most common way to assess cardiorespiratory fitness is to measure maximum oxygen consumption, or $\dot{V}O_2$max. $\dot{V}O_2$max will increase with training, reflecting increased functional capacity.

Adaptations to Aerobic Exercise Training

Remember that metabolism is the sum of all chemical reactions in living cells to provide energy for all essential physiological activities. The cardiorespiratory system supplies O_2 and carries CO_2 to the lungs for expulsion from the body.

Cardiovascular Adaptations

Because active muscles need more O_2 and nutrients, the cardiorespiratory system adapts to exercise in the following ways:

- Heart size increases.
  - Cardiac muscle undergoes hypertrophy as a result of endurance training.
  - The left ventricle experiences the greatest change.
  - Myocardial wall thickness also increases.
- SV increases.
  - The left ventricle fills more completely during diastole.

- In addition, HR of a trained heart is lower, allowing an increase in diastolic filling time.

- Increased muscle mass results in a more powerful contraction.

- Resting heart rate (HR) decreases. The actual mechanism for this decrease is unknown, but there appears to be an increase in parasympathetic activity accompanied by a decrease in sympathetic activity.

- Submax HR decreases. Following a six-month endurance training program of moderate intensity, decreases in HR of 20 to 40 bpm (at same intensity) are common.

- MHR either remains unchanged or decreases slightly with training. This probably allows for greater SV and therefore greater Q.

- The HR recovery period is shortened by endurance training. This fact is the basis for some tests of cardiovascular endurance (e.g., the YMCA bench step test).

- SV increases.

- Q increases at high intensity.

  - Increases at rest or submax exercise are small; however, a dramatic increase is seen at maximal rates of work.

  - Results from increased SV

  - Max Q in untrained individuals—14-20 liters of O_2/min

  - Max Q in trained—25-35 liters of O_2/min

  - Max Q in endurance athletes—+40 liters of O_2/min

- Blood flow becomes more efficient.

  - More capillaries in muscles—moderate endurance training = 20%-30% increase in muscle capillary density.

  - There is a greater opening of existing capillaries in the muscles.

  - There is more effective hemodynamics, or movement of blood to areas where it's needed.

- Blood pressure (BP) decreases, though it changes little during exercise itself.

  - Resting BP is greatly lowered in those with borderline hypertension (HTN) who exercise regularly.

  - The decrease averages about 10 mmHg (systolic) and 8 mmHg (diastolic).

- Blood volume increases.

  - Exercise increases the release of antidiuretic hormones.

- There is an increase in albumin, the plasma protein that increases osmotic pressure, resulting in increased plasma volume.

The increase in blood volume is one of the most significant training effects. Why? Because

- as plasma volume increases, so does blood volume;

- more blood enters the heart, so SV increases; and

- more SV means delivery of more O_2 to working muscles.

Respiratory Adaptations

We know that the heart and lungs work together to supply the essential currency of energy production in the body, oxygen, which the body requires for life. During exercise, the body's oxygen demands increase dramatically. We know that the heart supplies oxygenated blood to the cells, but how does the blood get oxygenated in the first place? That task falls to the lungs.

- **Pulmonary ventilation** is basically unchanged at rest and at submax levels but can increase dramatically at maximum effort to supply the oxygen that the body requires.

- The **arteriovenous difference** (a-$\bar{v}O_2$ diff), a measure of how much oxygen is extracted by the body's tissues, increases, which shows that the cells are pulling more oxygen out of the blood, as would be expected.

- As noted previously, $\dot{V}O_2$**max** is the best measure of cardiorespiratory fitness. An increase of 15% to 20% is typical for average person who was previously sedentary and trains at 75% of max three times a week for 6 months.

Metabolic Adaptations

The heart and lungs are the major players in the energy-production game, and with training other changes occur in the body that make it possible for it to perform at a higher intensity, for a longer time, or both.

- **Lactate threshold.** We've all experienced the searing burn that signals a buildup of lactic acid during anaerobic exercise. (If you haven't, put this book down and go run as hard as you can for about a minute. I'll wait.) With training you can perform at a higher rate of work without raising blood lactate over resting levels. This adaptation is a major factor in the performance of endurance athletes like elite

69

marathon runners who amazingly can sustain a 5-minute mile pace for 26+ miles.

- **Mitochondrial enzyme activity.** The mitochondria are the cells' energy factories, so it's not surprising that we would see some changes inside their tiny walls. Moderate activity training for 2 to 4 months results in a 20% to 40% increase caused by greater size, number, and efficiency of mitochondria. With more mitochondrial enzyme activity, more energy can be produced.

- **Respiratory quotient.** The respiratory quotient (RQ) measures the substrate being used for activity. With training, it reflects that more fat is being used to provide energy. When pure glucose is being burned, RQ will be 1.00. As it gets lower, that means more fat is being used to provide energy.

Designing the Cardiovascular Component of the Client's Program

Most people know that they need to do cardiovascular (CV) exercise in addition to resistance training. In fact, the understanding that "exercise" means something other than just CV exercise is a relatively recent development.

As we have seen, CV exercise improves the ability of the lungs to provide oxygen and the heart and vessels to supply blood to the tissues; therefore it improves the body's ability to use oxygen ($\dot{V}O_2$max). Consistent CV exercise increases the amount of oxidative enzymes in the muscle cells, which improves the ability of the muscles to extract oxygen from the bloodstream. Trained individuals have more and larger mitochondria and more capillaries supplying the cells. All of these metabolic adaptations mean that trained individuals have lower levels of lactic acid at the same fixed submaximal work rate than untrained people. To achieve these remarkable improvements, a person needs to work large muscles in a continuous, rhythmic fashion for a prolonged period (20-60 minutes per bout of exercise). Examples include, but are certainly not limited to, walking, jogging, running, in-line skating, cycling, stair stepping, rowing, and cross-country skiing. Remember that training is all about the SAID principle: specific adaptation to imposed demand. The take-home message is that the body adapts to that which is consistently repeated (3-5 days a week).

Benefits of CV Exercise

- Increase in $\dot{V}O_2$max
- Decrease in maximal and resting heart rate and increased SV (more blood pumped per heartbeat)
- Decrease in body fat (assuming overall calorie deficit)
- Reduced blood pressure
- Increased high-density lipoprotein (good) cholesterol
- Improved glucose metabolism
- More efficient transport and utilization of oxygen
- Improved ability to burn fat

Planning for Progress

ACSM has identified three stages of progression in CV fitness programs:

1. Initial conditioning
2. Improvement conditioning
3. Maintenance

In the initial conditioning stage, which usually lasts 4 to 6 weeks, the client should do low-level aerobic exercise every other day for 10 to 15 minutes. It's important during this stage to err on the low side of intensity to allow your client to adapt to the new demands exercise places on his body and prepare him for the improvement stage. Once your client has gotten to the point that he can do five 30- to 40-minute workouts per week at the initial intensity, without injury or excessive fatigue, he is ready to move to the improvement stage (Roitman et al. 1998). During the improvement stage (4 to 5 months), you can begin to increase both the intensity and duration of your client's CV sessions.

Depending on how well your client adapts to increased demands, you can increase the duration of each CV session by up to several minutes every 2 to 3 weeks. If he handles increased time with minimal difficulty, gradually increase intensity, too, so that at the end of this stage your client has reached a targeted level of intensity (usually 60% to 90% of MHR) and is able to maintain this pace for a minimum of 20 minutes. During maintenance (6 months after beginning and beyond), most clients will be satisfied with their level of CV conditioning but might occasionally need a tune-up, or a review and reassessment of their goals and objectives. Perhaps you might introduce new methods and types of exercise to eliminate the risk of boredom and dropping out.

What should you tell your clients about how much they will improve, and what happens if they stop exercising? Most healthy adults can expect to improve their aerobic capacity by up to 30% after 6 months of consistent training. If a person stops doing CV exercise, he or she will lose approximately 50% of these gains within 4 to 12 weeks (Roitman et al. 1998).

Principles of CV Training Design

All of your clients' programs should include CV exercise, but just as with resistance training, each client's CV exercise must be designed especially for him. Following are the principles that should guide your design.

Frequency

I aim for a minimum of three sessions per week and suggest as many as five for clients seriously intent on losing large amounts of body fat in a minimal period of time. Occasionally, clients want to know if it's OK to do CV exercise every day. The answer is usually yes, with an explanation. Though it is perfectly all right to do some type of CV exercise every day, it's not advisable to do a high-intensity, long CV session every day. Such zealotry can lead to overtraining, injury, and illness. (For many clients, wondering if it's all right to do CV every day will be the least of their problems. Finding time to do it even three days a week can be a challenge for many clients, what with careers, travel, and family demands.)

Intensity

Since most of you don't have access to a lab where you can do a $\dot{V}O_2$max test, you will have to employ more primitive, but no less effective means to get the information you need. Use a test that you're familiar and comfortable with to establish your client's baseline level of CV fitness and to decide where to begin and what your short-term and intermediate goals are. Your client's current resting heart rate (RHR) is a good indication of CV fitness. Think about it: A stronger heart doesn't have to pump as many times a minute to supply the body with the oxygen it needs at rest.

You'll also need to compute your client's target heart rate (THR) and maximal heart rate (MHR). Most of you are familiar with the formula

$$THR = \text{heart rate reserve} \cdot \text{desired intensity} + RHR .$$

In this equation, heart rate reserve is the difference between MHR and RHR. The desired intensity referred to is the percentage of MHR that you select given your client's current condition and desired objectives (that 60% to 90% of MHR referred to previously). Isolating your client's specific RHR and then adding it back provides a more accurate, customized result than simply taking a percentage of MHR.

Recently, there has been concern that the predicted MHR of 220 minus the client's age is less than an absolute formula. Aerobics pioneer Ken Cooper suggests that for fit males, 205 minus .5 times age is a more accurate way to calculate MHR. Some have suggested that for women, who have smaller hearts, it makes more sense to use 226 minus age. Regardless of which equation you use, keep in mind that if you obtain the client's predicted MHR from an equation rather than from a maximal stress test conducted in a lab, it is only an estimate. One expert has suggested that these guesstimates can be as much as 11 bpm too high or low for 30% of the population!

If you're primarily interested in promoting weight loss in a beginning exerciser, I suggest that you start with 60% of the MHR and eventually move up to 70%. These weight-loss CV workouts should last 40 to 60 minutes. Experienced exercisers who have established a base of conditioning and want to improve their CV fitness should aim for 70% to 80% of MHR. Clients seeking to improve athletic performance—for example, those who are planning to compete in a local 10K race—need to do at least some of their CV training in the 80% or greater range. These should be interval sessions during which the client varies between very high and moderate intensity.

You should also encourage your client to monitor her rate of perceived exertion (RPE), a subjective measure of how hard she is working. On a 1 to 10 scale, 4 to 6 corresponds to 60% to 70% MHR, whereas 7 to 8 is more like 75% to 85% MHR. This type of monitoring can be surprisingly accurate. It also has the advantage of increasing your client's body awareness.

Most important of all, remember that heart rate is not only a function of intensity level and duration. Factors such as temperature, humidity, altitude, inadequate rest and resulting overtraining, and time of day affect any individual's heart rate on any given day. For example, in a hot or low-airflow environment, heart rates may be 10 to 20 bpm higher at the same intensity (Roitman et al. 1998). When you also consider that the 220 minus age formula is inherently flawed, the bottom line is that the THR you and your client determine is a goal, but a flexible one. Educate your clients about the use of heart rates to determine duration and intensity, and encourage them to listen to their bodies.

Duration

The lower the intensity of the exercise, the longer your client will be able to continue. Elderly, extremely overweight, or otherwise compromised clients will be unable to sustain anything beyond the lowest-intensity activity for more than a very few minutes, and you might need to begin with less than the 20-minute minimum recommended by ACSM. If this is the case, your goal should be to maintain intensity while gradually increasing the number of minutes per session until your client can do 20 minutes nonstop. As mentioned earlier, eventually you'll want these clients to do sessions of 40 to 60 minutes at 60% to 70% of their MHR.

Appropriate Method

Obese, elderly, or poorly conditioned clients need to do low-intensity CV exercise without any complicated movement patterns. Walking fits this bill perfectly and is therefore usually the best form of CV exercise to recommend to them. Once a basic level of conditioning has been achieved, you should plan some higher-intensity CV exercise for all clients. Some clients enjoy group activities and might want to participate in an aerobics class. Others enjoy working out at home and will be more likely to do CV exercise consistently if they purchase a piece of equipment (stationary bike, treadmill, or stair stepper) for the home. Discuss the factors with your client and come up with the method that he is most likely to do consistently. The best CV exercise for your client is the one that he likes enough (or at least finds tolerable enough) to do frequently.

Consider Each Client's Unique Situation

Consider this example. I know someone whose road to hell, or should I say fat, was paved with good intentions. Week after week, month after month, he'd go through phases of excellent compliance with CV exercise. He'd get up at 5:45 A.M. and walk on the treadmill in his den for 30 minutes. This "being good" would last about 3 days, when he felt it was time to take a rest day. That "rest day" would turn into a couple of weeks before the whole hideous cycle would start again. He just couldn't make himself do it. It was right there across the hall, but convenience wasn't the issue. Even the TV wasn't a big enough distraction to make it bearable. He was tired at that hour, and he hated exercise. Then in a single day, everything changed. This same guy now gets up every morning without complaint no later than 5:20 A.M. and enthusiastically goes for a 2-mile outdoor walk. What happened? He fell madly in love, and this new girl demands that he do it. She won't take no for an answer. Not only that, but she is beautiful, and when he looks into her big brown eyes, he's a goner. He is tired but still delighted as he snaps the leash onto her collar and off they go, her tail up and wagging.

Many people have been dragged on the end of a leash into CV fitness. It works because of love and commitment, which are powerful motivators. So is the desire not to let someone else down, whether that someone is four-legged or two-legged. This is the reason that having training partners works well for many. You might suggest your client find a coworker who would enjoy a lunchtime or after-work walk or jog several days a week.

Another powerful motivator is social interaction, which is why some people find aerobics classes fun and make time, even when they claim they don't have any, to go to them consistently. Strategize with your client over what's convenient, what's worked for other people she knows, and what you think might work for her.

ACSM Guidelines for Designing CV Exercise

- **Frequency of exercise.** 3 to 5 days per week
- **Intensity of exercise.** Physical activity corresponding to 40% to 85% of $\dot{V}O_2$max or 60% to 90% of MHR
- **Duration of exercise.** Fifteen to 60 minutes of continuous or discontinuous aerobic activity per session

Preserving and Progressing CV Programs

Have your clients keep logs of their CV exercise and review these logs periodically. When your client is progressing through the stages of conditioning, especially the very important improvement stage, it is essential to have the information on her energy levels, perceived exertion, and exercise heart rate that the log will provide. In addition, simply being accountable to the log—a surrogate you—will provide that needed nudge on days when your client is tempted to skip her time on the treadmill or in the pool.

Make sure that the CV exercise you recommend is challenging but not too difficult. The goal is progressive but not excessive overload. Obviously, you need to suggest that your client work hard enough to obtain the many benefits of CV exercise, but if you demand that he work to the point of exhaustion during every CV workout, he will dread doing it, eventually so much so that he will stop doing it altogether! It's better that your client work out consistently, even at a lower level of intensity, than only intend to work out, think about working out while lying on the couch, or otherwise avoid doing a routine that's difficult, painful, and makes him feel like a failure at a higher intensity. A good rule of thumb is to increase only one of the variables—intensity, frequency, or duration—during a given session. For example, if your client has been doing 30 minutes per CV workout, increase sessions by 5 minutes but suggest that he continue exercising at a THR of 70% of MHR. Have your client record both his rate of perceived exertion and exercise heart rate, and keep these in mind when you design your routines.

Be aware that boredom is a constant lurking danger with CV exercise and suggest strategies to avoid it, including alternate types of exercise. Give your client an advantage by warning her that it's natural to be bored with CV exercise sometimes, and remind her that keeping the benefits in mind and varying the method will keep her on track. I find it helps some people do their CV workouts if they have some sort of distraction to keep them from getting bored. Reading (my personal favorite), watching television, listening to music, even returning phone calls can keep your client on that bike for the full 30 minutes she needs.

I've also found that it's useful to have clients use heart monitors during their CV workouts. The purpose of using the heart monitor is to give the client not only an objective measure of how hard he is working, but also a subjective feel for how hard he should be working. It will also give clients a gadget to play with, which some find motivating. Don't underestimate the effectiveness of gadgets in overcoming boredom. With some clients, this will make the difference between three CV sessions per week and three missed sessions.

The Flexibility Component

Flexibility is the ability of a joint to move through a range of motion. Despite the widely held belief that stretching reduces the incidence of injury, there is scant research to back up this claim. At least one study suggests that it does not (Pope et al. 2000). Still, flexibility is important, especially as we age. It helps clients maintain good posture and enhances their body awareness. It is relaxing, and it feels good! Unfortunately, flexibility tends to be the aspect of fitness most often sacrificed to lack of time. Time-pressed clients congratulate themselves for consistently doing their aerobics and resistance training and think, *Enough already! I have a life!* when it comes time to stretch. You can probably empathize with these feelings, but you should encourage your clients to stretch regularly, and you should include flexibility training as part of every (or almost every) session.

Principles of Flexibility Training

The best time for flexibility training is at the end of a session, after the muscles are warmed up and their tightness, as well as that of the connective tissue, is reduced. *Never* stretch a cold muscle! This is asking for injury.

Discourage your clients from engaging in bouncing, or ballistic, stretches. As you know from your anatomy and physiology training, when a muscle is stretched too quickly, it tightens as a protective reflex. The body is making sure that the muscle does not get overstretched or torn. Suggest that your client take the muscle into a perceptible but not painful stretch and hold it for a minimum of 20 (preferably 30) seconds. I strongly recommend that you time these stretches. You'd be amazed how 30 seconds can seem like an eternity when you're holding a stretch, and if it doesn't seem like an eternity to you, it will to your client. I've noticed this distorted time sense is especially acute in beginning stretchers, I suspect because stretching feels so unnatural, and maybe almost painful. Reassure your client that stretching, like everything else you're doing together,

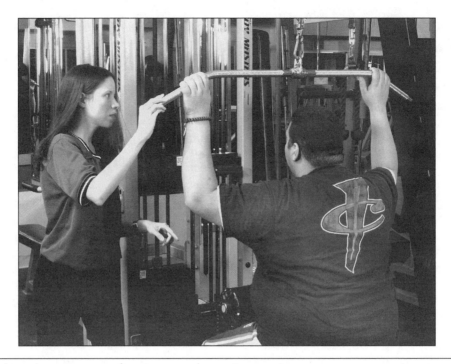

Each client has his or her own range of motion on each exercise.

will get easier, but not unless she holds the stretches at least 20 seconds. Some research suggests that four sets of 15 to 20 seconds per stretch will produce the greatest increases in flexibility.

Each joint has its own range of motion. Don't assume that a client with an extremely flexible upper body has equal flexibility in the low back and hamstrings. Also, remember that women tend to be more flexible than men, and well-conditioned clients more flexible than sedentary people.

Does Pre-exercise Stretching Prevent Injuries?

A randomized sample of 1,530 Australian male army recruits (17-35 years of age) were divided into two groups, a control group and a stretching group. During the standard warm-up period before training, the stretchers did a series of stretches for calves, hamstrings, quadriceps, hip flexors, and hip adductors. The control group did the warm-up only (jogging and stepping). The training period was 12 weeks, and the stretchers held their stretches for 20 seconds per stretch. There was no statistically significant difference in the number of injuries between the two groups (Pope et al. 2000).

The take-home message is that you should not tell your clients that "stretching prevents injury." Instead, recommend stretching to preserve flexibility and proper posture.

Stretching Guidelines

- Warm up before stretching.
- Hold stretches for at least 20 seconds, and preferably 30 to 60 seconds, or do each stretch three to four times and hold for 15 to 20 seconds.
- Avoid stretching without the prior consent of a physician if
  - you have a recent fracture or sprain,
  - you have suspected or diagnosed osteoporosis,
  - you have inflammation around a joint, or
  - you experience sharp, stabbing pain during stretching.

The Nutritional Component

Many clients will come to you to help them lose weight, so of course, nutrition is an important issue. As you know, as terrific and essential as exercise is, it is one of those things that is necessary but not sufficient in itself where the issue is weight loss. That's one reason so many people who exercise on their own become very frustrated. They expect the adipose tissue to fall off in buckets the minute they start walking three or four times a week. The reality is that to lose weight, most adults need to modify their diets. Don't get me wrong; exercise *does* improve the body's capacity to utilize fat for fuel through several important adaptations that take place:

- more mitochondria in muscles;
- more aerobic enzymes, the enzymes that facilitate fat mobilization and burning;
- more free fatty acid mobilization across the muscle cell membrane (McArdle, Katch, and Katch 2000); and
- more oxygen delivery to muscles, which facilitates more fat burning because it enables people to continue exercising longer at a higher intensity.

As mentioned before, you must be cautious about giving advice about anything beyond your expertise, including nutrition. You should refrain from giving clients special diets that claim to treat disease or other medical problems. In some states it is illegal for people without the required credentials to give nutritional advice (e.g., Illinois Dietetic and Nutrition Services Practice Act). Unless you are a registered dietitian, limit your nutritional advice to general concepts of good nutrition, such as the following:

- **We want our clients to eat diets low in fat and high in complex carbohydrates.** We also want them to consume alcohol and simple sugars such as honey, syrup, and candy and other empty-calorie foods only in moderation.

- **Remind them that even though it's easy to binge on doughnuts and other processed baked goods, it's nearly impossible to binge on apples.** That's because the fiber in fruits and vegetables helps people feel satiated, and they eat many fewer calories. Most nutrition experts recommend 25 to 30 grams of fiber per day. A side benefit is the many phytochemicals and nutrients contained in fruits and vegetables.

- **Explain that there are 3,500 calories in a pound, and that to lose a pound of fat, a person must create an energy deficit of 3,500 calories.** The best way to accomplish this objective safely and for the long term is to do it by increasing the energy expended (exercise) and creating a *slight* deficit in

energy intake. The ideal amount would be a 300- to 500-calorie daily deficit accomplished by burning 200 to 250 calories through exercise and consuming 200 to 250 fewer calories than needed. Although this protocol is ideal, it is difficult for people to sustain it precisely because it takes time. We live in an instant-gratification society, which accounts for the popularity of the low-carbohydrate, high-protein diets that resurface every few years like Jason in one of those hockey-mask movies. Because they don't provide enough carbohydrate to nourish the central nervous system, these diets force the body to cannibalize its muscle tissue to make glucose in a process called gluconeogenesis. The weight lost through these diets is mostly water, released when the body uses up its stored glucose (Katahn and Pope 1999) and tries to dilute the acidic by-products of ketosis. Despite what your clients may have heard about "excess insulin" making people fat, this is baloney. High insulin levels don't make people fat. It's the other way around; that is, fat, sedentary people's bodies produce more insulin because they are insulin insensitive (Bryant, Peterson, and Conviser 2001). This water leaches minerals from the bones, which is why these diets may increase the risk of osteoporosis (Manore and Thompson 2000). Discourage your clients from trying these ineffective and potentially dangerous diets.

- **Remind your clients that "fat-free" does not equal "calorie-free,"** and it's calories that count.

- **Speaking of calories, dispel the widely believed myth that people burn more fat while doing lower-intensity exercise.** The most important factor in using exercise as an adjunct to weight loss is the total amount of energy expended, not the substrate (fat vs. carbohydrate) used. So, the key to "burning fat" is to exercise at the highest intensity one can for the longest duration.

- **Remind your client that change is a process,** not a one-time event (see chapter 8).

In addition to explaining these guidelines, you can recommend books to your clients so that they can learn more about good nutrition. See the recommended resources in the suggested readings section (page 243). You should also consider networking with one or several registered dietitians to whom you can refer your clients and from whom you can get referrals.

75

Designing the Resistance Component of the Program

Questions we'll answer in this chapter:

■ What adaptations does resistance training cause in the body?

■ How do the laws of physics and mechanical forces affect body movements?

■ What causes muscles to contract?

■ What factors do I need to take into account when designing my client's program?

■ Why are certain exercises contraindicated?

■ How do I decide how much resistance is appropriate?

■ How do I increase the intensity of the resistance training?

■ What can I do about postural abnormalities?

It is no longer in doubt: Everyone should do some form of resistance training to prevent sarcopenia, the loss of muscle mass associated with aging. Resistance training helps people avoid injury, increase metabolism, improve sports performance, and, most important, help us maintain function as we get older. We know now that resistance training is also an important way to help people avoid "creeping obesity," the tendency to gain 2 or 3 pounds a year, which most American adults do between ages 25 and 50. The reason that resistance training is the key to lifelong leanness is that 60% to 75% of the calories that a person burns in a day is burned by resting metabolism. Since muscle requires more calories than does fat to simply exist, a person with a higher percentage of muscle burns more calories even when he or she is sleeping!

Resistance training, also known as strength training, is deliberate activity designed to increase, strengthen, and condition muscle tissue using equipment, such as weights, machines, or elastic tubing; or the body's own weight, as you do when you do calisthenics like pushups. Of course, as with all the other components of your client's program, you should understand the basic science behind resistance training. So before we get into the specifics of designing the strength training program, let's consider the physiology and the mechanics of resistance training.

Physiology of Resistance Training

You are the expert on muscles and how they grow stronger, at least in the eyes of your client, so you need to understand the underlying physiology. Think how impressed your client will be when he asks you, "How does my bicep know it's supposed to flex?" and you start throwing words like "acetylcholine" around? In all seriousness, it's important for all health professionals to have foundational knowledge about the workings of the body, so they can not only respond to client questions, but also be able to understand why and how their clients' bodies are changing.

Basic Structure of Muscle

Skeletal muscle is one of three types of muscle in the human body. (The others are cardiac and smooth muscle.) There are about 430 voluntary muscles in the body, which contract to produce body movement. A single muscle cell is called a muscle fiber. The number of fibers varies from muscle to muscle. For example, small muscles may have as few as several thousand, while a larger muscle like the gastrocnemius may have more than a million.

Each muscle fiber is surrounded by a plasma membrane called the sarcolemma. Within the sarcolemma, smaller subunits, the myofibrils, which are long, rodlike structures, rest in a gel-like substance called sarcoplasm. The sarcoplasm contains glycogen, fats, proteins, and minerals as well as organelles. Another important subunit within the sarcolemma is the sarcoplasmic reticulum (SR). The SR stores calcium, which is essential for muscular contraction. Figure 6.1 illustrates these structures of the muscle fiber.

The most basic functional unit of a myofibril is called the sarcomere. It is composed of actin and myosin filaments. The actin and myosin filaments are in a "staggered" arrangement, with their ends somewhat overlapping at rest. The thin actin filament is composed of three different protein molecules, actin, troponin, and tropomyosin. Actin provides a backbone on which the other two proteins can rest. Tropomyosin strands twist around the actin. The troponin molecules are attached at regular intervals on the tropomyosin strands like beads on a necklace.

Muscle fibers are innervated by motor neurons. A motor neuron and the muscle fibers it innervates are referred to as a motor unit.

How Do Muscles Cause Movement?

Muscular contraction results from a series of steps. A nerve cell, or motor neuron, releases a neurotransmitter, acetylcholine (ACh), which causes an electrical charge, called an action potential, to be generated in the muscle fiber. The action potential triggers the release of calcium from the SR. The calcium binds to the troponin on the actin filament, and the troponin pulls tropomyosin off the active binding sites. This allows the myosin to attach to actin and actin and myosin filaments to pull toward each other, increasing the overlap between them (see figure 6.2). This results in a shortening of the muscle fiber. ATP supplies needed energy. This theory of muscular contraction is called the sliding filament theory.

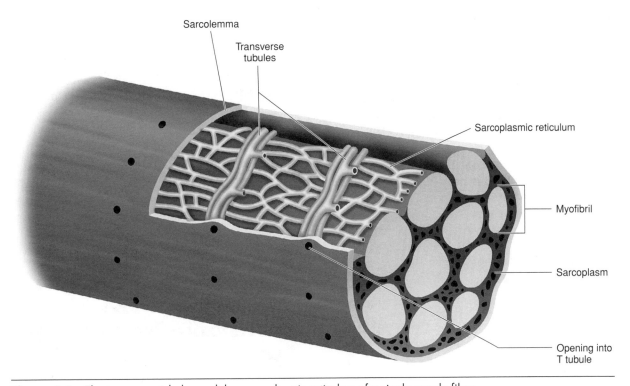

Figure 6.1 The transverse tubules and the sarcoplasmic reticulum of a single muscle fiber.

Reprinted, by permission, from J.H. Wilmore and D.L. Costill, 1999, *Physiology of Sport and Exercise,* 2nd ed. (Champaign, IL: Human Kinetics), 30.

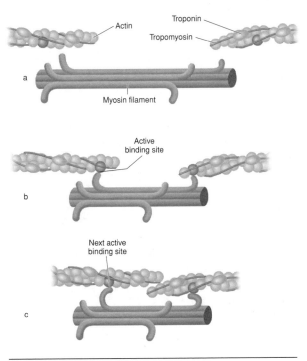

Figure 6.2 A muscle fiber *(a)* relaxed, *(b)* contracting, and *(c)* fully contracted, illustrating the ratchetlike action responsible for the sliding of actin and myosin filaments.

Reprinted, by permission, from J.H. Wilmore and D.L. Costill, 1999, *Physiology of Sport and Exercise,* 2nd ed. (Champaign, IL: Human Kinetics), 36.

Muscle Fiber Types

There are three types of muscle fibers:

- **Type I-SO:** slow oxidative (slow-twitch), for endurance
- **Type IIa-FOG:** fast oxidative glycolytic, for moderate intensity, duration
- **Type IIb-FG:** fast glycolytic, for power and speed

The proportion of these types in any individual's muscles is determined genetically (although some moderate enzymatic changes may occur with training).

Muscle Fiber Recruitment

Motor units contract at their max when stimulation threshold is achieved, which is referred to as the "all-or-nothing response." They don't contract at 50% intensity. Once they are fired, they are fired 100%. The practical implication of this fact is that when more force is needed, more muscle fibers must be activated.

Adaptations to Resistance Training

Just like the cardiorespiratory system, the muscles adapt to the increased demands of training. This is how the body "learns" the complex choreography that results in a smooth, controlled movement instead of the herky-jerky style exhibited by beginners. Think of someone trying to do a flat dumbbell press for the first time, even with very light weights. The weights wobble erratically through the air, the arms flail about, and every repetition is an adventure. Enzymatic changes allow muscles to store more glycogen and, therefore, to be able to perform movements longer.

Neuromuscular

Here are the neuromuscular adaptations that normally occur with strength training:

- Enhanced activation of motor units
- Greater synchronization (although some scientists dispute this theory)
- Early gains in strength resulting from enhanced neural activity; later gains resulting from not only this adaptation but also hypertrophy
- Hypertrophy, or increased fiber size
  - Increased contractile proteins
  - Increased enzymes and stored nutrients

It is possible that hyperplasia, or an increase in the number of muscle fibers, may occur. Studies on cats show hyperplasia with heavy resistance training, but research is conflicting as to whether it occurs in humans.

Metabolic

These metabolic adaptations occur with strength training:

- Glycolytic enzymes increase.
- Intramuscular fuel stores of glycogen increase.

Delayed-Onset Muscle Soreness (DOMS)

Remember the following points about delayed-onset muscle soreness:

- It is caused by minute tears in muscle and related inflammation.
- Eccentric exercise (exercise when the muscle is lengthening against resistance) is most likely to produce the most DOMS.
- The reason DOMS occurs is that although eccentric energy requires less energy, more force can be generated during it and fewer fibers are recruited.
- During recovery from soreness, strength is reduced by up to 50%.
- One strategy to reduce DOMS is to do concentric exercise to fatigue first, then do eccentric exercise.

Basic Biomechanics, or Everything You Ever Needed to Know About Resistance Training You Learned in Sixth-Grade Science

Understanding human movement is critical to designing effective programs and instructing your clients about how to do their workouts correctly. Remember that the body is a system of pulleys and levers. When you use a wrench to loosen a nut from a bolt, you exert a force against the lever (the wrench), which is connected to a fixed pivot point. Similarly, during movement, the bones (levers) move around fixed pivot points, the joints, when a force is exerted against the lever by muscle. Why is this important to understand? First, understanding the axis of rotation and the lever being moved directs your attention to the targeted muscle or muscle group. Second, once you focus your client's attention on the targeted muscle, you can keep your eagle eye on making sure he's not using other muscles or committing other form flaws that reduce the effectiveness of the exercise.

Biomechanics is the effects of the laws of physics on the body and the objects with which it interacts. It is a complex and interesting discipline that I recommend you study in depth. When you do take biomechanics, I strongly recommend that you get your hands on a copy of Peter McGinnis' excellent and extremely user-friendly text, *Biomechanics of Sport and Exercise*, published by Human Kinetics in 1999. For our purposes here, we need only understand the very basic concepts of biomechanics. Please refer to the suggested readings section for a list of additional excellent references that will help you learn more about biomechanics.

Newton's Laws of Motion

Newton's three laws of motion, from his 1686 *Principia,* specify how forces act on objects, including our bodies. Let's take a look at each of them.

- **Newton's First Law, the Law of Inertia.** "Every body continues in its state of rest, or of uniform motion in a straight line, unless it is compelled to change that state by forces impressed upon it." The most basic of these basics, in other words, is that in order for movement to occur, force must be applied (McGinnis 1999).

- **Newton's Second Law, the Law of Acceleration.** "The change of motion of an object is proportional to the force impressed and is made in the direction of the straight line in which the force is impressed" (McGinnis 1999). That is, forces have both magnitude and direction. The amount of *net* external force will determine the direction and speed of motion.

- **Newton's Third Law, the Law of Equal and Opposite Reaction.** "To every action there is always opposed an equal reaction." Or, as McGinnis states, "Forces exist in mirrored pairs." Of course, this does not mean that the effect on two colliding objects will be the same. That depends on whether they have the same mass or different masses. An example of this concept would be a car colliding with a bicycle.

Biomechanical Questions You Should Be Able to Answer

Whenever you include any resistance exercise in a client's program, you should be able to answer the following questions about it. Doing so will focus your attention on which muscles you are working, which ensures a balanced workout, and will remind you of the proper form for each exercise, something you want to have firmly in mind when you instruct your client.

What Are Linear and Rotational Forces?

Forces can act along a straight line, as when a bowling ball rolls down an alley. When an object moves in a straight line, the force has been directed through the object's center of gravity. Most personal

trainers are more concerned about the force exerted by muscles that cause body movement, and these are rotational forces. The key to creating these rotational forces is that the body's muscles work in pairs, acting through the pivot point and away from the center of gravity.

What Is the Pivot Point?

The pivot point is the point on the axis of rotation (a line in space around which rotation occurs)—in biomechanics, the joint that the bone rotates around (see figure 6.3). This is not simply a matter of academic interest; it has major practical implications for your client's form on every exercise. In a barbell curl, for example, the pivot point is the elbow. Since this is a single-joint movement, the shoulder joint is not also a pivot point. The practical implication is that the upper arms must stay stationary against the body throughout the range of motion.

Another important practical implication of the position of the axis of rotation is that the amount of torque increases the farther the resistance is from it. Think of a dumbbell side raise. If you hold your arms straight out to your sides, the exercise will be much more difficult than if you perform the exercise with your elbows bent to 90° of flexion (figure 6.4, a and b).

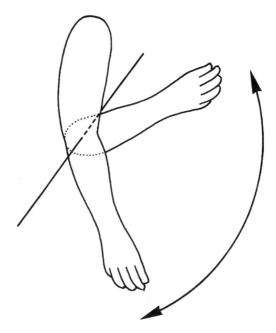

Figure 6.3 Rotation of the forearm and hand about the elbow joint.

Reprinted, by permission, from J. Watkins, 1999, *Structure and Function of the Musculoskeletal System* (Champaign, IL: Human Kinetics), 6.

81

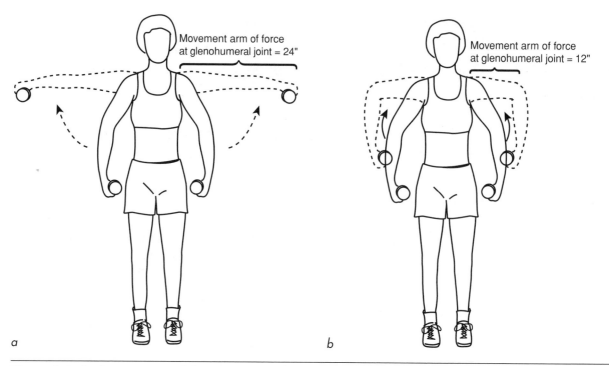

Figure 6.4 It takes twice as much force to overcome the weight's torque when *(a)* arms are extended than when *(b)* arms are bent at the elbows.

Is This a Single-Joint or Multijoint Movement?

We use the terms single-joint and multijoint to refer to the primary axis (or axes) of rotation and to help the client visualize how to perform movements with proper form. Some single-joint movements actually involve more than one joint, but not as a primary axis. For example, we refer to the dumbbell fly as a single-joint movement. During this exercise, the primary axis of rotation is the shoulder, so you should emphasize to your client that he should not flex and extend at the elbow. Single-joint movements are rotary (curved) movements, whereas multijoint movements are linear (straight). Single-joint movements are most effective in isolating a particular muscle, wheras multijoint movements involve several muscles.

This information is vital to your program design. Awareness of single-joint and multijoint movements will help you teach (and clients practice) correct form. Clients who understand that a triceps push-down is a single-joint movement also understand that they must keep their upper arms stationary to avoid shoulder extension. In general, it's best to do a multijoint movement before a single-joint movement involving one of the active muscle groups. For example, a client should do a dumbbell bench press first, working pectorals, anterior deltoids, and triceps, and then do dumbbell flys to isolate the pectorals. (This assumes you aren't working with an advanced client who wants to pre-exhaust the pectorals first.)

Where Is the Center of Gravity?

In some exercises, it's critical that the client have her weight distributed in a particular fashion. For example, when instructing a client on doing a squat, you should explain the importance of shifting weight onto the heels to make sure she drops her gluts and flexes at the hip, thereby taking stress off the knees. On other exercises, such as lunges, it's important to keep the center of gravity in the power core (low back and abdominals) for balance.

Which Muscles Are the Prime Movers?

You need to know which muscles are prime movers so you can focus your client's attention on the targeted muscle or muscle group and help him make the mind-muscle connection that makes the exercise more effective. This information can make each repetition a focused, effective effort instead of a ballistic, flopping waste of time.

What Is the Plane of Motion?

Since the body is three-dimensional, anatomists divide the body into fixed reference points called body planes to describe its structure. Taking a cue from them, I use the phrase "plane of motion" to explain the proper position of body segments during specific exercises. As you can see in figure 6.5, visualizing these "slices" through the body allows you to understand, and to explain to your client, the relationship of different body segments to one another during exercises. This is important because your client needs to remember to keep the moving body part in the proper alignment so that the targeted muscle will do the work. For example, if he is doing a dumbbell shoulder press, he needs to keep his arms in the same plane as his head to avoid the tendency to move them forward into an inclined position where pectorals, rather than the targeted deltoids, do most of the work.

What Is the Relationship of the Involved Joints to Each Other?

In some exercises, it is important to keep the joints in the proper position to work the targeted muscle in its own distinctive line of pull. For example, beginners might have a difficult time understanding that it is possible to move the upper arms without also elevating the scapula. By educating your client about the distinct nature of these two structures, you can dramatically improve her form on multijoint upper-body movements. Keeping these relationships correct can also prevent injury to your client. For example, in the squat, your client should flex not only at the knees, but also at the hips to avoid excessive knee flexion.

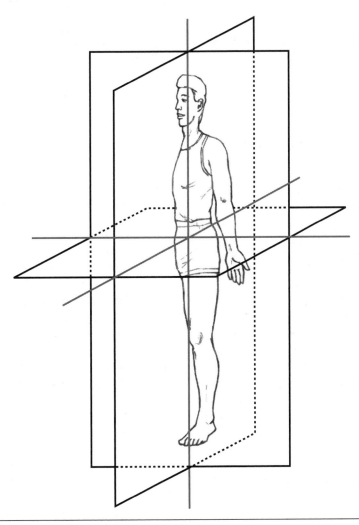

Figure 6.5 Cardinal anatomical planes and axes of the body.

Reprinted, with permission, from P. McGinnis, 1999, *Biomechanics of Sport and Exercise* (Champaign, IL: Human Kinetics), 26.

Designing the Resistance Component

Now that you have reviewed the science of how the muscles and joints work with each other, it's time to put it to good practical use for your client. Here are the keys to developing an effective resistance component.

Objectives of a Good Wellness Program

- Condition all major muscle groups
- Increase and maintain flexibility
- Avoid injury
- Maintain consistency
- Develop a strong sense of self-efficacy
- Develop body awareness
- Achieve and maintain functional posture
- Incorporate healthful nutrition and activity habits into the client's lifestyle
- Improve or maintain health

Identify Your Client's Unique Goals and Needs

Of course, designing the resistance portion requires that you give some thought to your client's specific objectives and needs. The catch is that, although he will probably have some idea of what he wants, it may be so vague that it is not very useful when it comes to designing a program. In addition, he may have some very definite needs (i.e., deficiencies that will have to be corrected if he's to get what he wants) that he's not even aware of. For example, many clients will come to you saying that they want to "'get in shape," by which they usually mean lose a few pounds and get firmer, which I would call "general conditioning." During your initial evaluation, you may learn that your client has been having trouble putting boxes up on a shelf, or has been having knee pain that he never had before. This information tells you that you need to work on strengthening certain muscle groups and stretching others to create muscular balance around the involved joints. When clients aren't very skilled at explaining what they want or need, the best way to find out is to ask open-ended questions like, "Why did you decide to call me?"

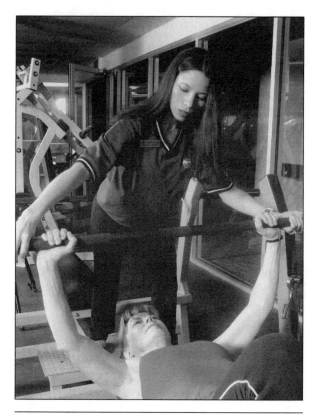

Strength training is an essential component of an effective fitness program.

"Why do you want to work with a personal trainer?" Then dummy up and let the client talk. She will reveal information that will tell you what you need to work on.

Two of the most important areas to ask about to help a client both identify and articulate her wants and her needs are lifestyle and medical issues.

Lifestyle Issues

One barrier that many clients need help overcoming is that whenever they try to begin exercising consistently, their lives get in the way. For example, many working mothers have difficulty fitting in exercise because they spend a lot of time in the morning preparing to leave for work and getting their children ready to go to school. When they return home, their good intentions to exercise are no match for the demands of dinner, homework, and sheer exhaustion. Many busy professionals have a difficult time with consistency because of travel and the long hours demanded by their careers. Thus, when designing an exercise program for this sort of client, you need to investigate the rest of her life.

Length of Session

Your client's lifestyle may dictate the length of your sessions. Fortunately, even short sessions of resistance training (10-15 minutes) can produce very desirable changes, especially in previously sedentary beginners. Some clients may find it more convenient to meet with you twice a week for 90 minutes. These folks can block out these two periods of uninterrupted time, but it would be impossible for them to meet with you more often. The aforementioned working mom might prefer five or six 10- to 15-minute sessions a week, some of which she might do on her own with suggestions from you about which muscles to work, which exercises to do, and in what order to do them.

Location

Convenience is a powerful benefit of in-home training. Many clients find that in the time that they can drive to the gym and back, they can complete an entire resistance workout at home. Many clients have tremendous success with in-home workouts, especially when they work with a talented personal trainer who can keep programs interesting even with limited equipment.

On the other hand, some clients are incapable of staying consistent with in-home workouts because they cannot overlook all the distractions that confront them everywhere. The working mom will have a tough time turning a blind eye to hungry children and piles of dirty laundry and marching

Some Corrective Steps for Common Postural Abnormalities

If your client's posture is less than perfect, consider these corrective steps:

1. Poor posture is the result of years of sitting, standing, and moving in less-than-optimal ways, so the first step to making things right is educating your client about proper alignment. Most people who walk around with hanging heads, collapsed rib cages, and winging scapulas have no idea that they are doing anything wrong. It takes constant vigilance for them not to fall into these dysfunctional patterns unconsciously. You can help by giving them visually vivid cues and constantly reinforcing proper posture and movement.

2. Identify the muscles involved. In most cases of postural dysfunction, one muscle or muscle group will be excessively weak and its opposing muscle or muscle group will be too tight; therefore, strengthen the weak muscle or muscles and stretch the tight ones. The following are some common muscle imbalances:

- "Bench press imbalance," in which the pectoralis major is too tight and the posterior delt too weak
- The upper trapezius, the large muscle in the upper back involved in shrugging motions, is too tight, and the deep neck flexors are too weak
- Levator scapulae, mentioned previously, and the serratus anterior, which is responsible for holding the scapula flush with the rib cage. When the serratus is weak, winging scapula will result.

3. Design a program of exercises and stretches that will address the specific imbalances you identified in step 2. If you are not clear on how to do this, consult John C. Griffin's *Client-Centered Exercise Prescription*, an extremely useful and informative reference that will help you design safe, effective programs. For bibliographic information on the book, see the suggested readings on page 243.

4. Do not permit clients to do exercises that will reinforce rather than correct dysfunctional posture or movement patterns. For example, if your client has an extremely tight and dominant upper trapezius, he will be nearly incapable of doing a lat pull-down without shrugging his shoulders. In fact, 99% of beginners (and, sadly, a large percentage of veteran weight trainers) will make this mistake when they are learning to do a lat pull-down. Instead of risking reinforcing this improper movement pattern, teach your client to depress his scapula while doing an easier exercise like a machine row. Once you have established the proper movement there, you can move on to the lat pull-down.

5. It may be necessary to have your client start over on exercises that he has been doing for some time, but doing incorrectly and in a potentially dangerous way. For example, people with severely tight necks and anteriorly tilted shoulders have no business doing regular push-ups. They risk shoulder impingements when they do. Instead, do exercises like dumbbell pullovers and push-ups against a wall with protraction to strengthen the serratus.

past them to her designated exercise area. It might be better for her to go the gym on the way home from work. There she'll find no distractions, lots of equipment, and maybe even some social support.

Medical Issues

With every client, investigate the answers to these questions:

• **Does this client have any medical or orthopedic conditions?** Some clients will have serious medical problems, and your program design will be constrained by what their doctors tell you is permitted and what is unacceptable for them. These are the easy cases. The more difficult ones will be those who have borderline serious problems, or vaguely described aches and pains. Typical areas of concern in deconditioned adults are the low back, the shoulder, and the knee. Postural problems underlie many other apparently unrelated difficulties. See "Some Corrective Steps for Common Postural Abnormalities" on the previous page for how to approach these all-too-common problems.

• **Any areas of potential injury?** Previously injured tissues are not as strong as those that have never been injured. This statement is particularly true of ankles and shoulders. An ankle that has been sprained is often less stable and more likely to be sprained again. Once dislocated, a shoulder is much more likely to pop out again. If your client tells you that he has suffered injuries to particular joints, you will need to be cautious with exercises involving them.

• **What energy system needs to be trained?** Remember, exercise is very specific, and the body adapts to the specific demands of training. That's the reason that even people who exercise regularly get very sore when they do something new. So, if your client wants to beat the guy in the next cubicle at the company 10K, he will need to train his anaerobic energy system by running fast during some of his training. On the other hand, a would-be marathoner needs endurance, so she would need to do some long-distance runs to be able to finish the race. The take-home message is to train what you're going to use.

Consider Whether This Exercise Is Safe for Any Client

As you know, certain exercises have earned the designation "contraindicated." This means that experts have determined that the risk of injury from doing them outweighs the potential benefit for most people. Thus, they should not be performed in any

circumstance. Some of these exercises are illustrated in figures 6.6-6.19.

Sometimes clients will say, "Why shouldn't I do this exercise? I've been doing it for years before I met you, and I've never had any problems." Although it's true that some people can do a contraindicated exercise for decades without any problems, these exercises earn their place on the no-no list because they are harmful to most people. Some people can also smoke for 50 years with no obvious ill effects, but no person knows until it's too late if he or she is one of the lucky few who won't pay a serious price. You might also mention to your client that some injuries that appear to be of the acute, sudden-onset variety are actually the result of that one stress too many that finally causes the tissue to fail. These injuries are not spontaneous at all, but rather the result of weeks, months, or years of poor technique or inappropriate movements. Is it worth the risk when there are safe ways to achieve the same benefits?

Consider Whether This Exercise Is Safe at This Time for This Client

A particular client might have a condition that creates a problem with training. Suppose, for example, that your client is a golfer who has suffered chronic elbow tendinitis. Wrist flexion and extension will aggravate this condition, as will gripping. Therefore, even though he might be able to move a heavier weight, you should err on the side of what the forearms can handle. (This rule might dictate your eliminating the exercise altogether.) Another example is a very poorly conditioned beginner who may have a difficult time doing a lat pull-down because of weakness in the low back and abdominals. She might not have the strength to hold her body at a 45-degree angle while doing the exercise. Her condition will dictate that you begin by strengthening the low back and abdominals and use a different exercise such as a dumbbell row or seated row to work the latissimus dorsi and rhomboids. Your initial evaluation will determine which exercises to eliminate or modify to protect your client from injury.

Select the Method of Training

Strength training doesn't have to involve hoisting heavy pieces of iron in a gritty gym. There are many ways to subject the muscles to increased challenge, each of which has its advantages and disadvantages. In most cases, you will decide to use more than one modality to achieve the results you and your client seek.

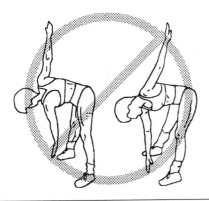

Figure 6.6 Unsupported spinal flexion, especially with twisting, places high-magnitude torque on the spine and the ligaments of the low back.

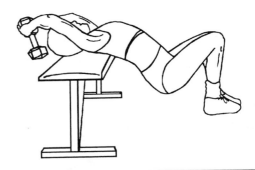

Figure 6.7 Pullovers across a bench leave the low back unsupported and hyperextended; the spine is unnecessarily subjected to high-magnitude compression forces.

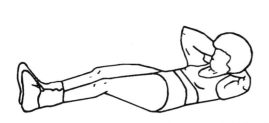

Figure 6.8 Straight legged sit-ups subject the spine to excessive compressive force.

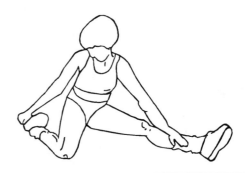

Figure 6.9 In the hurdler stretch, the knee is twisted and hyperflexed, which places excessive strain on the ligaments and may stretch them beyond their normal range.

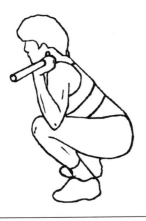

Figure 6.11 Barefoot exercise is very dangerous because of the risk of stubbed toes or other contact between vulnerable toes and feet and heavy equipment.

Figure 6.10 Deep squats cause excessive knee flexion, which can cause shearing of the patella.

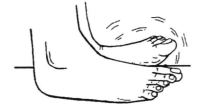

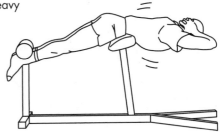

Figure 6.12 Bouncing hyperextension of the low back imposes excessive stress on the ligaments of the spine.

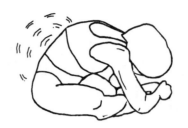

Figure 6.13 Bouncing flexion of the lower back imposes excessive stress on ligaments of the spine.

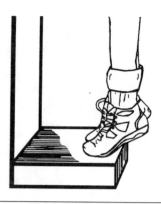

Figure 6.14 Ankle weights subject the ankle joint to external stress that could cause ligament sprain; they change the biomechanical relationships at the joint, which can distort foot plant and cause stress to the knee and hip.

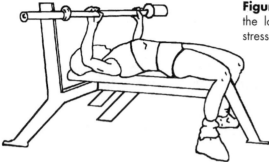

Figure 6.15 Bridging subjects the cervical spine to high-magnitude compressive forces and the lumbar spine to both compression and tensile forces.

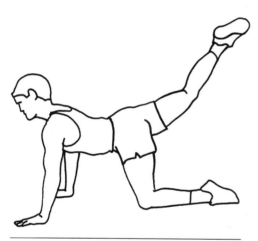

Figure 6.16 Lifting the leg above the body when on all fours compresses the spine.

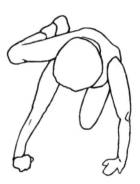

Figure 6.17 With fire hydrants, the tendency to twist the spine subjects the vertebrae to excessive shearing force.

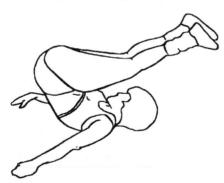

Figure 6.18 With the plow, most of the body's weight resting on the cervical spine causes excessive compression forces on this vulnerable area.

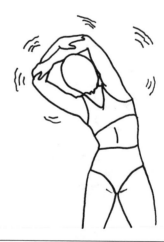

Figure 6.19 With ballistic movements, injuries may result from muscles and connective tissues trying to control the excessive forces produced by gravity. It is an ineffective way to improve strength, endurance, or flexibility.

Factors to Consider When Designing Your Client's Program

- Age
- Previous training
- Previous injuries
- Health history
- Medical restrictions
- Current physical condition
- Time available per week
- Time available per session
- Equipment available
- Client's desires
- Client's goals and objectives
- Client's life situation
- Client's personality

Free Weights or Machines?

Frequently you will be asked whether it's better for someone to train with weights or machines. As you've probably guessed, there is no single right answer. Each type of equipment has advantages and disadvantages for each individual. The short answer is that in general, most people need to use free weights at least some of the time to gain functional strength, that is, the type of strength we use in daily activities. Think about it: When you have to carry a bag of groceries, you use not only the directly involved muscles, but also the deep muscles that stabilize your limbs and joints. When you lift a free weight, these stabilizers have to do some work. When you use a machine, it does the stabilizing; you just have to push, pull, or curl using the muscles targeted by the exercise. Free weight movements are generally more challenging and more advanced. Consequently, some unconditioned clients might need to begin on machines with certain movements until they develop a good base of strength to prepare them for the challenge of free weights.

Clients who are rehabilitating from injuries might need to limit their work on certain muscle groups or joints to machines until they are pain free. With sedentary beginners, especially those over 40, I usually begin with machines (if available) on the multijoint exercises for large muscle groups—for example, the bench press. After three or four weeks, I introduce the free weight version of the exercise

using very light resistance. But this is not a hard-and-fast rule that you should apply to all of your clients. As in every other aspect of your duties as a professional, you must use your knowledge and judgment.

Bands, Balls, and Body Weight

As you know, dumbbells, barbells, and resistance training machines aren't the only tools you can use to help your client get stronger. Any device or modality that requires muscles to contract against resistance will do the job. The following methods have their advantages, so you should always consider whether they should be a part of your client's program.

- **Bands.** Resistance bands and tubing are extremely versatile and handy little pieces of equipment. Clients who have limited space for equipment will love that they can tuck them in a drawer and pull them out when they are ready to work out. Travelers can pack a couple in a bag and use them to do quick in-room workouts when they get to their destinations. With a common accessory, they can be placed between doorjambs and used just like the cable on a universal machine. Lest you think they are only for senior citizens or physical therapy patients, they come in strengths from tissue to suspension bridge, so even your strongest, most macho client can use them to do a challenging workout.

- **Balls.** Medicine balls, which were popular at the turn of the century, have made a comeback in recent years. They are extremely useful for sport-specific programs in which you are trying to develop speed and agility. For example, to improve club head speed, which is critical for performance in golf, your client needs to train through the specific range of motion of the golf swing against resistance. He can do that by holding a medicine ball and swinging away. The same analysis applies to basketball or any other skill and agility sport. Clients who aren't interested in sport-specific training can also use medicine balls for variety, such as holding a medicine ball during crunches to add intensity to their abdominal programs.

- **Body weight.** For years people have strengthened their muscles using body weight. Just ask Charles Atlas. For example, performed correctly, push-ups are one of the most effective ways to strengthen the upper body. So are chin-ups, although most deconditioned people can't do a single one. Many of these clients, though, can use a step to get into chin-up position, then do a negative chin-up, which is a terrific way for them to get stronger.

Use caution when suggesting body weight exercises for extremely overweight or deconditioned clients. Having these clients use their body weight as resistance is like piling plates on a bar: It's too much resistance for them. Asking a 300-pound (136 kg) person to do a set of dips is asking for trouble!

Select the Appropriate Intensity

Intensity is a function of several factors (amount of resistance, number of sets, number of repetitions, and amount of rest time). The first step in determining intensity is selecting the amount of resistance.

How Much Weight Should I Use?

Selecting the appropriate weight is both an art and a science—it requires the creativity and flexibility of an artist as well as the precision and sound judgment of a scientist. During your initial assessment of your client, you will do a series of strength tests that will give you some information to guide you in selecting appropriate weights. Table 6.1 shows general guidelines for selecting beginning weights expressed as a percentage of body weight. Note that gender, upper body versus lower body, and whether the exercise involves single joints or multiple joints are the factors that must be considered. Following are the other considerations you must think about before assigning a weight within each range that is given.

I don't believe in giving one-repetition maximum (often called one-rep max) tests to beginners, and it should be obvious why. Beginners do not have the experience and body awareness to lift heavy resistance safely. Instead, you can approximate a one-rep max test by using the following method.

Select a resistance that you think your client can lift eight times. The last two reps should be challenging enough that you might have to give your client a little spot. Multiply the resistance by 1.27 to get an approximation of your client's one-rep max. A beginning client should be able to lift a resistance at least 12 times under control with the last two or three reps being challenging. Generally, this will be 75% of the one-rep max. Although you can get a rough estimate of your client's one-rep max for a particular exercise using either method, I suggest using the 12 repetitions for beginners because it will be easier for them to maintain proper form with lighter weight. This is extremely important at the beginning stages of a program.

Remember, though, these are only guidelines. The results of any formula or other method for obtaining the appropriate weight for any exercise with any client must be evaluated in the light of common sense, the individual's unique physical characteristics and circumstances, and the following very important cautions:

- **Although a given amount of weight—say, 30 pounds (14 kg)—is always the same, it might not always require the same amount of force to move.** The number of pulleys, the design of a particular

Table 6.1	General Guidelines for Selecting Beginning Weights					
		Upper body			**Lower body**	
Male		Warm-up	First set		Warm-up	First set
Free weight	(SJ)	15-20%	25-30%		30-50%	50-70%
Free weight	(MJ)	10-20%	30-40%		50-70%	100-120%
Machine	(SJ)	15-20%	25-30%		20-30%	30-60%
Machine	(MJ)	20-25%	30-50%		50-60%	100-150%
Female		Warm-up	First set		Warm-up	First set
Free weight	(SJ)	5-10%	10-12%		20-30%	40-50%
Free weight	(MJ)	15-20%	20-30%		40-50%	70-100%
Machine	(SJ)	10-15%	15-25%		15-20%	30-50%
Machine	(MJ)	20-25%	25-40%		40-50%	80-100%

Note: Percentages refer to percentage of body weight. These percentages are only guidelines for selecting appropriate resistance, based on my work with a diverse client base. Every client has individual needs. Be sure to consider principles of good program design and the objectives of the client's program when selecting appropriate weights. Adjust the resistance after the warm-up to make sure the client can perform 8 to 12 repetitions (upper body) or 12 to 15 repetitions (lower body) with good form.

SJ = single-joint

MJ = multijoint

machine, and the quality of maintenance will affect how hard it is to perform one rep. Don't assume that your client should use the same weight at every club or machine.

- **Initially select a weight that is about 25% less than you think will be manageable for your client,** because the first few times performing a new motor activity are often awkward, jerky, and uncomfortable. Lifting weights is no exception.

- **Beginners should never lift heavy weights,** defined as a resistance so heavy that the client cannot control it alone, or do at least 10 repetitions without the help of a spotter. Lifting excessive resistance, especially in the beginning stages of a program, can result in tendinitis or other injury.

> Always err on the light side. You can always make the weight heavier, but the time to find out it's too heavy isn't after your client is lying in a heap on the floor!

- **Take the client's whole body and its condition into account,** not just the muscles and joints involved in the exercise. Consider the squat, for example. I often share this gym mantra with my clients: "The squat is the king of exercises." The squat earned this lofty title by effectively working so many muscles with one movement. This efficiency doesn't come without a price, though. The weightlifter performing the squat must be conditioned not only in his hamstrings and quadriceps, but also in his abdominals and low back. He must also have sufficient flexibility in his shoulder (rotator cuff, specifically) to hold a bar behind his neck and enough arm and shoulder strength to keep the bar from rolling down his back. Your new client's quadriceps and hamstrings may indeed be strong enough to flex and extend his knee, especially with a very lightweight bar, but are his abdominals and low back strong enough to support his spine in the proper alignment and to allow him to do the exercise with correct form? Is his rotator cuff flexible enough to allow him to hold his shoulders in abduction and external rotation for the time needed to do the exercise? You get the idea. Don't think of your client as a collection of muscles and joints, each with a given ability to generate force. Consider the whole human being!

Repetitions and Sets

Once you have determined the appropriate amount of resistance, the next thing you need to decide is how many times you will ask your client to move it.

A Numbers Game

The optimal number of repetitions depends on the desired objective. If you're trying to develop pure strength, generally you will want to use heavier resistance and fewer repetitions; however, this protocol is appropriate only for advanced weight trainers. Beginners should train in the 8- to 12-repetition' range, since this is the optimal number for increasing strength and endurance and improving overall conditioning.

How Many Sets?

Standard strength training protocols recommend three sets, but some research suggests that beginners can get the same benefit from one set of each exercise as they can from three. This one-set protocol can remain effective for approximately 3 months, so if you decide to use it, be sure to revisit the issue of number of sets after this time.

Increasing Difficulty

In order for exercise to continue to help your client make progress toward her goals, it must be progressive; that is, it must continue to challenge her muscles to get stronger by imposing greater demands on them. In the beginning, nearly every exercise will be challenging, but after a few weeks or months (everyone is different), you will need to ratchet up the intensity to keep things moving in the right direction.

There are five ways to increase the difficulty of an exercise:

1. Increase the amount of resistance.
2. Shorten the amount of rest between sets.
3. Increase the number of repetitions.
4. Change exercise order.
5. Increase the distance from the axis of rotation to the location of resistance.

Heavier Is Not Necessarily Better

The most obvious (but not always the best) way to increase the intensity of an exercise is to increase the amount of resistance. Do so cautiously. Remember that it takes longer for tendons to adjust to the demands of heavier resistance. If you increase the amount of weight too dramatically, your client might develop a nasty case of chronic tendinitis that will retard her progress for months. To avoid this risk, begin with a weight that your client can lift with good form for 12 repetitions. The last two or three repetitions should be challenging. When this weight is no longer challenging, increase weight no more than 5% and have your client perform eight repetitions. When this weight is challenging, increase another 5%, and so on.

Time Is the Tyrant

It amazes me to see trainers not monitoring the rest intervals that their clients take between sets. Decreasing the rest period from 1 minute, which is fairly typical, to 40 seconds will increase intensity dramatically. Try it yourself—you'll be amazed. (The one certain exception to this rule is abdominals, where you should keep the rest short, just 10 to 20 seconds. The key to effective abdominal training is working them very intensely for a short time.) I use a watch with a timer to keep track of rest intervals. It's important to have a system for keeping track of time, because during the rest interval you and your client will be reviewing form points or just generally gabbing away. I've found that decreasing the rest interval is a very effective way to increase intensity without some of the risks inherent in increasing the amount of resistance. Consider using this method with smaller muscle groups such as arms, where tendinitis is always a possibility.

More Reps?

Increasing the number of repetitions is a safe, effective way to increase training effort and strength stimulus. The time will come when that 12 repetitions with a given resistance that was so difficult for your client is now a piece of cake. You need to make the exercise more challenging, but it might not be appropriate to do so by dramatically increasing the amount of weight. For example, where the muscles you are strengthening are very small, it will be almost impossible to preserve good form with heavy amounts of resistance. The muscles of the rotator cuff and forearms are good examples of this phenomenon.

Changing Exercise Order

A typical workout routine is designed to work muscles from large to small; that is, legs, back, chest, shoulders, triceps, biceps, and forearms, doing multijoint exercises first, then single-joint isolation movements. (Abdominals can be done before or after the routine.) This order has its advantages (e.g., that the biggest muscles are worked in the beginning when energy levels should be highest), but it has one notable disadvantage: The large muscles are best worked by basic multijoint exer-

cises, which involve not only the prime mover but also smaller helper muscles. For example, the targeted muscle in the bench press is the pectorals, but it's impossible to perform the exercise without a lot of other role players: deltoids, triceps, and the rotator cuff. When confronted with resistance, these smaller muscles fatigue much sooner than the larger pectorals. Once the triceps are done, your client is done bench pressing. But the pectorals are thinking, *Whew, that was easy. Dodged a bullet there. I could do at least four more repetitions.* What if instead you had your client perform an isolation exercise for the pectorals first, and then do the bench press? The triceps and shoulders would still be fresh, but the pectorals would go into the bench press like an NBA team on a 12-day road trip, pre-exhausted. That is, in fact, what this technique is called—pre-exhaustion. It's a terrific way to increase intensity, but it should be used only with advanced trainees, not beginners.

Increase the Distance From the Axis of Rotation to the Location of Resistance

This strategy is usually applicable when a very weak and deconditioned beginner who could not do an exercise in the standard way starts out by doing a modified version, and is eventually strong enough to do the more advanced version. For example, a very deconditioned older woman who could not do a single push-up might begin by doing one with her knees bent. Bent-knee push-ups are easier because the force arm of the resistance (the body's weight) is shorter in this position than when the exercise is done with the legs straight. When she gets strong enough to do 15 bent-knee push-ups, you might decide to have her try doing the exercise with her legs straight, which will make it more challenging. This strategy would never be appropriate if the involved joints were vulnerable because of previous injury, dysfunctional posture, or inherent structural weakness. For example, one should never impose high-magnitude forces on the low back by moving the location of the resistance. In all low-back exercises, the resistance should remain close to the body to reduce torque on the vulnerable ligaments in the spine.

Instruct Your Client in Correct Technique

One of the most important reasons that people hire personal trainers is to teach them how to lift weights properly. Despite the number of books and videos around, it's extremely difficult to learn resistance training without some hands-on instruction and a knowledgeable adviser to answer your questions. You will be that adviser for your clients.

Ensuring Correct Form

For every exercise, it is important that you understand and are able to explain to your client all of the following:

- Pivot point or points (the joint or joints that are the axis or axes of rotation)
- Lever (the bone or bones being moved)
- Plane of motion (frontal, sagittal, horizontal)
- Puller or pusher (the muscle or muscles providing the force for the movement)
- Position (the relationship of the joints to each other)

If you do understand and explain these points to your client, you will be able to correct form mistakes and make the workout more effective.

I periodically give my clients little pop quizzes before certain exercises just to help them learn and understand these critical elements for every exercise. I might say, "Mary, can you describe the relationship between the shoulders and elbows in this movement?" or, "What is the axis of rotation in this exercise?" You need to constantly reinforce your client's knowledge.

Pace of Repetitions

You've probably seen someone in the gym writhing and contorting, practically doing a back bend, while a blur of something passes in front of him. After a few seconds, you realize that the blur is actually a barbell that he is hurling up and down with the momentum of his undulating spine. Effective? Yes, if the objective is to see how much weight he can move without regard to which muscles do the moving or to the potential for injury. The more momentum used to move a resistance, the greater the risk of injury, the greater trauma to joints and surrounding structures, and the less work performed by the targeted muscle. To avoid this sort of thing, I suggest to my clients that they maintain a slow, steady pace, especially on the negative portion of the exercise.

One exception to this rule: If you are coaching your client with a view to improving her performance in a sport in which speed matters, you need to add some fast-paced training to her regime. This type of training is safe and effective if done with extremely low resistance (body weight segments, a golf club, a medicine ball) under control.

Range of Motion

In general, you should instruct your client to move the resistance through a full range of motion (ROM). There might be situations in which you will find it desirable to limit the range of motion of a particular exercise. For example, if your client has been experiencing some shoulder tendinitis, he should limit his range of motion on the flat dumbbell press by refraining from lowering his upper arms below the plane of the bench, at least until he is pain free and has medical clearance to resume full ROM.

You'll be able to tell when your client is reaching momentary muscular failure because he will start voluntarily (he might even say it's involuntary—"I swear I can't help it!") limiting his ROM. Encourage him to maintain his perfect form despite fatigue and muscle-searing lactic acid. When he can't do so any longer, the set is over.

Vary the Routine

Some chronic injuries that bedevil weight trainers, especially those over 30, are the result of repetitive motion. For example, tendinitis and more serious conditions can result from performing the same movements constantly, especially with heavy weights. You increase this risk dramatically by not conditioning both sides of a joint, thereby creating dangerous strength imbalances. To avoid this potential problem, do the following:

- **Change your client's routine periodically.** Vary aspects of your client's routine. Beginners' routines should change every 6 to 8 weeks. More advanced clients can benefit from short (2- to 4-week) phases focusing on particular muscle groups or on achieving gains in strength or power.

- **Rotate exercises within phases.** Design your routines so that the client does different exercises for all major muscle groups. Unless she is preparing for a bench press contest, for example, no client should bench press every time she works out. This is asking for a shoulder problem. Plan a workout that is all single-joint isolation movements or one that gives your client a break from weights and uses different types of resistance (medicine balls, bands). In my experience, this sort of variety not only helps avoid injury, it keeps workouts interesting and fun, and thereby beats two motivation killers, boredom and burnout.

Troubleshooting

There are a number of problems you could run into, as I'll describe in the following section.

- **Discrepancies in muscle size.** Every multijoint exercise is a team effort, but not every member of the team is the same size. One muscle or muscle group is smaller than all the others and must use a greater percentage of its force-generating ability to move the resistance than a larger muscle will. For example, if you do a lat pull-down with 100 pounds, you are using your latissimus dorsi, rhomboids, posterior deltoids, biceps, and forearms. Your back looks at this 100 pounds and says, "That looks like a good, challenging resistance to move," but your forearms say, "You want me to move what?!"

- **Discrepancies in the rate that body structures strengthen.** You need to consider not just muscles, but also tendons and ligaments when you select exercises and weight amounts. I cannot emphasize enough the importance of remembering that muscles get stronger much more quickly than tendons and ligaments! Tendons and ligaments transmit the force generated by the muscles to complete movement and maintain the integrity of joints. They will get stronger, just as muscles will, but take more time. Excessive amounts of weight, especially used by beginners and older, poorly conditioned clients, can result in severe tendinitis or the related condition, tendinosis, in which through years of use, tendons have become frayed and pitted. Unlike tendinitis, tendinosis is not an inflammatory condition but an overuse syndrome, which has a more gradual onset and much longer recovery time.

- **Conditioning in the power core.** Sometimes trainers exhibit the unfortunate shortsightedness that has often plagued businesses and governments. As in the case of these institutions, the results can be disastrous. Specifically, these trainers focus on developing specific muscles or muscle groups and neglect the important need to strengthen the power core, or the abdominals and low back (see figure 6.20). Resist the tendency to emphasize the Hollywood muscles—the biceps, triceps, chest, and deltoids—to the exclusion of these vital trunk muscles. Beginners especially need to develop strength and flexibility in the abdominals and low back. If you include plenty of basic multijoint movements in your client's program, the smaller, show-off muscles will reach a level of basic conditioning that will prepare them for the more specific, intense workouts to come. The patience and long-range thinking reflected by your intelligent program design will be

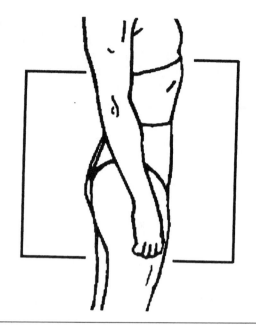

Figure 6.20 The power core.

rewarded when your client's strong power core provides a stable base for arm and shoulder movements.

- **Pay close attention to aches and pains.** Often, chronic injuries begin insidiously. A slight twinge on shoulder abduction after performing a set of machine shoulder presses can be the beginning of a serious injury. Take these things seriously. If a client tells you over and over again about a persistent ache or pain, especially when doing a particular exercise, redesign your routine to avoid stressing the area. If rest doesn't result in significant improvement within two weeks, strongly recommend that your client consult a physician. Never attempt to diagnose injuries on your own! What might seem like tendinitis to you could be some underlying pathology that will benefit from immediate medical intervention.

> Failure is a good thing. It's not only OK to be negative—I encourage it.

Failure Can Be Good

I always tell my clients that the gym is the only place where failure is the result you actually hope for, and that it's OK, even desirable, to have negative thoughts. By that I mean that we want to work to the point of momentary muscular failure on the last rep or two; that is, take the muscle to the point of complete fatigue so it will come back stronger. Normally, I think negative thoughts are nothing short of poison to the spirit and the mind, but I actually encourage my clients to think negatively when it comes to weight training. I want them to use the negative: Lowering the resistance slowly, resisting the effects of gravity while the muscle is lengthening, makes the muscle produce much more force and dramatically improves the effectiveness of resistance training. I suggest that you have your client perform the positive part of the movement to a count of two and the negative to a count of four.

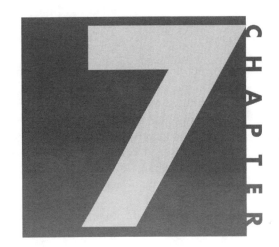

Conducting the Workout and Conducting Yourself

Questions we'll answer in this chapter:

- ■ What should I do before I begin a workout with a client?

- ■ What should I say if a client tells me he or she doesn't want to warm up?

- ■ What are some general rules of conduct and courtesy that all personal trainers should observe?

Once you've designed your client's program, now what? Here are some suggestions about how to conduct client workouts and how to handle some typical situations that may come up when you do. Because I've already covered how to assess, prescribe, and progress the cardiovascular workouts you'll be assigning your clients, I will not discuss those issues in this chapter. Just be sure that you reserve time in each workout session to check in with the client about both progress and problems in her cardiovascular work and to discuss any changes or solutions that she needs to take action on.

Conducting the Workout

When you begin working with a new client, you should set up a record book for her. I suggest that you use three-ring binders containing

- workout record forms (see appendix A);
- copies of goal inventories, homework, and related materials that you have given your client;
- any notes of special importance such as medical information relating to this client; and
- emergency contact information for this client.

Plan Everything

Before the scheduled session, you should plan everything about the workout—the exercises, sets, and reps—basing your plan on your previous experience with this client, or, if this is your first workout together, your best estimate based on the results of your fitness assessment. Remember to *always* err on the conservative side! You can increase the amount of weight or number of reps on the second or third set if necessary. Make a habit of noting these adjustments in the workout record. Then before you begin, determine whether any of the information you got in this pre-exercise exchange dictates that you should change any aspect of the planned workout. Be flexible in your plan. What if you have an upper-body workout planned, but your client tells you when you arrive that she hurt her wrist? You never know when you will have to change everything, and you should be prepared to do so without advance warning.

Before You Start

Before beginning a workout (including the warm-up), go over the MAPP. After exchanging pleasantries when you greet the client, always ask

- Are you taking **M**edication?
- Do you have any **A**ches that might affect your ability to exercise?
- Do you have any **P**ain, and if so, where?
- Do you have any other **P**roblems that might affect your workout?

The Warm-Up

Sometimes clients will arrive late for a workout. "C'mon—do I have to warm up?" they plead. "Let's just get started." It is at this point that my ability to tell people things they don't want to hear comes in quite handy. A general warm-up is essential before beginning the workout. It decreases the risk of injury by raising the temperature of muscles, thereby making them contract more efficiently. It also makes muscles more pliable. It reduces the risk of tearing tendons and ligaments. It increases blood flow to working muscles, including that all-important muscle, the heart. It improves oxygen consumption and prepares the body for the increased demands of exercise.

Now that I've convinced you that a warm-up is essential and provided you with ammunition to combat your clients' protestations that they don't have time to warm up, please understand that you don't need to overdo it. You don't want your client so wiped out by the warm-up that he is unable to do a single resistance exercise. I recommend a minimum of 5 minutes of moderate CV exercise, usually on a stationary bike, before beginning the workout. You can tell that the client is warmed up when he breaks a sweat.

In addition to the general warm-up, you should have your client do a specific warm-up for the muscle or muscle groups being worked with approximately 50% of the weight of the first set prior to working it. This warm-up set is especially important for exercises involving the knee, low back, and shoulder.

The Resistance Portion of the Workout

After your client has completed his general warm-up, it's time to head for the weights (or machines, bands, or other equipment) and take him through the resistance exercises that you have planned.

After each set, it's useful to ask the client how difficult the set was for her to complete. You can use these responses to decide whether to decrease the rest interval or increase reps or weight, or even to determine whether your client feels the muscles contracting the way she should. Rather than simply asking, "How hard was that?" and having the client say, "Not too bad," or "Really horrible," I've found I can get a much more specific, informative response by asking, "On a scale of 1 to 10, if 1 is like lying on the couch watching *X-Files* reruns and 10 is like trying to lift the Sears Tower, how would you rate the difficulty of that last set?" I call this the client's subjective intensity rating (SIR) for this set. Record these for each set, or at least for the last set of each exercise. When you do your postsession review, use these numbers to plan the next session.

Subjective Intensity Rating

1	Like lying on the couch watching *X-Files*
2 to 3	The effort required to walk to the fridge
4 to 5	Almost broke a sweat
6	Moderately challenging
7 to 8	Last two or three reps were really tough
9	Like trying to give a piggyback ride to a sumo wrestler
10	Like trying to lift the Sears Tower

In most cases, you want clients to rate the exercise in the 7 to 8 area.

The Cool-Down and Flexibility Training Portions of the Workout

The cool-down portion of a CV session consists of slow, low-intensity (30-40% MHR) activity such as pedaling with low or no resistance or slow treadmill walking. The cool-down helps prevent venous blood pooling and lowers the probability of cardiac arrhythmias. It's easy to understand why when you remember that during exercise, the contracting muscles help to move blood back to the heart. When you stop exercising, blood can tend to pool in the extremities, which can cause blood pressure to drop and even irregular heartbeat or arrhythmia. Be sure to explain the importance of cool-down to your client since he will probably be working out on his own, at least from time to time.

Since it's not advisable to stretch when muscles are cold, stretch after the workout when they are warmed up and in optimal stretching condition. (If your client prefers, he may stretch after his general warm-up, but never before!) If your workout with your client consists of resistance training only, stretching will serve as the cool-down portion. Plan the flexibility training so that you give priority to joints that need the most work. Remember that when it comes to stretching, halfway is no way. If you don't hold a stretch long enough, it does not improve flexibility and range of motion in the joint. When you're stretching, especially stretching joints that have limited range of motion, 20 to 30 seconds will seem like forever, and your normally astute sense of time will desert you, so time the length that your client holds his stretches and use these prolonged intervals to check proper form. On especially tight areas, it's advisable to perform each stretch three to five times and to include stretches for these areas in the client's homework. See the Resistance Workout Guide for stretches for particular muscles and joints.

The Reinforcing Good-Bye

There are some clients you will see only once a week, once every two weeks, or once a month. With these clients, it's important that you send them off with praise for their successes during today's workout and specific instructions about what they need to do before your next session.

- **Positive feedback and reinforcement.** Find something positive about your client's performance and point it out. If her form on an exercise you've been working on has improved, tell her! Say it loud, say it proud! Sometimes we assume that our clients know that they're improving, but we forget the natural human tendency to discount improvement and focus on the things that aren't getting better.

Praise their successes!

99

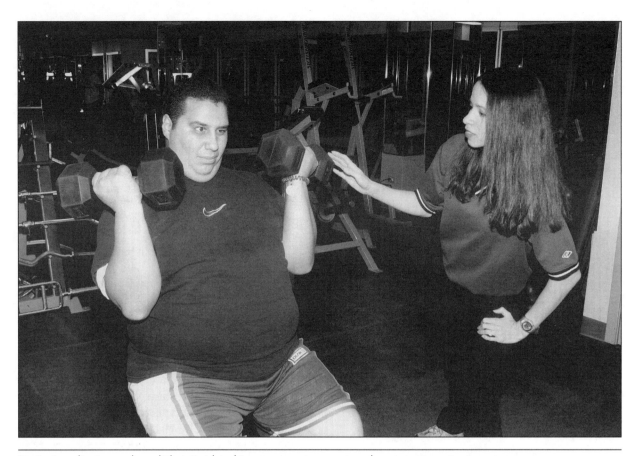

Beginning clients may be a little intimidated in a gym environment, so be as encouraging as you can.

• **Homework**. It's wise to assign your clients some specific activities to do before your next session. For beginners, often it is only their CV sessions and stretching, but even in these cases, give them a target time and intensity and a list of stretches to do. More advanced clients should get more detailed workouts with specific exercises, sets, reps, and rest intervals. Be sure to explain everything that you give a client to do on his own! Never assume that he understands what he is supposed to do just because you've done it together a hundred times. Often clients suffer from sensory overload during your workouts together, and when left on their own, their memories of the specifics are as fuzzy as a well-worn polyester shirt. If you decide to give your clients homework, I recommend that you come up with a short list of general guidelines to remind your clients about general safety precautions. Give them these guidelines along with a list of exercises you want them to do, noting special precautions and form points for each. Giving clients homework helps reinforce the idea that exercise and healthful lifestyle behaviors are not just something that happens during the few hours a week that they see you, but are a natural part of life.

Reinforce Information

The first few times you do an exercise with a client, and periodically thereafter, you should explain all of the following:

• The name of the exercise (Your clients probably won't remember most of these names. Every time you say, "seated dumbbell triceps extension," your client is likely to say, "You mean dumbbell behind the head?")
• The muscle or muscle groups being worked
• The muscle or muscle group's function
• The pivot point
• Body position and correct center of gravity
• Form points
• Common mistakes in form made by beginners

Keep Accurate Records

There will come a day when your client will ask, "How much weight did I use the first time I did a bench press?" or, "What's the most I've ever done on the leg press?" Your client might also tell you that his right knee has been very sore for about 3 days and ask you why. You've got to be able to answer these questions, not only to be responsive to your client, but also because information about your client's progress is vital in designing his program. That's why it's so important to keep accurate records.

Sometimes it's hard to remember to write everything down while you're trying to talk to your client, watch his form, and focus on the workout, but it's very important to do so. You should write down any aches, pains, or problems at the beginning before you begin the workout. As for keeping track of the volume of work, the best way to make sure you keep an accurate record is to write down the number of reps after each set. By the way, counting reps is important. Sometimes when you're trying to watch your client's form, correct mistakes, and give encouragement, you tend to lose count; therefore, you might suggest to the client that he count, too, or give him a target number of reps so that he can let you know when he gets there. (A sample workout record form is provided in appendix A.) Before you say goodbye, make sure to give your clients ample opportunity to ask you any and all questions that may occur to them.

The necessity of accurate record keeping also means that the session doesn't end when the client leaves. After the session, go over your notes; client SIRs for each exercise; and your overall annual, semiannual, or quarterly plan for this client. Make additional notes about specific areas you want to work on at the next session or subsequent sessions.

Each workout is more than just another day at the office. At the end of several weeks or months, when you both look at the transformation that has occurred and celebrate your achievements, recall that it happened one workout at a time. So approach each session as the important thing it is: a small step toward the goals that you and your client have determined to reach.

Conducting Yourself in the Gym

Although some people don't seem to realize it, we're trying to have a civilization here. To that end, it would help if we all observed some simple rules of courtesy with our fellow human beings. The gym is no exception. Here are some simple rules that you should always observe.

Be a Good Citizen—Follow the Rules

There are some rules of gym etiquette—good manners for the weight room—that are known to bodybuilders and weight trainers throughout the world. You should always try to comply with these standards when you are working with clients. Being a good gym "citizen" will make the experience more pleasant not only for you and your client but also for other gym members. Keep in mind that your client will probably be someone who hasn't spent any time in a gym and who looks to you to set an example about how to behave. Make sure you set a good one. These, then, are the "rules."

- **Respect other members.** When you approach a bench with a towel on it, or a pair of dumbbells resting on the floor nearby, or other evidence that suggests that someone might be returning to finish a set, ask people standing around if anyone is working there. Few things are more annoying to weight trainers than their fellow gym members just walking up and taking over their spot or the equipment they're using. Always ask. Often several people will be using a particular piece of equipment, so you'll have to be courteous and work in (see next point) with other gym members.

- **Politely ask to work in.** The custom of "working in" is accepted in weight rooms all over the world (really—I once worked in with someone in Japan). In case you're unfamiliar with the term, working in means using a piece of equipment while another gym member is resting between sets. Let's say you're working with your client Nancy Novice and you want to use the 10-pound (4.5 kg) dumbbells. Unfortunately, as you approach the weight area, you discover that someone else is using them. Waiting until she is finished with her set, you say politely, "Is it OK if she (indicating your client) works in with you with the 10s?" Ninety-nine point nine percent of the time the person will smile and say yes. When he or she doesn't, you're probably dealing with a dysfunctional person.

- **Beware of rude people.** Every gym, school, and workplace has some of these. Unfortunately, gyms may have more than their share because of the hideous and well-documented psychological side effects of anabolic steroids. Once you are around a particular gym or club for a while, you will get to know who these people are. They're the ones who strut around as if they own the place, bellowing unsolicited comments about other members and anything else that enters their minds. They don't converse so much as broadcast their opinionated bleating to the entire room. In my experience, some of these people find your very presence a threat. After all, why should a client hire you to get advice on exercise when she could just ask him? He's a lot more muscular than you'll ever be, right? If you have the misfortune to encounter one of these individuals, understand that they live in their own world. If they're rude to you, resist the temptation to respond in kind by telling them to put it where the sun don't shine. Remember that you are a professional and you have your client to think of. A confrontation will only make you look bad. Just get your client out of harm's way. Clubs and gyms don't want troublemakers either. So make a note of exactly what happened or was said in any untoward incident and inform the gym's management in writing, being very specific: Documentation may come in handy.

• **Be friendly.** One of the reasons your client likes working with you is that you are a friendly, pleasant person. Your client will appreciate your being friendly and polite to other gym members, too. Introduce yourself to other members and learn their names. Saying, "Hi, Steve. Mind if she works in with you here?" instead of "Hey you—can we work in?" will smooth the way for your client.

• **Help your client get acclimated to the gym environment.** It may come as a surprise to you, since you find the clanging of barbells and the grunts and groans of sweaty hulks as natural as breathing, to learn that many clients will feel as out of place in this environment as they would at a stag party in Sunday school. I can remember a client, a middle-

aged woman who had previously been very sedentary. Her eyes grew as large as saucers the first time she saw—and, more importantly, heard—a tattooed young man struggle and strain doing battle with a pair of 100-pounders . He had barely completed his last rep when, with a triumphant cry, he allowed the dumbbells to crash to the floor. She visibly slumped, as if trying to hide from what clearly was a frightening situation. If you put yourself in her place, her feelings won't seem that unusual. Have empathy for your client, and try to make her feel at home in the gym. Introduce her to fellow members that you know, and explain that those guys, scary as they look and sound, are really harmless.

• **Mind your own business.** A day never passes that I don't see things in the gym that give me nightmares. Some of the gyrations that pass for proper form are injuries waiting to happen. In law, there is a term called the "officious intermeddler," which is someone who sticks his nose in a situation without invitation. I won't bore you with a bunch of legal mumbo-jumbo. Suffice it to say that almost no one appreciates unsolicited advice, no matter how good it is. Be like me: Walk around with little red teeth marks on your lip, but say nothing.

• **Avoid distractions.** During and immediately after the workout, your attention must remain riveted on your client. If you do a lot of your workouts in the same gym or club, you'll get to know lots of people there, and though being friendly is always a good policy, don't let your desire to be sociable interfere with your number-one priority, your client. For example, don't get caught up in a conversation with another gym member and leave your client left out, standing around awkwardly wondering what to do next, wondering whether you've

Bite Your Lip

Still not convinced to mind your own business? Read on.

Is it worth $5,000 to you to prove that you are the smartest person in the room? That's what a volunteer spotter ended up paying another club member who got injured. Here's what happened: One club member was doing an incline bench press and another walked over and volunteered to spot him. As is often the case, there were several pairs of dumbbells on the floor. When the weightlifter went to place one of his dumbbells down, his index finger was crushed when the weight he was holding collided with one of the weights on the floor. A lawsuit was filed, based on the claim that the defendant-spotter had assumed the legal duty to not be negligent. In the case of the spotter, the court looked at the standards of the National Strength and Conditioning Association to say that ordinary care requires a spotter to make sure the areas surrounding the bench were clear. The case was eventually settled. The guy got $20,000 for his crushed finger, $15,000 from the club and $5,000 from the volunteer spotter.

The take-home message is that when you volunteer to do something, you assume a legal duty when one previously did not exist. My advice: Don't do it.

forgotten he is there, and wondering why he is working with you in the first place! After saying hello, introducing your client by name to your gym pal, excuse yourself and move to the next exercise.

• **Get there first, or the importance of punctuality.** How many times have you been late for something because a semi jackknifed and spilled frozen green beans all over the expressway, a 300-car freight train was between you and your destination, or some similar catastrophe? When a client is waiting for you, even one time is too many. *Never* be late for a workout! Always assume that some unforeseen event beyond your control is going to happen, and leave 5 to 10 minutes earlier than you think you have to. If you're going to a new place, I suggest that you drive there in advance 2 or 3 days before the scheduled appointment and figure out the best way to get there and just how long it takes. Then you won't be surprised, or more important, late. Oh, and one more thing: When you schedule your day like this, you will probably arrive before the client. That's ideal because it gives you time to go over the workout again, think about the specific instructions you're going to give the client during the workout, and generally be well prepared.

| Never be late for a workout! |

Special Considerations of Home Workouts

Home workouts have become quite popular, as the vast assortment of home fitness equipment will attest. It's no wonder. The convenience of home workouts is tough to beat. The only downside for some would-be fitness buffs is the lack of knowledgeable instructors. That's where you come in. When someone invites you into her home, even as a paid professional, she is making a statement about the confidence she has in you. Let's face it: Most of us wouldn't let just anyone into our homes. It's a special trust, one placed in you because of your professionalism and competence. Of course, going into a client's home is much like going into anyone else's home—good manners are always in style. In your capacity as a professional, there are some other things to think of.

Remember: You Are a Guest

Never enter a client's home without permission. Sometimes clients will tell you that they will leave the door open for you when you come, and in these cases, of course you should let yourself in. Until your client tells you this, though, you should always just ring the doorbell and wait patiently to be let in. If you knock on the door and ring the doorbell and get no answer, be sure to leave a note in the door, stating you were there and saying that you're sorry you missed her. Go out to the car, phone and leave a message on the machine, then wait 5 minutes in your car before leaving. Though this happens rarely, it's important that the client know that you did show up when you were supposed to.

It's desirable, but not essential, that the phone be in the same room that you and the client are using to work out. If not, make sure that it's accessible to you in case of an emergency. Yes, sometimes clients look twice at you when you say, "OK, before we get started, I need to know where the phone is, and whether this area is served by a 911 system." Be prepared for your client to look a little disconcerted and say, "Why? Are you going to push me until I have a heart attack?" They feel quite reassured when you reply that even though you've never hurt anyone, you want to be prepared for any contingency. If, like many on-the-go people today, you have a cell phone, I recommend that you keep it charged and handy when you are conducting a session with a client.

When You Go

When you go to a client's home, be sure

• you either bring your cell phone, with batteries charged and sufficient minutes left, or

• you know the location of the client's phone; and

• you know whether the town or village is on a 911 system, and if not, the phone number for emergency medical service.

Treat your client's furniture with special care. If she offers you something to drink, be sure to use a coaster before placing a glass on a table. You may have to ask for one, and she may say, "Oh, you don't have to use a coaster on that table. It's from a garage sale," but make sure you ask first.

Ensure that the workout area is safe; that is, that there is no loose carpet, water, extension cord, or other object or condition that might cause your client (or anyone else in the area, for that matter) to slip and fall. As you complete an exercise, pick up and put away equipment. Don't leave the area littered with objects.

Since you are not in control of the workout equipment or area, it's advisable to use a special waiver when you work with your client at home. A sample waiver form for home workouts is in appendix A. As always, and as with the other waiver form, it is provided as a starting point for you and your attorney to use in preparing a waiver for you that will comply with the current requirements of your state's law.

Children

During your initial consultation, talk to your client about how you can ensure that you have an hour of uninterrupted time for the workouts. Often stay-at-home parents can find this hour while their children are at school or napping. The important thing is to make sure that the client can concentrate on working out without worrying about having to drop everything to deal with children. Once the importance of being able to focus on the workout is explained, this isn't usually a problem.

What can sometimes be a problem is children coming into the workout area and causing a potentially dangerous situation. We try to minimize this risk by suggesting that the client keep the workout area off-limits to children during the workout. Sometimes clients assure us that their children have been instructed about safety in the workout area and stay there all the time while they are working out, and their presence won't cause any problems. In these cases, you should permit the children to stay, but use extra caution about moving bars and weights. Before you begin an exercise, check on the children's locations and advise them

to stay out of the way. With children, it's especially important that you pick things up and keep the area reasonably clear of potential trip-over hazards. If the situation becomes dangerous, you will have to discuss it with the client before continuing with your workouts.

Pets

Many clients have pets, usually cats and dogs. You probably won't have to deal with them much, other than petting them if they greet you at the door. (Like every other general rule, this one has its exceptions. I remember the time when one client's three huge dogs got a bit testy with one another, and eventually ended up in a teeth-bared, snarling fight! Or the time I rescued a client's dog by dislodging a plastic toy from its throat. Or the time a client's dog got a tad frisky and bit me, unintentionally I think. In all cases, everything turned out fine, I'm happy to report!)

If you and your client have agreed that you let yourself in, be sure that the door is closed behind you and that all pets are present and accounted for before you leave the entryway.

Be cautious conducting workouts in the presence of pets. Always know where they are before you move equipment or begin an exercise. A rambunctious dog underfoot adds nothing to a workout, except maybe an injury and a lawsuit!

In the introduction to this book, I told you that details would separate you from the pack and let everyone know that you are a professional. The little pearls in this chapter are examples of what I was talking about: They may seem like small things, but your clients will notice and marvel to their friends at being able to find a treasure like you!

Motivating Your Client

Questions we'll answer in this chapter:

- How do I help my client get in touch with his or her personal motivational touchstone?

- How do my client and I work together to achieve powerful goals?

- How can I earn the respected title "coach"?

A wise person once said that almost anyone can spot a wrong answer, but it takes a creative mind to spot a wrong question. Clients hire fitness professionals to solve a problem, but what problem are they really asking us to help them solve? Many fitness professionals assume the obvious answer: that our most important job is to design safe, effective exercise programs for our clients and to teach them how to execute them.

As important as it is to teach someone the correct way to do a bench press, or to decide whether he should even be *doing* a bench press in the first place, let's think this through. Otherwise you'll end up like the young soldier who was preparing to make his first skydive. His commander told him (1) to jump when given the order, then (2) pull the rip cord, and if the chute didn't open, (3) pull the second rip cord, and (4) when he got down, a truck would take him back to the base. He jumped out of the plane on command and pulled the rip cord. When nothing happened, he pulled the second rip cord. Still nothing happened. "Oh great," he said to no one in particular. "I'll bet the truck won't be there either!" To have the life-changing impact on your clients that you are capable of having, you need to ask the right questions in the right order; to take the analysis to the next level; and, most of all, to see the big picture.

One of America's greatest philosophers, Yogi Berra, once explained that "90% of the game is half mental." Well, we all knew what he meant. Unfortunately, some personal trainers have given little thought to the mental side of their work with clients. They show up with their dumbbells and their fat calipers, and jump in doing a fitness assessment so that the workouts can begin. But what about the mental fitness assessment? What about the character assessment? Why be a glorified spotter, counting sets and reps, when you can change someone's life, dramatically, at a gut level—and I'm not just talking about their waist size—for all time?

Maintaining your clients' motivation to exercise is one of the biggest challenges you will have. Let's face it: You can't be with them every single day. (Even if a client could afford this, he probably would tire of it in a very short time.) Motivation must come from within. Each client will have his own reasons for beginning and staying with your program. Many are motivated by the desire to change their looks. Some want to improve their health or avoid lifestyle-related diseases. Others may need to relieve stress. Understanding why your client called you in the first place and what he expects to get from your program will help you design a program that addresses his needs, values, and expectations—in short, a program that he will stick with.

Clarity: Your Client's Personal Motivational Touchstone

If I ask you to picture the color "green," do you see the same thing I see? We use the word to communicate a description of a color, but say it to 10 people, and they might have 10 different pictures in their heads of what it means. Similarly, it might seem that almost every client who calls you is interested in one thing, and one thing only: losing weight. Getting in shape is a close second. What do statements really mean, anyway? When a client tells me that she wants to lose weight, I've been known to reply, "A person could lose a lot of weight in a hurry by cutting off one of her legs, but I'm not sure that she would be much better off, are you?" Of course, this is ridiculous, but I think it makes the point. Your client doesn't really want to lose weight. She wants to change her body composition, to have more lean tissue and less fat. She wants to fit into those form-fitting jeans that have been hanging in her closet mocking her for several months. "Getting in shape" usually means the same thing to her. At least that's what I think she means, but what I think isn't important: What she thinks is. Push your clients to be specific about what they desire and what they expect (not always the same thing) from the program. Only by getting in touch with both of these will your client reach that perfect Zen state that we can call "clarity," that place where all the mental chatter and "shoulds" fall away, and she finds that clear and compelling understanding of her special and personal "why." Now you are ready to get serious.

A key to providing targeted motivation to clients is understanding what they believe about their own abilities, exercise, and fitness level and what they value. Psychologists speak of the concept of outcome expectancy, the belief that something will lead to a desirable, valued outcome. In order to sustain your client's motivation, you will need to keep him focused on something he values and educate him about his ability to get it by continuing the program. Some clients have no doubt that exercise can do all of the wonderful things that you say it can but don't believe that they can do it. ("Me, an athlete? What a laugh! I've been uncoordinated and unathletic my whole life!") These people need more work on bolstering their self-confidence about their ability to do the things you tell them they need to do. Create simple, very small goals that present opportunities for success. Build on these successes to eradicate their former impressions of themselves. Other clients need education about the benefits of exercise and good nutrition. They may not know, for example, that exercise can reduce their risk of adult-onset diabetes or stroke. For these clients, who have no interest in looking "buff," motivation comes from understanding that the payoff is long-term good health and independence. The bottom line: Tailor your motivation strategy to your client's beliefs and values so that she will have a ready answer whenever that little voice in her head, which usually pipes up just in time to hit the snooze alarm, says, "What's the point?"

Goal Setting: Your Client's Vision

You know that your clients look to you for inspiration, knowledge, encouragement, and—most of all—results! You might say that results are like one Supreme Court justice's memorable comment about obscenity: You know them when you see them. This approach might seem tempting at first because it frees you of the responsibility of doing the hard work that is really the essence of professionalism in every field, that is, thinking and planning. Personal training is no exception. Like any professional, you will not be able to escape responsibility if your client doesn't achieve whatever constitutes results to him. Once you and your client have a clear understanding about the reasons he hired you in the first place, you need to work together to create a vision of what "results" will look like. How will you know that you've achieved what you set out to do? How do you define "success" in this joint endeavor? How do you know when you're "there"?

"If you don't know where you're going, you might end up where you are headed."

Dr. Rod Gilbert, sport psychologist

Albert Einstein said, "The world we have made as a result of the level of thinking we have done thus far creates problems we cannot solve at the same level of thinking at which we created them." In

other words, the day of the stereotype of the greased-up guy or the perky, Lycra-clad instructor with million-dollar bodies and 10-cent brains, long on enthusiasm and short on knowledge, is over. To really help our clients be their best, we need to raise the level of thinking beyond simply focusing on sets, reps, and exercises. We need to use insight and creativity to address the real barriers to positive lifestyle change. We need to become more than trainers. We need to be coaches. Coaches understand the power of goal setting. They understand that every achievement is created twice—once when it's actually accomplished, but first in the hearts and minds of its creators.

Setting specific, measurable, realistic goals for your client is an indispensable part of your job. Often clients come to us with a vague, poorly defined idea of what they hope to get from working with a personal trainer.

Why Are Goals So Important?

Most people pay lip service to setting goals in all areas of life, but few have given much thought to why goal setting is important. In my years of working with clients, I have discovered that goal setting is a fundamental part of personal training. Here's a list of some of the benefits you can get from effective goal setting. Goals

• **make overwhelming tasks manageable.** Anyone who has run a marathon knows it's a lot easier to envision running one more mile (or in that last five, one more block) than to think of running the full 26.2. If your client needs to lose 15 pounds (6.8 kg), you want to take her attention off losing the whole 15, especially if she has failed to do so in the past. Rather, get her to think in terms of losing 1 pound (.45 kg) a week for the first 3 weeks. As Robert Schuller often says, "By the yard, it's hard, but inch by inch, it's a cinch."

• **clarify what your program will and won't do.** Many clients who ask us to help them get in shape don't have extensive knowledge about the risks and benefits of exercise or realize that exercise adaptations are very specific. You would not want your client, the Masters swimmer, to be surprised to discover that weight training will not improve his time in the 800 meter. If improving performance in his sport is a high priority for him, you should discover this in your initial goal-setting conferences. With this information, you can not only design a better program, but also clarify your client's expectations.

- **create realistic expectations about progress.** One question we usually get from new clients is "When will I see results?" This is a golden opportunity to explain the best result he can hope for and the fact that results are a function of compliance with the program. For example, speaking to a woman who has come to you to get in shape for a Christmas trip to Hawaii, you might say something like this: "If you consistently stick 100% to the number of workouts per week and the nutrition plan we discussed, you should be able to lose .5% to 1% body fat per month. By your trip to Hawaii next Christmas, that would have you down to the 22% body fat goal we set. If you can't manage to stick to the whole program 100% of the time, your results will reflect that. We'll be checking your progress every month, so we can see if we need to make any adjustments to help you get in bikini shape in time." Trust me: Nothing sours someone on a program like unrealistic, and therefore unmet, expectations.

- **provide a structure to keep your client on track.** People today are so deluged with information about exercise and nutrition that they often feel overwhelmed, ready to throw up their hands and scream, "I give up!" The goals you and your client set will help combat this feeling by giving her specific actions to take every day, week, and month to stay on track.

The Goal-Setting Process

These days goal setting has become almost a cliche, more blah blah blah from helmet-headed "gurus" in late-night infomercials. That's a shame, because nearly every important accomplishment begins as a goal. A wise person once said that a goal is a dream with a deadline. That definition is an especially good one for fitness goals, which should be measurable and specific.

Questions for Clients

Your client needs to think about and answer these questions:

- What do I want to accomplish?
- Why do I want to accomplish this goal?
- Am I willing to pay the price?

I work with my clients to define two types of goals: process goals and outcome goals. Think of these as means and ends. The process goals are the means. They are the map, the path you take to get to your destination. Outcome goals are just that—the ends, the destination.

Step 1: Define the Vision—Find Your Client's Fitness Dream

Notice that previously I said that I work with my clients to define their goals. Goal setting must be a team effort. The client's input is key. He must feel that he has a personal stake in both the process and the outcome. Otherwise, he won't be able to sustain the commitment necessary to stick with his program during the inevitable plateaus and even occasional setbacks.

We begin by getting the client to focus on his fitness dream. What is his idea of ultimate fitness? What was the vision that brought him to you in the first place? The goal inventory helps your client gather his thoughts (see page 222 in appendix A). I have found it useful to send these forms to clients in advance so that they can take the time to sit down in a quiet room and think before responding. After he has filled it out, go over it with him. During this conference, encourage your client to talk. And I mean really talk! Long, rambling, stream-of-consciousness monologues are fine. By listening, you'll learn a lot about your client—not only what he wants to accomplish, but his personality and his attitude about exercise. Does he seem like a driven, compulsive, list-making type A, or a more laid-back sort? What impression do you get of his commitment to making lifestyle changes?

After listening to your client describe his fitness dreams, it's time for you to narrow the focus from the global and general to the narrow and specific by asking the right questions. We want the client to understand the lifestyle changes he will have to make to reach his goals and to do a cost-benefit analysis. There's nothing like being hanged in the morning to focus a man's attention, and there's nothing like hearing that he will have to give up alcohol and desserts for the next 12 weeks to make him reevaluate whether he really wants that six-pack stomach.

Step 2: Gather Information

Where does your client plan to work out? What type of equipment is available to him? How many days a week can he work out? For what length of time at each session? Does he travel frequently? Does he have a high-stress job? A physical job? How disciplined is your client about his diet? If dietary discipline is a problem, does he feel he can overcome it, at least temporarily? Without answering all of these questions, you will not be able to come up with specific, measurable, and realistic goals for your client.

In addition to understanding the time and equipment parameters you're working with, you need to know something about your client's current condition. Progress is a relative term, which is another way of saying that in order to see how far he's come, your client must know where he started. I suggest that you do a thorough fitness assessment on every new client, but you and your client might decide to focus on only one component of fitness, such as body fat, in which case it won't be necessary to perform all your standard tests each time you set new goals.

Step 3: Formulate Specific Goals

Walter Payton, legendary Chicago Bears running back, often described the tremendous motivation that Bears head coach Mike Ditka provided the team by setting a specific goal. Payton recalled that lots of other coaches said, "We're going to play well," or "We're going to win some games," but Ditka was the first to say, "We're going to win the Super Bowl." The specificity of this goal, combined with a specific date and its attractiveness, was powerful. It gave the team a focus, something to hang onto when the going got tough. Armed with your data about time, equipment, and your client's current condition, as well as your gut feeling about the type of program that would work for this particular client, you are ready to write specific, measurable goals and to answer the questions "What am I working so hard for?" and "How am I going to get it?"

Take a look at the sample goal map in figure 8.1. This summary is the result of a discussion with a typical, albeit hypothetical, client, a 42-year-old housewife named Connie Client. She has come to me wanting, like most women, to lose weight. After measuring her body fat, we decide that a realistic goal will be for her to lose 5% body fat in 4 months. This is an ambitious goal, but Connie is extremely disciplined and committed, and she has enough time to work out frequently during the week. The objective of the goal map is to provide a good framework for Connie to reach her goal. First, it is very specific. Second, it tells her what she needs to do daily, weekly, and monthly. Third, it leaves no room for Connie to fool herself. This program is not a cakewalk, but if she wants to reach her body fat goal, she will need to make some sacrifices.

Step 4: Goal Conference With Your Client

I suggest that you send or give the client his copy of the goal map in advance and make plans to discuss it at your next appointment. There are several reasons to go over the map together. First, and most obvious, you want to answer any questions your client might have about the things he needs to do. Second, given the reams of paper we each receive every day, there is an unfortunate tendency to just accept that one more we receive with a smile, only to find it weeks later crammed under the car seat. Not that you have to bring in a brass band, but the introduction of these goals and objectives should be an occasion, a notable occurrence that your client understands you take seriously and hope that he takes seriously as well. Third, you want to create some positive self-talk for your client about these goals. Focus on question 5 on his goal inventory ("When I reach this goal, here's what I will get and how I will feel") and help him create a vivid visualization of the benefits he will receive from doing all the arduous things on the goal map. For example, Connie Client responded to question 5 on the goal inventory by saying that when she accomplished her goals she would feel "healthy, powerful, and in control." These are very empowering images that will help her focus and give her strength on days when she is tempted to blow off her routine.

At this time, also reassure your client that you will be there to provide support and information to help him stick with the process goals, by helping him figure out food labels, for example. I suggest that you ask the client to initial the goal inventory and the goal map to reinforce the importance of the goals and the understanding that you are a team committed to a common purpose.

In their remarkable book *First Things First*, Stephen Covey, Roger Merrill, and Rebecca Merrill (1994) write, "Done well, traditional goal setting is powerful because it accesses the power of two of our unique endowments, creative imagination and independent will" (p. 140). Encourage your client to use his creative imagination to visualize the best he can be, and support and strengthen his independent will by providing information and feedback. When you do, you will discover that goal setting is one of the most effective tools you can use to make your clients' routines productive and your work satisfying.

Goal Map

Assume that on January 1, 1997, Connie Client has 28 percent body fat. She would like to reduce her body fat to 23 percent in time for the annual party at her husband's office on April 30, 1997.

Outcome Goal	How Measured	Target Date
Body fat at 23 percent	Calipers	April 30, 1997

PROCESS GOALS

Daily

Consume no more than 25 g fat
Consume no more than 1500 calories
Consume no alcohol
Consume no simple sugars

Weekly

Minimum of four cardiovascular exercise sessions, at least two at high intensity and two of longer duration
Minimum of three 40-minute resistance training sessions per week

Monthly

Two days a month eat a few extra calories (2000 maximum) as a reward
Two days a month eat a "forbidden food"—a glass of wine, candy, cookie, or similar sweet (300 calories maximum) as a reward

REALITY CHECKS

Daily

Food diary with accurate amounts of every food, beverage, and other item consumed, including gum, supplements, cough drops—anything taken by mouth

Weekly

Weight recorded at the same time and on the same day

Monthly

Body fat measurement (calipers) and anthropometric measurements (tape)

_____ Client's initials

Figure 8.1 Sample goal map.

Focus: How to Keep Your Client Motivated and Moving

You have been given a unique opportunity. You have the power to change every life you touch, permanently and for the better. Let's discuss how you can get there.

Once you and your client have clarified the "what's the point?" and have developed a vision that's so tempting and enticing that she can almost taste it, it might seem that your work is done. Surely he doesn't need more than that to stay motivated! As John McLaughlin might say, "Wrong!" The most important service that you can do for your client is coaching; that is, encouraging him by reminding him of how far he's come, keeping his eyes on the prize by constantly refreshing that precious vision, and sometimes reminding him that whining never got anyone anywhere. Lest you think this is more work than you bargained for, rest assured that there's plenty in it for you as well. Personal trainers who become coaches don't have clients. They have evangelists.

Essential Principles in Any Important Relationship: Are You Coachable?

Back when I was doing one-on-one personal training, my initial meeting with a potential new client often wasn't what he was expecting. He was thinking he'll get to know me and decide if he wanted to hire me. I viewed it as an interview for both of us. You should adopt this attitude, too. Obviously, it's important for the client to satisfy himself that you are the sort of coach who can help him reach his goals. It might be less obvious, and sometimes people are surprised to learn, that not only are they making a decision about you, but you are making a decision about them as well. Specifically, is this person someone you can coach?

To be coachable, in my opinion, a person must accept and commit to certain essential values and principles. I've discovered that those who succeed demonstrate a high degree of understanding and dedication to these principles. Those who fail usually have not even thought about them. Your first job as a coach is to focus your client's attention on these three principles during your initial meeting: commitment, integrity, and trust.

Commitment

A major problem that people have achieving success, in fitness and in life in general, is understanding and making a real commitment. Nietzsche said that man can endure any *how* if there is a *why*, and that tends to be true. As we've discussed, when you are faced with a difficult task, it is absolutely essential that you have a clear, tangible vision of the reason that you're doing all this hard, painful stuff. I often say that for every part of your program you must be able to answer the question "What's the point?"

Now, your clients can probably think of lots of good reasons to avoid eating high-fat, high-sugar foods, and getting up an extra hour early to fit exercise into their days. Knowing that they should do certain things is not a challenge. The challenge is

being able to remember those reasons when the alarm goes off at 5:30 A.M., and more important, to actually do them. Commitment is a 5:30 A.M. kind of thing. You need to explain to potential clients that you don't intend to waste your time, which is very limited and precious, on people who are not prepared to make a genuine commitment, no matter how much they want to pay you. It's not about the money. It's about changing lives.

Integrity

In the abstract, most of us realize that commitment is inextricably connected with integrity. Maybe that's why it is so scary for so many people. When I was doing one-on-one training, I realized that many of the people who came to me didn't like themselves very much, and I knew why. They understood that, no matter what others thought of them, they were not the people they were capable of being. They backslid. They were lazy. They often didn't do what they say they were going to do.

"The first key to greatness is to be in reality what we appear to be."

Socrates

Think about the word "integrity." It has the same root as "integral," and for good reason. Integral means belonging to a whole. Integrity means devotion to principles, but not just some of the time. It's not enough to be honest here and there. You must be committed to do what you say you are going to do, and you must recognize how important it is to do so. Nothing less than your self-esteem depends on it. More important, your client's self-esteem depends on it.

Let me explain. It seems today that we worship self-esteem and we attribute every type of self-destructive or stupid behavior to a lack of it. Yet, when we turn the volume on brains up and lower the emotional noise, I think it is apparent that in many cases, what we really worship is an ersatz self-esteem. It is more in the nature of self-congratulation. If you *feel* good about yourself, if you *love* yourself, than it really doesn't matter if you deserve to. Unfortunately, eventually the charade of liking yourself no matter what you do breaks down, and it's hard to even pretend you like yourself anymore. It's at this point that people sometimes lapse into self-destructive behavior, in an effort to avoid facing their self-contempt. Every time you say that you're going to do something and then fail to do it, especially when you make lame excuses for not doing it, you reinforce in your own mind your self-concept as a backsliding liar. It should be obvious that this type of behavior is death to your self-esteem because, as Dr. Nathaniel Brandon, one of the most thoughtful experts on the subject, has written, "Self-esteem is the reputation that you have with yourself." As I am fond of saying, maybe your self-esteem isn't what it should be because you're a good judge of character. Potential clients must understand that they can expect nothing less than absolute integrity from you and that you expect nothing less from them.

Trust

This one should be a no-brainer. No one will take advice from someone she doesn't trust. That's the reason that all important relationships can exist only in an atmosphere of absolute mutual trust. Trust is the glue that holds these relationships together. The trainer-client relationship is no exception. Your knowledge, integrity, and commitment will inspire trust in your clients.

I'm Your Vehicle: Your Role in Your Client's Life

Over the years I've found that analogies involving cars are very useful in explaining concepts that might otherwise be difficult to grasp. Perhaps that's because most of us have cars and enjoy the freedom they provide. Or maybe it's all those "Knight Rider" reruns we've seen. Whatever the reason, it works. When I ask, "If I gave you a beaker of fluid of unknown origin or composition and suggested that you pour it in your car's gas tank, would you do it?" Without hesitation, the listener reacts with surprise, or even something bordering on outrage: "What do you think I am, stupid? Crazy? Of course not!" From there, it's easy to make the point that many people who react with horror at the thought of unwholesome substances coming near their precious autos enthusiastically ingest equally unhealthy food and drink.

When you think about your role as your client's coach, perhaps a similar vehicular analogy applies. Like the car's guidance system, you provide the map and help him chart his course. Like the steering

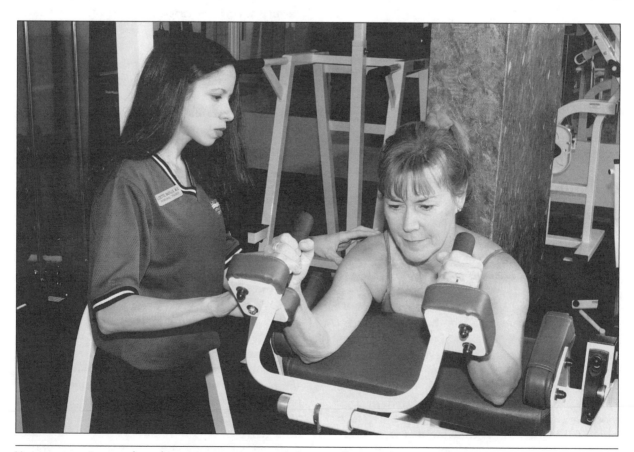

Your encouraging words and inspiring presence can help your client get that extra rep.

wheel, you set him on the right path. When he is overcome with irrational exuberance, you are the brake, helping stay within his safe limits. Like the rearview mirror, you show him what's behind him (how far he's come) and help him stay alert to potential dangers (distractions, temptations, and other program derailers).

Be a Coach, Not Just a Personal Trainer

Great personal trainers recognize that lifestyle change happens in the brain, not the biceps. They are not only personal trainers who are interested in improving cardiovascular fitness and muscular strength, although of course, they do know how to accomplish those important goals. In addition, they are coaches. Coaches recognize that the difference between success and failure is often measured in millimeters, not miles, and that the key to making that little extra effort that changes everything is attitude. These outstanding professionals train the mind, understanding that the body will follow. Contrast those personal trainers whose professional development stops at the level of staying completely focused on the body. They don't deserve the title "coach." Their idea of "motivation" is to drive a client harder and harder, even when a knowledgeable coach would understand that real, long-term progress results from knowing when to push the envelope and when to back off. They don't have the intelligence, expertise, or empathy to know any better.

Here's an acronym to help you remember what your client needs from you:

- **C** is for communication. Great coaches know that communicating is the essence of coaching because we get from people what we expect from them. A coach uses her communication skills to teach and to convey expectations about the great performances to come.

- **O** is for opening doors, which is what you will do when you show your client the terrific achievements that are possible for him, achievements he may never have imagined were within his grasp. With your belief in him and your skillful instruction, you show him the way.

- **A** is for accountability, something that many clients find a powerful prod to keep them compliant. They might be willing to blow off a workout if no one is looking but are loathe to face your withering stare when they have to admit it to you. There's nothing worse than letting your coach down!

- **C** is for challenge, the challenge that you provide by designing workouts that are doable but still tough, and the tremendous high you both share when she completes them.

- **H** is for health, which is ultimately what fitness is all about—not just short-term health and wellness, but lifelong function, independence, and dignity.

Exceed Expectations Every Day: Customer Service

Questions we'll answer in this chapter:

- How can I be a premier service provider?

- What are the elements of effective communication?

- What are the top 10 mistakes personal trainers make?

When I was practicing law, lawyers would joke—at least I think they were joking—"Practicing law would be great if it weren't for the damn clients." And, of course, the joke there is that without clients, there would be no practice of law, and therefore no jobs for lawyers. I can just hear all your sympathetic sighs now. No tears, please! There will never be any shortage of work for lawyers, but as in any service business, there will be some lawyers who excel and others who don't.

These two guys, George and Harry, set out in a hot-air balloon to cross the Atlantic Ocean. After 3 hours in the air, George says, "Harry, we'd better lose some altitude so we can see where we are." Harry lets out some of the hot air in the balloon, and the balloon descends to below the cloud cover. George says, "I still can't tell where we are; let's ask that guy on the ground." So Harry yells down to the man, "Hey, could you tell us where we are?" And the man on the ground yells back, "You're in a balloon, 100 feet up in the air." George turns to Harry and says, "That man must be a lawyer." "How can you tell?" "Because the advice he gave us is 100% accurate, and totally useless." (That's the end of the joke, but for you people who are still worried about George and Harry: They end up in the drink and make the front page of the *New York Times*: "Balloonists Soaked by Lawyer.")

Recently I was interviewed for a magazine, and the writer was fascinated by my career change. In his mind, being a lawyer and being a personal trainer were miles apart, until I explained that really there are more similarities than you'd think. People come to both lawyers and personal trainers for the same reason: to solve a perceived problem. Granted, the types of problems are different, but we're still both problem solvers. In both professions, you sometimes have to tell people things they don't want to hear, and even get them to like it. Like lawyers, personal trainers are in a service business, which is another way of saying we exist to serve our clients, not to give advice that is 100% accurate and totally useless, not to prove we're the smartest people in the room, but *to serve our clients*. The difference between success and failure is understanding and keeping that objective always in mind.

Appreciate the Specialness of Every Client

One of the most enjoyable things about being a personal trainer is the opportunity to meet a variety of interesting, wonderful people. You'll be a much better motivator if you get to know your client as a person rather than just a collection of joints and muscles.

Two Clients, Two Approaches

Compare these two hypothetical clients: Client 1, a middle-aged sedentary woman whose exercise routine since high school gym class has consisted of walking to and from her refrigerator during commercials; and Client 2, a 30-something professional who participated in sports all through college and has continued to be active in a variety of sports since leaving college, is very knowledgeable about physical fitness, and comes to you for help in improving his performance. Now, it's obvious at the first level that their programs are going to be very different. That's a no-brainer, but what might not be as obvious is how to interact with each particular client on a personal level. For example, Client 1, the sedentary woman, in addition to needing some very basic education about her body awareness and physiology and all the technical matters that people come to trainers about, is also going to require some reassurance on an emotional level. "Am I doing this right? Do I look like a klutz? Is everyone staring at me because I look so uncoordinated?" These are the kinds of concerns that you're going to have to anticipate as a part of the uniqueness of this particular type of client.

Client 2 is probably going to want to interact with you on more of a peer level. Your biggest concern is to avoid his thinking you're talking down to him and not giving him his propers as a fellow athlete.

And this even extends to what words you use. If you say "iliac crest" to a client who is a physician, that's going to make perfect sense. If you say it to someone like Client 1, she might think you're talking about the place you went on your ski vacation. The point is you're going to be interacting with individuals and you need to make sure you understand not only what they need in terms of physical fitness, but also what they need at an emotional level and how to speak their language.

It's called empathy. Check into it. Empathy means being able to put yourself in another person's position. In the case of personal trainers, it's a matter of being professional and caring at the same time.

Respond to Each Client's Changing Needs

Recently a longtime client told me what he liked best about my company's service: "You always seem to know exactly when to push me and when to back off." That's another aspect of appreciating the uniqueness of clients. There seems to be a notion afoot in our industry, sort of a macho mentality, that the way to be a good trainer is to (a) scream at the top of your lungs, and (b) push people until they either throw up or have a stroke. Now, as to the first one, I think we all know screaming is not coaching or training. And, as to the second one, not only is that a recipe for possibly seeing your name with the word "Defendant" after it, for most clients it's going to be a *complete* turnoff.

A real professional understands that even clients who like to be pushed should have some workouts in which they don't dial it up to the max; you and I both know that no one makes progress if all his workouts are high intensity. That's another problem with this macho routine. It says that everyone out there needs to be told to get off their lazy butts, but some people actually need a personal trainer to pull back on the reins and tell them to back off in the short term once in a while so that they can make progress in the long term.

Enjoy your clients as people. Get to know them, their interests, their dreams. Your life will be enriched and your relationships with your clients will develop into friendships. Why is your client in your program? What motivates her to continue? In addition, you should have something to say as well. Be a well-rounded person. Be able to talk about something other than exercise if your client so desires, but be sure to remember that tact and diplomacy are always important.

Rx for Trouble

As our mothers told us, it's not nice to play doctor, so don't. And don't play dietitian. Don't play anything that you aren't. If you're doing this right, clients will trust and respect you as a health professional. They are probably going to ask you questions about their aches, pains, and injuries. Of course, you want to know about those things anyway, and certainly there is no problem giving them general advice such as treating injuries with RICE (rest, ice, compression, and elevation), but you should never attempt to diagnose a client's injury unless you're a medical doctor, nor should you be advising them about medications. You should not be telling clients to take a particular pain reliever, for example, nor should you give them vitamins, supplements, or any other products to ingest.

The key point here is not to exceed your area of expertise, but that doesn't mean you have to be like a potted plant and do nothing. Remember, clients

Speaking of Supplements . . .

What about being a supplement salesperson? I personally have a very strong bias against personal trainers selling supplements, although I know it's widely done, and I know that many trainers sell supplements because they frankly believe in the products. That's a personal decision and one that I won't argue with, but for my own personal practice, I think it's a conflict of interest, one that's awfully hard to avoid when you have a financial incentive to sell particular products.

come to us to solve a problem. In the case of clients, they come to us for help in improving their health and fitness, and that's one of the things that customer service is all about—problem solving. In the case of injuries, the way you can help solve that problem professionally is to refer clients to competent physicians. Some trainers think if a client asks them about an injury, declining to diagnose it and suggesting that the client see a doctor makes them look bad or incompetent, but it's just the opposite. Clients will respect you and consider you all the more professional if you refer them to a competent physician.

As a professional personal trainer, you should be networking with other professionals in the field. You should make it a project to develop a book of competent doctors, dietitians, physical therapists, and other allied health professionals who you think can benefit your clients. In this way, when a client asks you a question, rather than exceeding your area of expertise, you can help solve the client's problem.

A side benefit of this type of professionalism is that physicians will begin to refer clients to you. Studies have shown that there is no more reliable referral than one that comes from a physician. If a doctor tells a patient that he needs to exercise and then gives him your business card, that is a guaranteed new client in 99% of cases.

Never Stop Learning

One of my pet peeves about certain retail stores, and maybe it's one of yours too, is that sometimes I feel I know more about the products than the people working there. Product knowledge is definitely a key to effective sales and effective customer service.

117

It's even more important where the product is personal expertise, and that's the situation we're in. We're selling our knowledge, expertise, and ability to solve clients' perceived problems and meet their needs, specifically, the need to get healthier and fitter. I sometimes joke that in my personal training practice, I work with all the smart kids, and that's both an advantage and a disadvantage. The advantage is, of course, that they learn the things I'm teaching them quickly and master them with little difficulty, but the downside is that they're always asking me hard questions. Your clients are going to ask you hard questions, too. That's why you earn the big bucks: because you can answer them. You can't be in the position where clients think they know more than you do!

Have you ever had the experience of learning a new word and then all of a sudden, you see that word everywhere? Well, once your clients start exercising and working with you, all of a sudden they are going to start paying attention to all of that health and fitness information on the news, in the newspaper, and in magazines that they may have not even heard before. They're going to be scouring those articles, highlighter in hand, and bringing them to you and asking you about HMB, creatine, elliptical trainers, or whatever the latest fitness fad or supplement is, or whether something they saw on an infomercial really works.

It's up to you to be able to provide them with some kind of a competent answer. You may think that when you're not working with clients you're not working, but that's not true. You're *never* not working. You have to be constantly aware of information or misinformation that is in the popular culture because a client might ask you about it at any time, and you have to either be able to give an answer or know where to find it.

Unfortunately, you won't be able to provide that kind of service unless you really stay on top of your game. Subscribe to publications in our industry— several of them, in fact— and read them when you're on the treadmill, on the stationary bike, on the train, even at traffic lights. Whatever you're doing, read, read, read. New research comes out every day. To be the best coach and fitness professional you can be, you must be on the cutting edge of knowledge in your field. All great coaches and teachers are lifelong learners.

Henry Ford said that anyone who stops learning is old, whether at 20 or 80, and anyone who keeps learning stays young. If you look around, you'll see that that is really true. And if you subscribe to this theory, when your clients look at you, they will see that you are the sort of professional they want to work with as well as recommend to all their friends.

The Business You're Really In: Communications

I suspect that most personal trainers don't think of themselves as being in the communications business, but like teachers, attorneys, and radio personalities, they are. What good is it to know precisely what a person needs to do to become the best he can be if you can't tell him in a way that he will understand? How can you really understand a client's vision of success, what he dreams of in his heart of hearts, if your listening skills are at a remedial level? How can you sell your prospects on all the wonderful benefits your programs offer if you can't find the words? I think I've made my point, so let's take a look at some important aspects of communication.

Never Stop Listening

Learning and active listening go hand in hand, so let's think about listening.

Why Listen?

Not only do people actually enjoy finishing their sentences, if you let them do so, you might learn something that will help you provide better service to your clients. And isn't that what you're here for? Being responsive is critical to providing excellent customer service, and you can't be responsive if you never listen! Once on my radio program I had a conversation on the air with a regular listener. I was lamenting the fact that he's such a big fan of the show but doesn't have access to e-mail or the Web page because he doesn't have a computer. He promised to get one, so I asked if he knew the e-mail address. Now, I repeat this address constantly on the show, but he explained, "I've heard you say it a million times, but since I couldn't use it anyway, I guess I didn't pay attention."

When your client talks, it's *always* something you can use, so you've always got to pay attention. Studies have shown that most people speak at about 125 to 150 words a minute, but people can listen at up to 450 words a minute. So, it's no wonder sometimes our minds wander. But when your client is speaking, *you can't let that happen.* Just as "nothing says lovin' like something from the oven," nothing says "indifference" like not listening.

Not only is the appearance of indifference the kiss of death when it comes to bonding with your

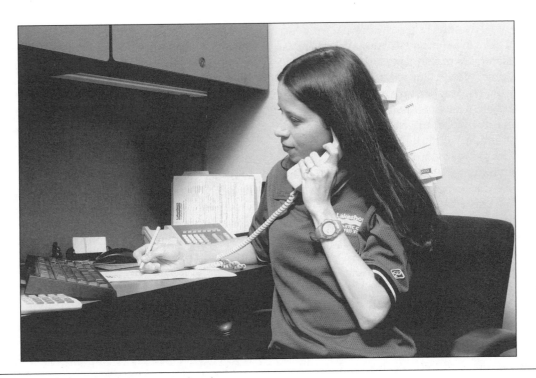

Great coaches are great listeners, even on the phone.

client, it's even simpler than that. You can't learn anything while you're talking. And if you don't learn what concerns your client, you don't have a prayer of effectively coaching him.

The Three Components of Listening

There are three components of effective listening. If you learn them and employ them regularly, your communications with everyone, not only your clients, will become a thousand times more effective. I mentioned earlier that personal trainers need to be effective, *active* listeners. These components will transform your listening from a passive, uninvolved activity to an active, interactive experience.

• **Mirroring.** Think of all the trouble that could be avoided if people didn't assume—didn't assume that they knew what other people were feeling, didn't assume they knew what other people were thinking, didn't assume that they knew what someone said when they didn't. Have you ever had a conversation with somebody who was afraid to tell you that he didn't really hear what you said and so he just responded to what he thought you said? You end up in one of those "Who's on first?" conversations that is not only a complete waste of time, but also makes that person, the one who assumed he knew what you said when he really didn't, look like a moron. And the last thing you want to look like in

front of your client is a moron. The first technique, mirroring, will help you avoid that unfortunate possibility. Mirroring is simply restating what you think the speaker said to make sure that you are both on the same page.

For example, if a client is telling you something and you don't really understand it, how would it sound if you said, "Oh, I know what you're trying to say." Now, you don't mean to offend anyone, but think about it. You're telling your client that she's a bad communicator and that even though she's too dense to say what she really means, you can figure it out. And that *is* offensive. So this is a good opportunity to use your mirroring technique. Ask, "Did you mean . . .?" and give her an opportunity to clarify at that point. You'll never go wrong by asking for more information and giving your client the opportunity to talk. If you're at all confused about what a client is saying, the worst mistake you can make is to assume you know what she means. You know the old saying: "When you assume, you make an *ass* out of *u* and *me*." It's really true.

• **Validating.** The second rule of effective listening is validating. Sometimes people get into trouble with this one because they assume (there's that troublesome word again!) that validating means agreeing, but that's not true. You can validate what someone says without agreeing. You are merely recognizing that they have a right to their own feelings, even if those feelings are different from the ones you'd have in a similar situation. Validating is making a statement of that fact.

For example, maybe you're like me. I'm not the biggest fan of cats. Maybe you even hate cats, especially your client's cat. But if your client says to you, "Gosh, I feel really bad, my cat just got run over," even if you might be thinking to yourself, *Yippee*, you should be able to honestly say, "I can understand how you must feel. You must feel terrible." Putting yourself in your client's place, the cat that you despised was a beloved friend, a member of the family. It was to him just like your pet is to you. If you think of it that way, you should have no problem validating your client's feelings.

- **Empathizing.** Remember empathy? Being professional and caring at the same time? Often, clients are going to tell you about things you really can't relate to very well—situations at work, even their personal problems—and you need to be able to put yourself in their place and reassure them. You do this by genuinely and effectively listening. When your client is describing some politically motivated demotion at work or some other problem that really has nothing to do with you, you have to remember that it *does* have to do with you because it has to do with your client, and *everything* that has to do with your client has to do with you.

Which is why you have to get in the habit of writing things down. Believe it or not, when your personal training practice gets hugely successful, you are not going to be able to remember everything about every client, or, even more important, everything that every client tells you. Clients will tell you something of tremendous significance to them that's happening in their lives, and then you might not see them again for an entire week. A lot of things can happen in a week, both to you and to them, so it's absolutely critical to keep in your client workout records a section for general notes—not only injuries, aches, pains, and other physical problems, but also those other things they tell you. For example, when your client tells you she's been extremely nervous about layoffs in her department, you might note "Situation at work" in her record. Then, before your next session with her, you'll open the book, see that note, and be reminded.

Think Before You Speak

Granted, we've just established that listening is more important than speaking. But that doesn't mean you shouldn't be concerned about how you speak! I like to think that once you have listened to your clients, understand what they are saying, and are ready to

communicate with them, you will think before you speak and choose the words you use. Words mean things, don't they? But sometimes, sadly, people are not very precise in the words they use. When it comes to your interaction with clients, using the wrong words can set you miles back in your relationship.

There's a true story of a conscientious young personal trainer meeting with her new client, an overweight middle-aged man. Approaching him with her calipers, she asked him to pull his shorts down. "What are you going to do?" he asked. "Oh, we're just going to do four skinfold measurements," she said matter-of-factly. Hearing "foreskin," he was out of there! He didn't stick around for the explanation, and I don't think he came back. So you've got to choose your words carefully.

Here are some other phrases you ought to banish from your lexicon if you want to provide excellent customer service to your clients:

- **"Hang on."** When you're on the phone with your client, don't say "Hang on." That's rude. Instead, say, "Do you have a second to hold on while I check?" It's a simple thing, but remember, details make all the difference. If you put yourself in the client's place, you'll understand completely.

- **"I can't do that."** This phrase conveys the impression that you are not willing to accommodate your client. How about, "Let me see how we can work this out"? If a client is looking for a schedule change that you don't think you can make, instead of saying, "Well, that's impossible," suggest an alternative: "I'm not going to be available at that time, but how about this time? Might that work for you?" Always try to make your communication with clients positive.

- **"No."** Try to avoid saying "no" as the first word of a sentence. Subconsciously, beginning your answer to a client with "no" suggests unresponsiveness and unwillingness to accommodate, and that's the opposite of what you want to convey. You want your clients to always think that you are bending over backward to make their life easier and solve their problems. So, rather than beginning a sentence with "no," begin by saying, "I might not be able to do that, but how about this?" Once again, offer a positive alternative and change your client's expectation. It's all part of effective communication.

The Telephone

I want to say something briefly now about telephone interaction. There are three things you must keep in mind any time you talk with a customer on the phone:

- **Stay focused.** If it's easy to become distracted in face-to-face communication when, ideally, you have eye contact and are very much a part of the conversation, it's a hundred times easier to become distracted in telephone interaction. We've all been on the phone with telemarketing people selling products we're not interested in, and while we're waiting for an opening to break in and say, "Excuse me, I'm not interested," our minds wander. We're thinking about the grocery list, the TV show we were watching when the phone rang, and 18 other things. But when you're talking to clients on the phone, you have to be even more attentive than you are during a face-to-face conversation, because any distraction will come through.

- **Know about the person you're talking to.** Before you initiate any client calls, it's very important that you pull out your record and take a look at what happened during your last interaction. There's nothing worse than calling a client to find out how she's doing and forgetting to ask her about the dental surgery she told you she was having the day after she saw you last. A client told me recently that one thing she really likes about my company's service is that when she talks to me, she feels as though she is our only client. The reason she feels that way is because we keep careful records and don't interact with her unless we are focused on what's going on in her life. As mentioned previously, an aspect of effective listening and communication is writing down what your clients tell you and reviewing it before you talk to them. Sounds simple, sounds obvious. You'd be amazed, though, at how few people actually do it, which is why you're going to be one of the outstanding performers when you do.

- **Always return your clients' calls promptly.** Actively and consciously demonstrate your concern for your clients by moving them to the top of your priority list during your day. In this age of instant communication, people expect to be able to reach others, particularly those who work for them, immediately, or close to it.

Establish a Businesslike Communication System

Have you ever seen that movie *The King of Comedy?* Robert De Niro plays an emotionally disturbed man, Rupert Pupkin, who stalks a late-night talk show host played by Jerry Lewis. Rupert fantasizes about being a famous talk show host like Jerry, and his fantasies aren't limited to daydreams. He constructs his own version of the talk show set in his basement, complete with life-size cardboard cut-outs of celebrities. One of his favorite activities is sitting in the host's chair and pretending to interview these cardboard "guests." Often when he is in the middle of acting out the role of host, you hear his mother, off camera, yelling to him, "Rupert, you're going to miss the bus," causing him to scream back at the top of his lungs, "Ma! I'm busy down here!" This yelling—"Ma!"—is incredibly grating and adds to the comic aspect of the film. In real life, though, it won't be funny if potential clients call and ask for you, and then have to listen to someone screaming "Ma!" as you come to the phone.

Remember that clients come to us to solve problems because we are professionals. Here are some phone foibles guaranteed to make you appear very unprofessional:

- **Kids answering the phone who are barely able to carry on anything resembling an intelligent conversation.** I think that because people find their own children so cute, they don't always realize how annoying it can be for other people to deal with them on the phone. If you're calling a business, the irritation factor goes up geometrically.

- **Roommates or family members who can't find a pencil and don't know when you're coming home.** (This works both ways. Once I called a client who lives with her parents. I had to endure about 15 minutes of "Oh, hold on, I can't find a pencil," getting more irritated by the second.)

- **Fax machines that don't work.** When a friend of mine recently went away on a trip, I tried about 700 times to send him a fax. The machine wouldn't answer. I was climbing the walls! When he returned, he explained that his cleaning lady had accidentally turned it off.

- **Anything that keeps your client from conveying information to you in a timely fashion.** The meaning of that word "timely" has changed in the last years or so. Recently I was in a retail store and I noticed that every time someone bought something with a credit card, the woman behind the cash register said, "That will be right up." The customer impatiently expected the charge slip to emerge from the machine the moment the clerk hit the "enter" key. When I got up to the register to pay for my purchases, also with a credit card, she said the same thing. "Don't you get sick of saying that?" I asked, and she replied, "Yes, but people are so impatient these days." And of course, we are. Technology has completely changed people's expectations about how long things should take. You need to be responsive to your clients, and these days "responsive" means being reachable virtually 24 hours a day, 7 days a week.

To make sure that none of the scenarios just described materializes, set up a professional telephone system devoted exclusively to your business. Given the affordability and availability of voice mail, there's no excuse not to have your phone answered in a professional way. Pagers are also cheap and available. These days people expect to be able to reach everyone at any time, or at least to leave a message. We're all too busy to get into a runaround. We want to make our call and check it off our list.

Will you ever get tired of having your pager on and getting client calls at any time of day or night? Maybe, but remember your goal is to run a profitable personal training business, and that means being responsive to clients. That's all that matters to them.

Do What You Say You're Going to Do

Television windbags, purporting to impart great insights to us little people, are incessantly waxing on the reasons that voters are "angry," or why the public is so cynical about everything. Assuming for the sake of argument that these observations are true (which I'm not saying, but go with me on this), most of us could tell them in one sentence why there's a lot of anger and cynicism out there: People get extremely annoyed when other people don't do what they say they are going to do.

Don't you? Is this surprising? The take-home message: Be reliable.

Exceed Expectations Every Day

"Underpromise and overdeliver" is a motto that will never let you down.

Commit Yourself to the Continuing Pursuit of Excellence

In their terrific customer service book *Customers for Life*, Carl Sewell and Paul Brown say that customer service is really about one question: How good do you want to be? That's the burning question you need to ask yourself every day. How good do you

want to be in every aspect of your business: in your demeanor, in your dress, in the eye contact you make with your clients, in the confidence you convey and the empathy you convey? Personal trainers need to remember the difference between doing things right and doing the right thing. Both are important.

Doing things right relates to your technical knowledge, your ability to figure out what a client might need based on a fitness assessment, a body fat test, a medical report from a doctor. But *doing the right thing* relates to doing what that client needs in his particular situation. If you commit yourself to the continuing pursuit of excellence, you'll not only do things right, because you will never stop learning (attending continuing-education seminars, reading everything you can get your hands on, watching and observing), but you'll also do the right thing because you'll appreciate the uniqueness of every client and you'll never stop listening. All these things together will happen if every day you remember the question "How good do you want to be?"

It's amazing how much more energy and persistence you can bring to a project that you have actually committed to accomplishing. Something about making that critical choice seems to provide the strength you need when the going gets tough. I hope this book will help you begin your business with the firm determination to be your best, and that the power of that commitment will propel your level of service into the stratosphere of excellence. Be your best!

Never Forget Who This Is About

The final rule of customer service, and maybe we could say the umbrella rule of personal training, is this: Never forget who this is about. It's about them, it's not about you. And when you keep that idea topmost in your mind, you can see that at least three guidelines are crucial:

1. **Maintain your enthusiasm.** Sure, you have a physical job, and sometimes you're tired. But one of our obligations is to maintain a really high degree of enthusiasm for the workout, and for life in general. Your clients are entitled to an energized motivator, not someone with the demeanor of a wrung-out dishrag. Enthusiasm is contagious; be a carrier.

Top 10 Mistakes Beginning Personal Trainers Make

1. **Overestimating the time available, especially with beginners.** Sure, you want to do a lot of exercises, but when instructing a beginner, that won't be possible. You may be lucky to get through two sets of three exercises in an hour, particularly if you are teaching complex exercises like the squat and lat pull-down. If you plan to do too many exercises, you will be tempted to shortchange your client in the instruction department and risk letting him learn to do it wrong, not right.

2. **Underestimating how intimidating exercise and gym environments are to many people.** Gym rats and other denizens of the workout room forget: a gym is a loud, scary place for many people who are accustomed to being around computers and photocopiers rather than Smith machines and squat racks. One of your most important jobs is to be the tour guide and facilitate your client's becoming comfortable in this foreign world.

3. **Including exercises that clients are not ready to do.** We know you're anxious to get started with the real heavy stuff, or at least with some sort of resistance training because you know how effective it is in helping sculpt lean, metabolism-boosting muscle. Unfortunately, many new clients who have been sedentary for many years need to spend some time correcting postural imbalances and strengthening underlying musculature. Be sure not to put the cart before the horse.

4. **Dressing like refugees from a bodybuilding magazine.** If you want to be treated like a professional, and paid like one, you need to dress like one. It's your business if you want to run around in spandex, sporting a do-rag or a moussed pompadour with ponytail, but don't blame me if *no one* takes you seriously.

5. **Focusing too much on the body while neglecting the mind.** When it comes to lifestyle changes, everything important happens in the brain, not the biceps.

6. **Talking too much, especially about themselves.** The old saying "empty barrels make the most noise" is applicable here. Why is it that the dumbest people in the world are determined to try to convince everyone that they are the smartest people in the room?

7. **Failing to be well-rounded people.** Clients, at least the high-income, high-achieving kind who can pay top dollar, enjoy the distraction of being able to talk about something other than a triceps pushdown. Make sure that you can.

8. **Allowing clients to continue faulty, potentially dangerous movement patterns.** If your client walks around like the typical computer buzzard, that's going to compromise what you're trying to accomplish in your sessions. Give clients suggestions about ways to achieve optimal and functional posture all day long, not just when they are with you.

9. **Recommending or selling supplements.** Taking supplements is a personal choice. Your clients may choose to do so, but they should not make this choice at your suggestion. If you sell supplements to clients, you run the risk of compromising your objectivity about whether clients should continue to use them, which is a clear conflict of interest. You also run the risk of being sued if the supplement doesn't agree with the client.

10. **Underpricing their services.** Remember, what is fungible is undervalued. Make yourself special, then charge what you're worth. And yes, you *are* worth it!

From Teri S. O'Brien, 2003, *The Personal Trainer's Handbook, Second Edition.* Champaign, IL: Human Kinetics.

2. **Keep your personal woes to yourself.** Maybe your personal life is not going very well, but you should save those stories for your clergyman or therapist. Your client doesn't want to hear this stuff, and you shouldn't be sharing it. I was in a store recently and the young man who waited on me started telling me about all the problems in his personal life. His dad kicked him out of the house because someone had gotten pregnant—I don't even remember who, because the whole time I was thinking, *This affects me how?* Don't get me wrong; I felt bad, I felt empathetic, but I'm a customer, and the experience is supposed to be about me and my needs and the problem that I came in to have him solve for me. And this was just an encounter in a retail store. When I was practicing law, we had a secretary in our office who was quite a character, and she not only enjoyed dressing in a flamboyant, even provocative way, but she also liked to tell us way too much about her personal life. It got to the point where I was afraid to ask, "How was your weekend?" for fear that she would tell me in excruciating detail. Do you think your clients are going to view the experience of being with you as a positive one if they are afraid to ask, "How are you?"

3. **Care about your client's concerns.** Clients are always thinking, *This affects me how?* It's a cliché, yet one that in my experience is often ignored: People don't care how much you know until they know how much you care. Clients aren't interested that you got an A+ in anatomy and can identify the origin and insertion of every muscle in the body. Those facts are beneficial to them if they help you design more effective programs, but ultimately, your clients are more interested in how you can help them solve their problems. If all your technical knowledge will do that for them, great. But if not, well, really they couldn't care less. Remember, we all have that little radio station playing in our heads, WIIFM—What's In It For Me. And that's all the more true where the person listening is paying for the benefit of having you around.

So, never forget that it's about them, it's not about you, and you'll never go wrong. As long as you keep this little phrase in mind, so many things will turn around: your attitude; your behavior; and most important, your success.

Finally, as a reminder of some of the biggest mistakes that beginning personal trainers make, with apologies to David Letterman, I've come up with my own top 10 list (page 123). It's no joke! I suggest that you consult it frequently. You might even want to post a copy in a prominent spot in your workspace so that you can refer to it frequently. It's not bad as a reminder of some of the most important lessons you've learned from this book!

Conclusion

People usually think of customer service as a counter they go to when something gets screwed up, but you need to think about it as the way you differentiate yourself in the marketplace. There are a gazillion trainers out there. The good news is that as an industry, we're doing a good job of eliminating the size-3-hat, size-17-shirt "trainers." In years to come, we will see a lot of competent knowledgeable personal trainers. That means competition, but that doesn't have to be bad news, at least not for you, if you're committed to unsurpassed customer service.

Resistance Workout Guide

(continued)

CRUNCH

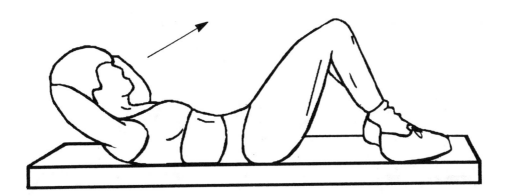

Primary muscle worked
Rectus abdominis

Secondary muscles worked
External obliques, internal obliques, transversus abdominis

Objective
To lift the shoulders off the ground

How to do it
Lie on your back on the floor or on a mat with your knees bent and heels close to your body. Your heels should be together; your pelvis should be tilted up and your low back pressed down to the floor or mat. Place your hands behind your head on your neck. Keeping your elbows behind your head and your chin to the ceiling, tighten your abdominals and lift your shoulders off the ground by contracting your abdominals. Continue lifting and lowering until you have completed the desired number of repetitions.

Remind your client
- Keep your pelvis tilted up and your low back pressed firmly against the floor or mat. There should be no space between your low back and the floor. Do not arch your back.
- Keep your chin to the ceiling. Do not flex or extend your neck as you complete your repetitions. Your head should rest in a relaxed position in your hands. Your cervical vertebra should stay in a neutral, not flexed, position. If your chin is scrunched up, *stop* and readjust it so that your neck is not flexed.
- Keep your elbows behind the plane of your head. That is, do not point your elbows toward your knees.
- Emphasize the need to do this movement slowly while keeping tension on the abdominal wall.

Trainer's pointer
If the client finds the exercise difficult to perform with hands behind her head, suggest doing it with arms crossed across the chest. If while doing the exercise in this fashion her neck becomes tired, she should use one hand to support the neck while completing the desired number of repetitions.

TWISTING CRUNCH

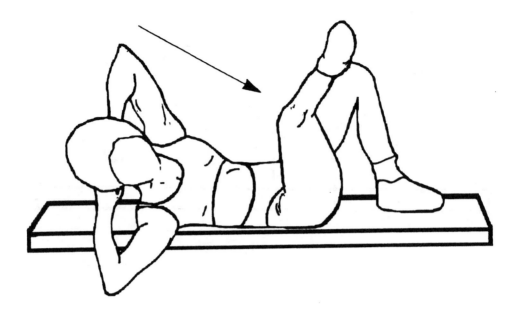

Primary muscles worked

Rectus abdonimis, internal obliques, and external obliques

Secondary muscle worked

Transversus abdominis

Objective

To lift the shoulder toward the opposite knee

How to do it

Lie on your back on the floor or on a mat with your knees bent. Place your right ankle on or in the vicinity of your left knee in a cross-legged fashion. Tilt your pelvis up and press your low back into the floor. Place both hands behind your head and, keeping your pelvis flat and square on the ground, lift your left shoulder toward your right knee. Repeat for the desired number of repetitions, then switch legs and shoulders.

Remind your client

- Do the exercise in a controlled fashion.
- Keep your pelvis flat and square on the floor. The twisting should come at the waist.
- Do not twist or pull on your neck during the exercise. Your chin should stay in line with the center of your body at all times.
- Do not arch your back.
- Keep your neck relaxed. If it is flexed so that you have a double chin, *stop* and readjust.

Trainer's pointer

Your client must keep her pelvis flat and in contact with the floor. The rotation should occur at her waist.

OBLIQUE CRUNCH

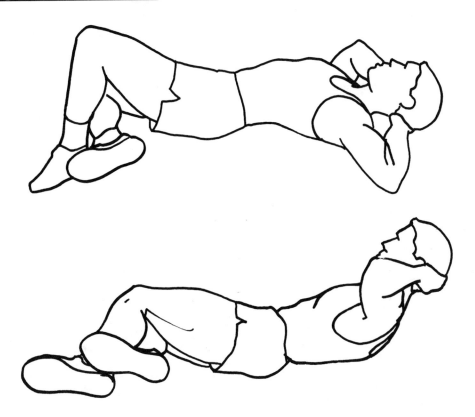

Primary muscles worked

Rectus abdominis, internal obliques, and external obliques

Secondary muscle worked

Transversus adbominis

Objective

To lift the shoulder off the ground

How to do it

Lie on your back. Place your hands behind your head. Bring your knees together and drop them to one side. Lift your shoulders toward your hips as if you were doing a crunch. After completing the desired number of repetitions, repeat with knees on the other side.

Remind your client

- Activate your transversus abdominis, the deepest abdominal muscle, by trying to pull your iliac crests (the two hipbones just below and to each side of your navel) together so they meet under your navel.
- Do not pull on your neck.

Trainer's pointers

- Do not allow your client to pull on his neck. Tell him to imagine that he has a cantaloupe between his chin and chest, and to keep his chin toward the ceiling. Also, suggest that he keep his elbows behind his head, which will also reduce the risk of neck pulling. If he has difficulty keeping his neck relaxed, try having him place each hand on the top of the opposite shoulder blade and rest his head in his crossed arms.
- Check activation of the transversus abdominis before and during the exercise.
- This is an advanced exercise that requires back and hip flexibility.

LYING LEG RAISE

Primary muscles worked
Rectus abdominis, psoas

Secondary muscles worked
Rectus femoris, transversus abdominis

Objective
To flex the spine and lift the pelvis toward the rib cage

How to do it
Lie on your back on the floor or on a mat with your knees bent and your feet flat on the floor. Tilt your pelvis up and place your hands under your glutes like a wedge to tilt your pelvis and support your lower back. Lift your feet off the ground and raise your bent legs until your thighs are perpendicular to the floor (90 degrees of hip flexion). Straighten your legs. Keeping your legs straight (your knees can be soft, i.e., not actively locked out and rigid, but not actively bent), try to touch the ceiling with your pointed toes. Concentrate on flexing your pelvis and lifting your gluteus using your lower abdominals.

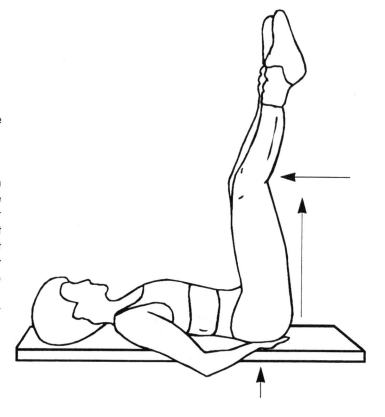

Remind your client
- Do not arch your back.
- Keep your pelvis tilted up.
- Keep your shoulders relaxed.
- Keep your wrists flat on the floor or mat.
- Do not flex or extend knees.

Trainer's pointers
- Suggest that your client think of this exercise as a pelvic tilt, the only difference being that the legs are off the ground.
- Tell your client to keep her transversus abdominis tight, and reinforce this during the exercise.

REVERSE CRUNCH

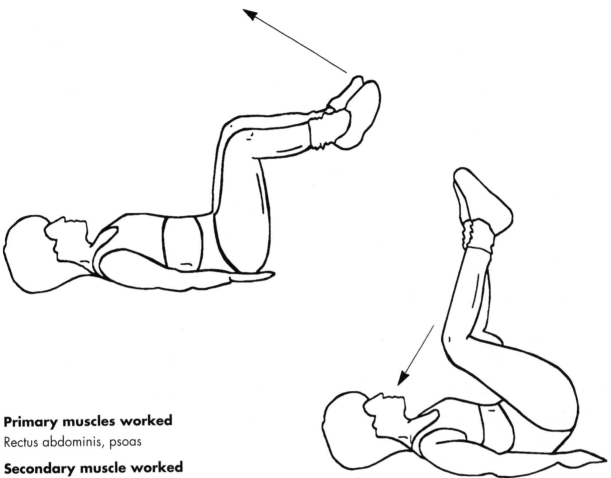

Primary muscles worked

Rectus abdominis, psoas

Secondary muscle worked

Transversus abdominis

Objective

To move the pelvis toward the rib cage

How to do it

Lie on your back with your feet on the floor and your knees flexed 90 degrees. Place your hands under your glutes so that they can act as a wedge to tilt the pelvis up. Keeping the knees at 90 degrees of flexion, lift your hips off the floor.

Remind your client

- Feel each vertebra lifting off the floor.
- Don't move the thighs back and forth; the objective is to lift the pelvis, not the legs.
- Keep the shoulders and neck relaxed.
- Keep the transversus abdominis tight.
- Lower the pelvis very slowly.

Trainer's pointers

- A useful cue: Tell your client that this movement is exactly like a pelvic tilt, except the feet are off the ground.
- Watch for the tendency to move the thighs rather than the pelvis. Emphasize the need to keep the knees flexed at 90 degrees throughout the range of motion.

SINGLE HIP FLEXION

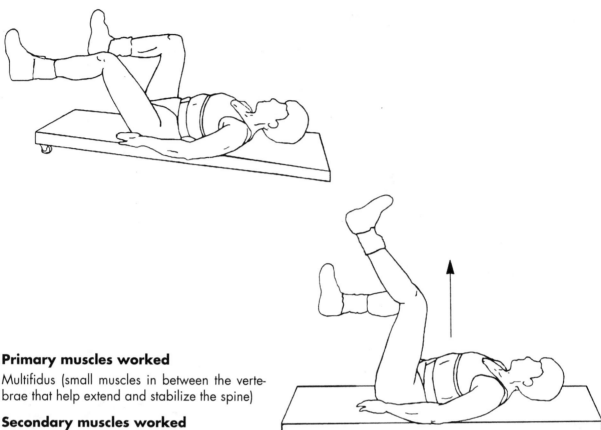

Primary muscles worked

Multifidus (small muscles in between the vertebrae that help extend and stabilize the spine)

Secondary muscles worked

Transversus abdominis, psoas

Objective

To lift and lower the leg by flexing the hip

How to do it

Lie on your back. Lift your feet off the floor and flex your knees to 90 degrees. Keep the natural curve in your low back. Don't press the low back down or tilt the pelvis. Tighten the transversus abdominis. Straighten the left leg to approximately 45 degrees of flexion. Keeping the left knee frozen, move the left leg toward the floor until the heel almost but doesn't quite touch the floor or mat. Return to the start position. Repeat for the required number of repetitions. Readjust the transversus abdominis muscle by tightening it, then perform the same number of repetitions on the other side.

Remind your client

- Keep your transversus abdominis tight.
- Keep the knee frozen. The axis of rotation is the hip.

Trainer's pointers

- This exercise works on the muscles in the low back that stabilize the pelvis.
- Before your client begins the exercise, check the activation of the transversus abdominis by placing your finger on his lower abdominals. It is critical that he maintain this activation throughout the exercise.
- Be sure your client maintains the natural curve in his back. He should not press his low back down.
- Beginners should do this exercise with the knee of the working leg flexed 90 degrees. The straighter the leg, the more difficult the exercise.

BICYCLE CRUNCH

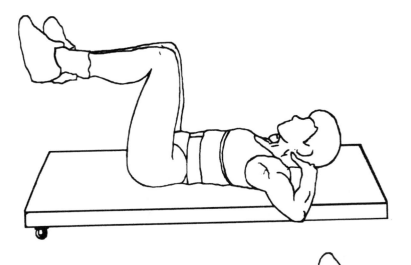

Primary muscles worked
Rectus abdominis, external obliques, internal obliques

Secondary muscle worked
Transversus abdominis

Objective
To lift and rotate the shoulder and the opposite thigh by flexing the spine

How to do it
Lie on your back with the knees bent. Place the hands behind the head. Lift the feet off the floor. Tilt the pelvis up and press the low back down. Begin with the knees at 90 degrees of flexion and the elbows behind the ears. Lift and twist the right shoulder while bringing the left knee in to meet it. Repeat for the required number of repetitions. Switch sides.

Remind your client
- Don't rotate or flex the neck.
- Keep the elbows back behind the head.
- Focus on rotating the spine. Visualize the flat, trim waist you're working for.
- Keep the transversus abdominis activated.

Trainer's pointer
Neck rotation is a real problem on this one. Suggest that your client try to keep his chin in line with his sternum.

STRAIGHT LEG U-CRUNCH

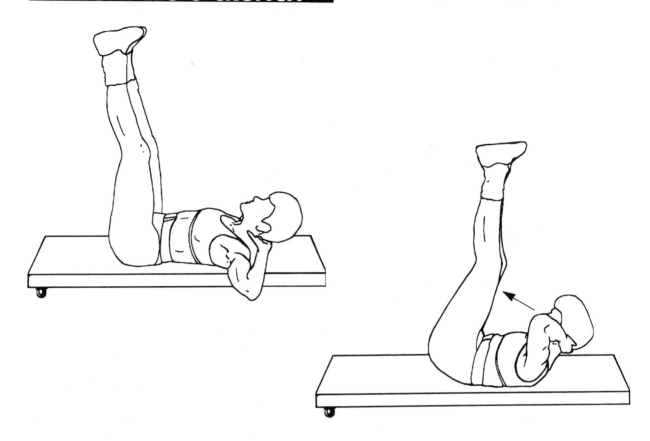

Primary muscles worked

Rectus abdominis, external obliques, internal obliques, psoas

Secondary muscle worked

Transversus abdominis

Objective

To lift and rotate the pelvis toward the rib cage while lifting the shoulders off the ground

How to do it

Lie on your back. Place your hands behind your head. Lift the feet off the floor and straighten the legs so that the heels are facing the ceiling. Tighten the transversus abdominis. Keeping the knees rigid, lift the pelvis toward the ceiling.

Remind your client

- Relax the neck and shoulders.
- Do the exercise slowly and under control. Don't bounce your low back off the floor (ouch!).
- Keep the elbows back behind the ears.

Trainer's pointers

- Encourage your client to think of lifting the pelvis and rotating it toward the rib cage, not just lifting the legs up and down. Suggest that she focus on feeling each vertebra returning to the floor as the pelvis lowers on each repetition.
- Watch for flexion and extension at the knees. They should stay frozen.

BENT KNEE U-CRUNCH

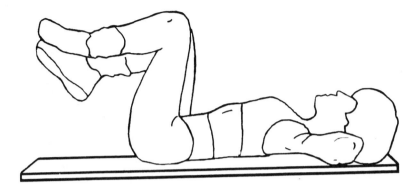

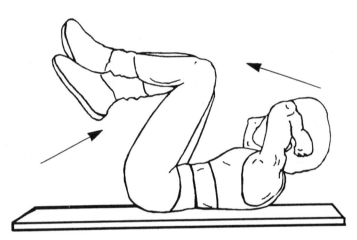

Primary muscles worked

Rectus abdominis, external obliques, internal obliques

Secondary muscles worked

Transversus abdominis, psoas

Objective

To lift the pelvis and rib cage toward each other

How to do it

Lie on your back. Flex your knees to 90 degrees and lift your feet off the ground. Place your hands behind your head. Simultaneously lift your shoulders and pelvis toward each other. Return to start position.

Remind your client

- Keep your neck relaxed.
- Do not bounce your pelvis off the ground. This should be a controlled lift.
- Keep the transversus abdominis activated.

Trainer's pointers

- Do not allow your client to pull on her neck. Tell her to imagine she has a cantaloupe between her chin and chest, and to keep her chin toward the ceiling. Also suggest that she keep her elbows back behind her head, which will reduce the risk of neck pulling.
- Make sure your client squeezes and tightens her abdominals at the top of the movement.

HANGING LEG RAISE

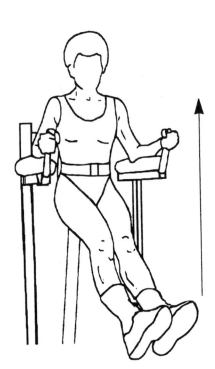
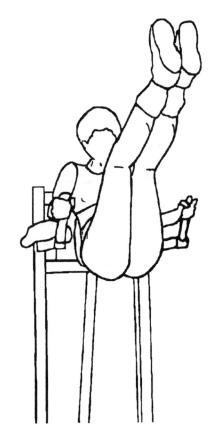

Primary muscles worked

Rectus abdominis, psoas

Secondary muscles worked

Rectus femoris, external obliques, transversus abdominis

Objective

To lift and rotate the pelvis toward the rib cage

How to do it

This exercise has three variations:

1. Hang from a chin-up bar by holding on with your hands.
2. Hang from a chin-up bar while supported under your upper arms using specially designed straps.
3. Rest your elbows and forearms on the pads of a specially designed elevated chair found in many gyms and clubs.

Begin with the legs straight, or with the knees only slightly bent. Keep your knees rigid and lift your legs until your thighs are at a 90-degree angle to your torso. Continue curling your lower body by lifting your pelvis up toward your rib cage. Actively contract your abdominal muscles. Return to the start position and repeat for the required number of repetitions.

Remind your client

- Don't do the exercise ballistically by swinging your legs up and down. Instead, focus on lifting the pelvis.
- Squeeze the abdominals. Feel the active contraction.

Trainer's pointers

- This is an advanced exercise. Your client should not attempt it until she finds lying leg raises and U-crunches no longer challenging. In addition, clients who have excessive body fat shouldn't attempt this exercise because the excess weight will put too much stress on the elbows and wrists.
- If your client cannot perform this exercise with good form, but you think she is ready for something beyond lying leg raises, try the bent knee version.
- Sometimes you see people using ankle weights while doing this exercise. This is not recommended due to the risk of excess stress on the ankles.

HANGING KNEE RAISE

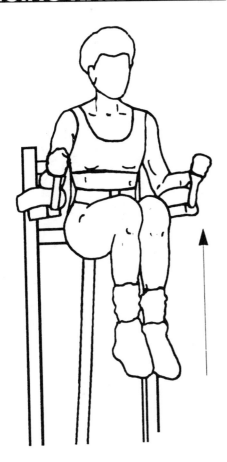 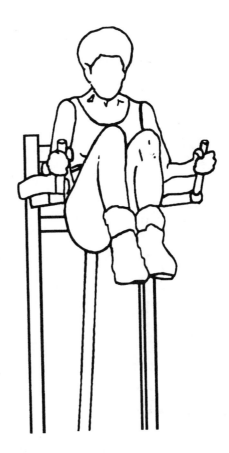

Primary muscles worked
Rectus abdominis, psoas

Secondary muscles worked
Rectus femoris, external obliques, transversus abdominis

Objective
To lift and rotate the pelvis

How to do it
The three position variations for the hanging leg raise can be applied here, too (see p. 136). Begin with the knees bent at 90 degrees of flexion. Keep your knees rigid and lift your legs and pelvis up toward your rib cage. Actively contract your abdominal muscles. Return to start position and repeat for the required number of repetitions.

Remind your client
- Keep the knees rigid. Focus on moving the pelvis.
- Actively contract the abdominals on each repetition.
- Don't swing the legs up and down. Move slowly and under control.

Trainer's pointer
It should be possible to lift the pelvis much higher in this exercise than in the hanging leg raise. Take advantage of this to help your client achieve a more powerful contraction.

LAT PULL-DOWN

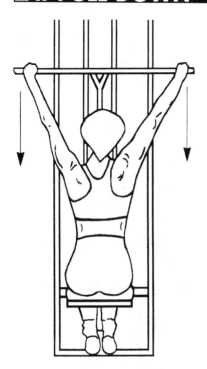 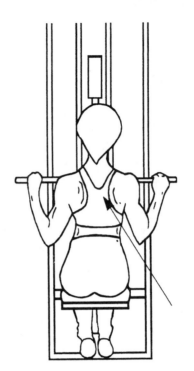 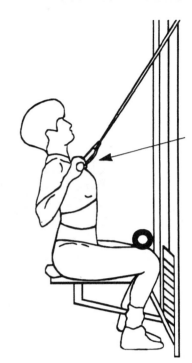

Primary muscles worked

Latissimus dorsi, teres major, posterior deltoid

Secondary muscles worked

Trapezius (lower division), rhomboids, biceps brachii

Objective

To pull the resistance down by squeezing the shoulder blades back and down

How to do it

Grasp the bar at a universal or other pull-down machine. Sit down. Let your latissimus dorsi (lats) stretch out. Pull the bar down to your sternum while simultaneously arching your back and sticking out your chest. Lean back at about a 70-degree angle. Pull the stack down in the following sequence: pull shoulder blades toward spine, flex elbows, depress shoulder blades (that is, pull the shoulder blades down and back).

Remind your client

- Do not hunch forward as you pull down. The shoulder should retract before the elbow flexes. Think of it like this: "Shoulder comes in, elbow comes in, chest goes out."
- Do not "turtle," that is, shrug your shoulder blades up toward your ears; your trapezius should be relaxed.

Trainer's pointers

Please note that this exercise and all the multijoint back exercises that follow (pull-downs and rowing) are very challenging for beginners, who tend to fail to move the shoulder blade before flexing the elbow (if they move it at all).

- Make sure your client pulls her scapula back ("retract") and then down ("depress"). Use the tactile cue described in "Pull-Down Behind the Head" (p. 140).
- Make sure your client's torso does not move back and forth in a rocking motion. Keep the abdominals tight and maintain the four-finger space between the pelvis and rib cage.
- If your client hunches forward as she pulls down, reduce the weight.

CLOSE-GRIP PULL-DOWN

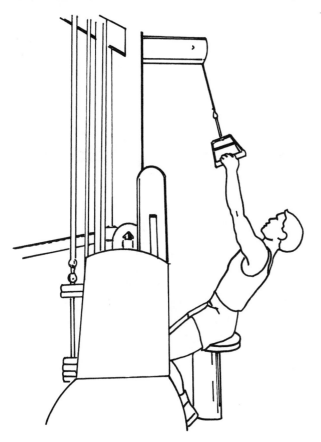 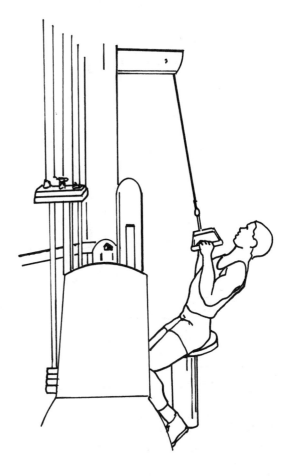

Primary muscles worked

Latissimus dorsi, teres major, posterior deltoid

Secondary muscles worked

Trapezius (lower division), rhomboids, biceps brachii

Objective

To pull the handle to your rib cage

How to do it

Grasp the close-grip handle attached to the cable of a lat pull-down machine. Sit down on the seat. Lean back and allow your lats to stretch out. Pull the stack down in the following sequence: pull shoulder blades toward spine, flex elbows, depress shoulder blades (that is, pull the shoulder blades down and back). Try to get your elbows back as far as possible.

Remind your client

- Don't turtle.
- Don't hunch forward.
- Don't rock the body.
- Keep the arms close to the body.

Trainer's pointers

- During the exercise, place your hands on top of the client's shoulders. If you feel clicking and popping, suggest that he depress his scapula and relax his neck.
- Watch for wrist flexion and extension. Your client's wrists should stay straight.

PULL-DOWN BEHIND THE HEAD

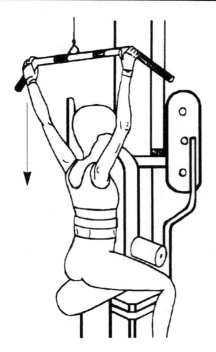 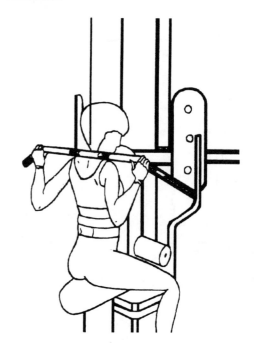

Primary muscles worked

Latissimus dorsi, teres major, posterior deltoid

Secondary muscles worked

Trapezius (lower division), rhomboids, biceps brachii
behind the head

Objective

To pull the resistance down by squeezing the shoulder blades together

How to do it

Grasp the bar at a universal or pull-down machine. Sit down. Let your lats stretch out. Pull the bar down behind your head until it touches the base of your neck by pulling the shoulder blades back, flexing the elbows, then depressing the shoulder blades.

Remind your client

- Make sure you pull your shoulder blades in and down *before* your elbows flex. Don't hunch forward as you pull down. Do not shrug your shoulders up toward your ears. Try to keep your upper trapezius relaxed while activating the lower trapezius. Think of it as "retract scapula, flex elbows, depress scapula."
- Do not bend forward at the waist.

Trainer's pointers

- Try to keep your client's upper trapezius relaxed while she activates the lower trapezius. I find it useful to put my fingers just below the inferior angle of the scapula and have the client activate the lower trapezius to get a feel for it so she'll know what to focus on when she pulls her scapula down.
- Caution: Because of the extreme external shoulder rotation in this exercise, it is inappropriate for people with rotator cuff problems. Some authorities believe it should be eliminated from all programs because of the risk of injury. Clients who have rounded shoulders should never do this exercise. When in doubt, substitute the lat pull-down.
- Place your hand at the back of the client's head to prevent her from whacking herself on every rep.

SEATED ROW

Primary muscles worked

Latissimus dorsi, posterior deltoid

Secondary muscles worked

Rhomboids, trapezius (lower division), biceps brachii

Objective

To pull the resistance by squeezing the shoulder blades in toward the spine

How to do it

Sit facing the low pulley of a machine with either a short straight bar handle or a close-grip handle. Grasp the handle and position your body so that your knees are slightly bent (about 150 degrees). You should be leaning forward in a beginning rowing position. Row the handle by straightening your body; pulling your shoulder blades in; and, finally, flexing your elbow, in that order. Squeeze your shoulder blades and stick your chest out in a military position and return to the start position.

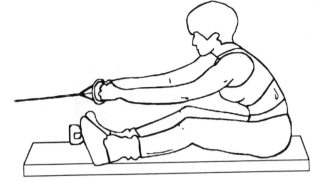

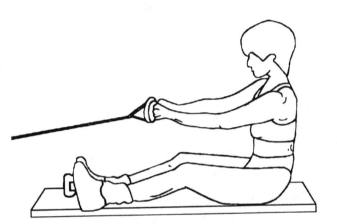

Remind your client

- Keep your back flat and your head up during the exercise.
- Do not flex your elbows until your shoulder blades have retracted into your spine.
- Remember to do the exercise under control, especially during the negative (return) portion of the exercise.
- Do not allow the stack to jerk your elbows into an extended position.
- Don't turtle—keep your upper trapezius relaxed.
- Don't flex or extend your knees. They should remain motionless.
- To achieve the right "military posture" in the last movement of the exercise, imagine a cadet standing at attention.
- Create and maintain the four-finger space between your pelvis and rib cage. Keep your back flat.

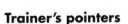

Trainer's pointers

- Make sure your client is not only retracting, but also depressing, her scapula during this exercise.
- Watch for flexion or extension at the wrists and knees or spinal rotation.
- Watch the position of your client's elbows. They should stay close to the body. If they flare out, your client is probably "turtling."

This exercise may not be appropriate for those with pre-existing low-back injuries or undiagnosed low-back pain. Consider substituting a rowing exercise on a machine that has a chest pad to prevent spinal flexion.

INCLINE DUMBBELL ROW

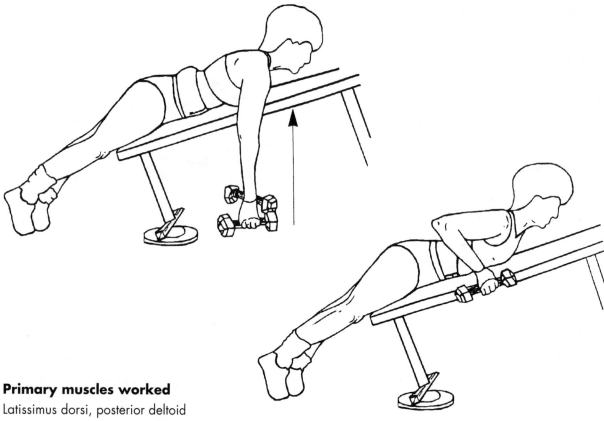

Primary muscles worked

Latissimus dorsi, posterior deltoid

Secondary muscles worked

Rhomboids, trapezius (lower division), biceps brachii

Objective

To lift the resistance by pulling the shoulder blades back and down

How to do it

Lie on your stomach on an incline bench or other elevated bench. Grasp a dumbbell in each hand. Reach out toward the ground. (You should feel a stretch in your lats.) The dumbbells should be at about a 45-degree angle to the bench. Pull your shoulder blades in toward your spine, then flex your elbows. Squeeze your shoulder blades together and arch your back.

Remind your client

- Make sure that you pull your shoulder blades in before you flex your elbows.
- Do not flex or extend your knees.
- Keep your neck straight and your back flat.

Trainer's pointers

- Watch your client's spine and make sure it doesn't twist.
- Make sure your client doesn't round her back.
- Make sure the weight isn't so heavy that your client cannot hold it straight. If you notice that she holds the dumbbell so it is hanging off her hand with one end lower than the other, this means that her wrist flexors and extensors can't handle this much resistance. Reduce the weight to avoid elbow tendinitis.
- I suggest that you place the bench against a wall for safety.

DUMBBELL ROW

Primary muscles worked

Latissimus dorsi, posterior deltoid

Secondary muscles worked

Rhomboids, trapezius (lower division), biceps brachii

Objective

To lift the resistance by pulling the shoulder blade in toward the spine

How to do it

Grasp a dumbbell in one hand. Stand next to a flat bench, lean forward, and place the opposite hand on the bench. Place the knee on the side of the resting hand on the bench to support your back. At this point, your torso should be parallel with the ground. Lift the dumbbell up by first pulling your shoulder blade and flexing your elbow. Your elbow should be very close to your side at hip level at the top of your movement. Squeeze your shoulder blades together.

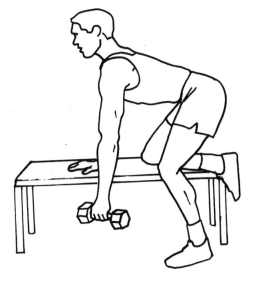

Remind your client

- Concentrate on pulling your shoulder blades in toward your spine and down toward your low back.
- Don't turtle.
- Don't swing the dumbbell.
- Keep your wrists straight. Do not allow them to flex or extend.
- Keep the knee of the supporting leg slightly bent, but rigid. Do not flex or extend the supporting leg to provide additional momentum in the exercise.
- Your weight should be resting on the supporting leg, not on the supporting wrist.
- Keep your back flat, not rounded. Keep abdominals tight to stabilize the spine.
- Do not twist your torso.
- Create and maintain the four-finger space between your pelvis and rib cage.
- Keep the neck straight to keep the cervical vertebra (vertebra in the neck) in a neutral position.

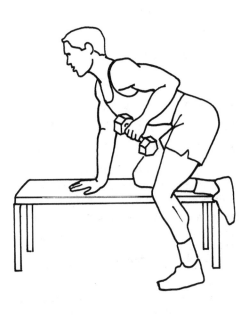

Trainer's pointers

- Keep your eye on your client's scapula. Make sure he's pulling it down and back, not up toward the ears. Make sure the scapula of the supporting side is in line with his spinal column.
- Make sure your client doesn't flex or extend his supporting knee.
- If your client can't keep the dumbbell straight in his hand, that is, if one end hangs down toward the ground, it's too heavy for his forearms. Reduce the weight.
- If your client has a hard time keeping his back flat, try doing this on an incline bench (supporting hand on incline portion, supporting leg on seat).
- Watch for spinal rotation, especially during the last few reps.
- Make sure the working arm stays close to the body. Excessive upper-arm abduction can put undesirable stress on the shoulder.
- Make sure the client's weight is on his supporting leg, not supporting wrist.

DUMBBELL PULLOVER

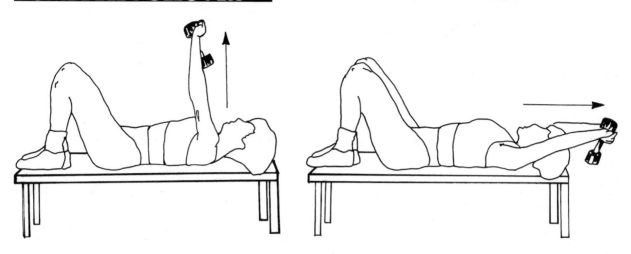

Primary muscle worked

Serratus anterior

Secondary muscles worked

Trapezius (middle division), biceps brachii, triceps brachii

Objective

To move the upper arms parallel with the head

How to do it

Lie on your back on a flat bench with your knees bent and your feet flat up on the bench. Hold one dumbbell with both hands around the plate portion at one end. Begin with your arms extended, elbows slightly bent and facing out (shoulders externally rotated), and the dumbbell at the level of your sternum. Move the dumbbell by lowering your upper arms toward your head. When the dumbbell is at the same level as the bench and slightly behind your head, return it to the start position.

Remind your client

- The axis of rotation is your shoulder joint. Keep your elbows slightly bent, but do not flex or extend them during the exercise. They should be rigid.
- Do not take the dumbbell farther back behind your head than the point at which you can bring it forward under full control. You should never lower the dumbbell past the point at which your arms are parallel with your ears.
- Your head, back, gluteus, and feet should always remain in contact with the bench.
- Do not arch your back.
- Do not flex or extend your wrists.

Trainer's pointers

- Spot your client by placing your hand near the bottom part of the dumbbell.
- Ask your client if there is any clicking or popping in her shoulders. Place your hands there and feel for unwanted snap, crackle, or pop.
- Watch for the tendency to rotate internally at the shoulder. The elbows should point out throughout the movement. If they don't, this means that there is probably a lot of tightness in the neck (computer buzzard syndrome) and round-shouldered posture that require attention.

CHIN-UP

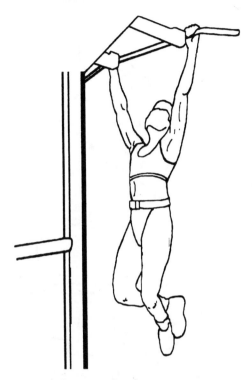 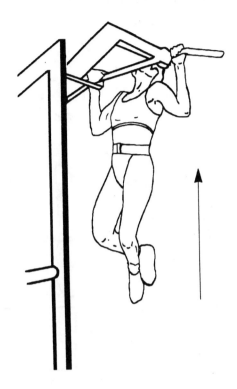

Primary muscles worked

Latissimus dorsi, posterior deltoid

Secondary muscles worked

Rhomboids, trapezius (lower division)

Objective

To lift the body with the arms and back

How to do it

Place a sturdy chair or bench in front of a chin-up bar. Step up on it and grasp the bar. Your grip should be slightly wider than shoulder width. Lift your feet off the bench. Keeping your head back, lift your body toward the bar. Try to touch your chest to the bar. Arch your back and feel for a peak contraction in the lats.

Remind your client

- Don't hunch forward. Keep the head up.
- Focus on the motion of the scapula, which should be back and down.
- Arch your back into exaggerated military posture at the peak of the movement. Feel your shoulder blades squeeze together.

Trainer's pointers

- Obviously, this is an advanced exercise and as such, it should not be done by unconditioned individuals, especially those who are overweight. Since most people fitting this description can't do a single pull-up anyway, this is an academic point, but still worth noting. Establish a good base of conditioning before it is attempted. Failure to follow this advice is sure to result in elbow and shoulder problems.
- Form is extremely important on chin-ups to keep the targeted muscles working.
- Some commentators suggest that it is safer to use a palms-facing grip (with the palms facing each other) to avoid the risk of injury from excessive external shoulder rotation.

PREACHER CURL

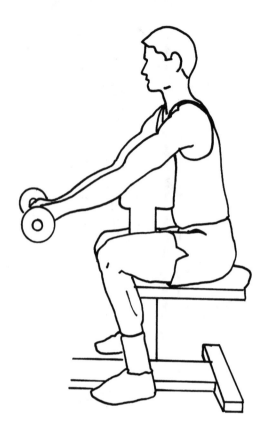 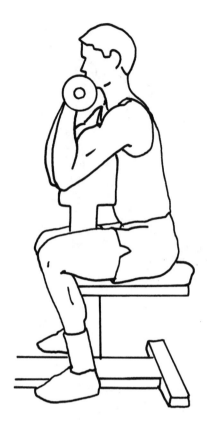

Primary muscles worked

Biceps brachii, brachialis, brachioradialis

Secondary muscle worked

Supinator

Objective

To flex the elbows

How to do it

Sit on a preacher bench. It should be adjusted so that the armpits rest on the top part of the bench and the feet are flat on the floor with the knees at 90 degrees of flexion. Lean forward and grab the bar, which may be angled or straight. Position yourself with hands shoulder-width apart and your armpits resting against the bench. The top of the bench should hit you at about collarbone level. Curl the bar up to your chin and lower the weight to repeat. Keep your wrists straight during the exercise.

Remind your client

Keep your shoulders and chest against the bench during the exercise. Move only at the elbow joints.

Trainer's pointer

Make sure your client goes through a full range of motion by straightening (but not hyperextending) his elbows on each repetition.

BARBELL CURL

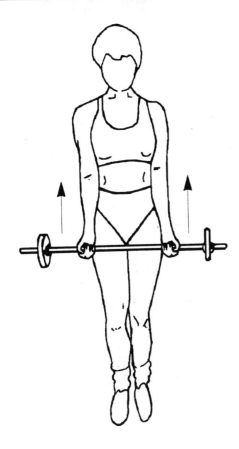
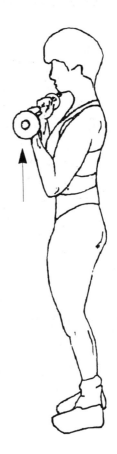

Primary muscles worked

Biceps brachii, brachialis, brachioradialis

Secondary muscle worked

Supinator

Objective

To flex the elbows

How to do it

Grasp a straight or angled bar with a shoulder-width (or slightly wider), palms-up grip. Position yourself so that your feet are firmly planted and your knees are slightly bent. Keeping your upper arms against the sides of your body, curl the bar up by flexing at the elbow joint.

Remind your client

- Keep your body still. Do not rock your back.
- Your wrists should remain straight during the exercise. There is no need to flex your wrists at the top of the movement.
- Remember to lower the bar to a count of four while raising it to a count of two.

Trainer's pointers

- If your client has trouble keeping her back from rocking, make sure she keeps her knees soft. If that fails, have her do this exercise standing against a wall, and reduce the weight.
- Suggest that your client lock her elbows against her rib cage.

SEATED DUMBBELL CURL

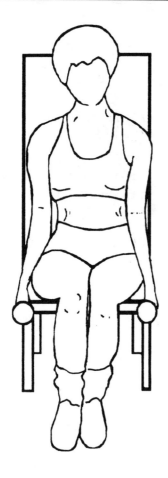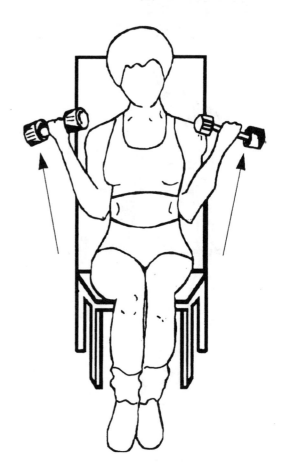

Primary muscles worked

Biceps brachii, brachialis, brachioradialis

Secondary muscle worked

Supinator

Objective

To flex the elbow and turn the hand

How to do it

Sit on a bench with a back support. Grasp a dumbbell in each hand, palms facing your sides. Curl the weight up by flexing at the elbow. Simultaneously rotate your forearm. At the peak of the movement, your palm should be facing up with the little finger higher than the thumb.

Remind your client

- Make sure your upper arm stays next to and slightly in front of the center of your upper body. Do not let the elbow move away from the body, because this takes the tension off the biceps and stresses the elbow.
- This exercise can be done one arm at a time or both arms at the same time.

Trainer's pointer

As your client fatigues, watch for the tendency for the upper arms to move forward. If necessary to keep the upper arms still and against the body, stand behind the client and hold them in place.

CONCENTRATION CURL

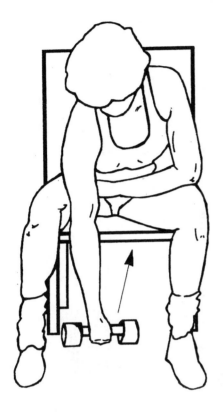 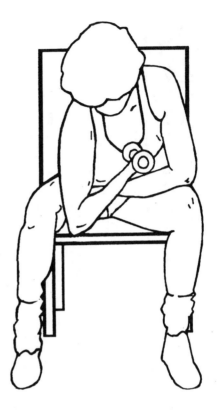

Primary muscles worked

Biceps brachii, brachialis, brachioradialis

Secondary muscle worked

Supinator

Objective

To flex the elbow and turn the hand so that the little finger is higher than the thumb

How to do it

Sit on a bench and grasp a dumbbell in one hand. Your knees should be apart, feet flat on the floor. Lean forward and place the forearm and elbow of the working arm (the one grasping the dumbbell) against the thigh on the same side of the body with the palm facing you. Curl the weight up by flexing at the elbow joint. As you flex your elbow, turn your forearm so that at the top of the movement your palm is up. Squeeze the biceps at the top of the movement and lower the weight to the starting position.

Remind your client

Keep your upper arm firmly planted against your thigh. Do not rock your body during the exercise.

Trainer's pointers

- Watch your client's shoulder on the side of the working arm. It should be relaxed.
- Make sure your client keeps her wrist straight while performing the exercise.

STANDING CALF RAISE

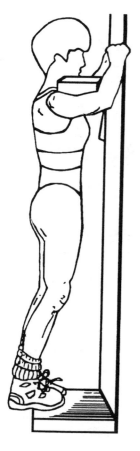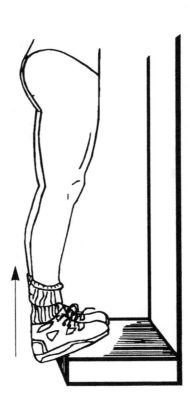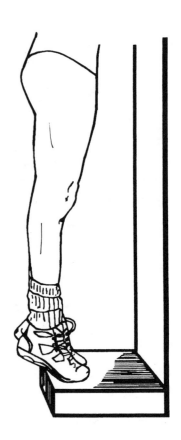

Primary muscle worked

Gastrocnemius

Secondary muscles worked

Soleus, plantaris, peroneus longus, tibialis posterior

Objective

To flex and point the toes

How to do it

Stand at the calf raise station of the universal machine or hold a dumbbell in your hand for resistance. If you are using a machine, crouch down under the pad and raise it by standing up straight. If you are doing the exercise with a dumbbell, stand on a bottom stair or a stable bench (maximum height of 6 inches [15.2 cm]) with your heels off the edge. Keeping your knees locked (but not hyperextended), rise up and lower down on your toes.

Remind your client

- Keep your knees locked but not hyperextended.
- Drop your heels in a slow, controlled manner as low as possible on the way down, and come up as high as possible at the top. Hold the peak contraction for a second when you are up on your toes.

Trainer's pointers

- Make sure your client goes through a full range of motion. There is a tendency to stop descending before the heels have dropped to their maximum depth.
- Try varying foot positions (parallel, toes in, toes out) to work all angles of the gastrocnemius.

SEATED CALF RAISE

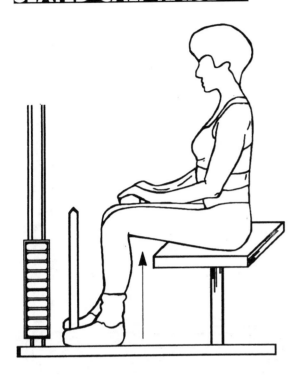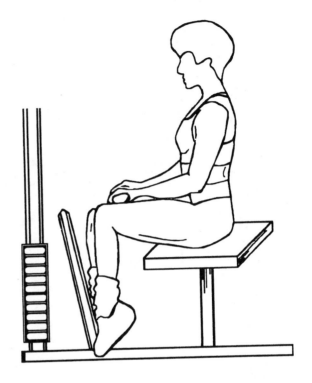

Primary muscle worked

Soleus

Secondary muscles worked

Plantaris, tibialis posterior, peroneus longus

Objective

To flex and point the toes

How to do it

Sit at a seated calf raise machine. Place your knees under the pad after adjusting it so that your knee is at a 90-degree angle while you are seated. With your feet firmly on the platform, release the stack and allow your heel to drop to its lowest range of motion. Press the stack up by flexing at the ankle joint.

Remind your client

Do the exercise slowly and under control. Your upper body should be relaxed. No bouncing, twisting, or similar histrionics (yes, it's supposed to really burn).

Trainer's pointers

- Your client should keep her upper body relaxed.
- Watch range of motion as in the standing calf raise.

BENCH PRESS

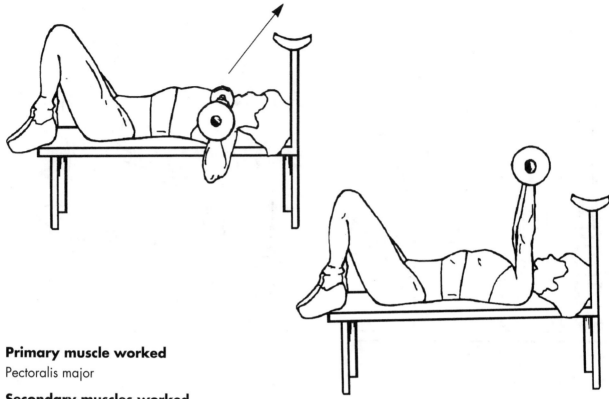

Primary muscle worked

Pectoralis major

Secondary muscles worked

Anterior deltoid, pectoralis minor, subclavius, subscapularis, triceps brachii

Objective

To straighten the arms and bring them toward the center of the body by squeezing the pectorals together

How to do it

Lie on your back on a flat bench with your feet up on the bench. Grasp the bar with your hands slightly wider than shoulder width, palms facing forward, elbows bent. Your elbows, shoulders, and wrists should stay in the same plane during the exercise. Press the bar straight up by straightening, but not hyperextending, your arms. Breathe out as you raise the bar. The bar should travel in a slightly diagonal line, that is, the angle formed by your upper arms and your upper body should be approximately 78 degrees, not 90 degrees.

Remind your client

- Control your wrists. They should stay straight and rigid and should not flex or extend.
- Do not bounce the bar off your chest.
- Your head, back, and glutes should stay in contact with the bench at all times. Do not arch your back!
- Keep elbows in line with shoulders.
- It is *strongly* recommended that you have a spotter when you do the bench press.

Trainer's pointers

- Remind your client to inhale while lowering the bar and exhale while raising it. Don't allow your client to hold her breath, as this causes serious increases in blood pressure.
- The bar should not touch your client's chest when she lowers it. Stop her just short of chest level.
- If the bench is too short for your client to comfortably put her feet up on it, place another bench at the end for this purpose.

INCLINE DUMBBELL PRESS

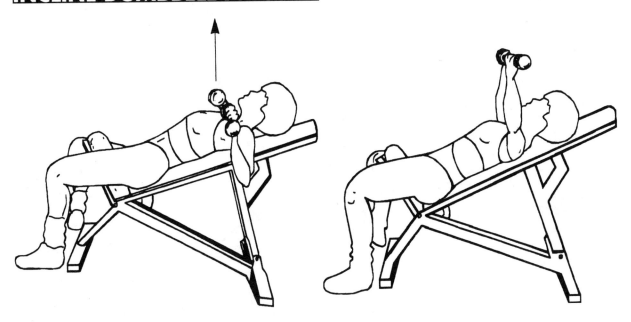

Primary muscles worked

Pectoralis major, anterior deltoid

Secondary muscles worked

Pectoralis minor, subclavius, subscapularis, triceps brachii

Objective

To straighten the arms and bring them toward the center of the body

How to do it

Lie on your back on an incline bench. Grasp one dumbbell in each hand, with palms facing forward, elbows bent, and dumbbells just to the sides of your shoulders. Your elbows and shoulders should be in a straight line. Press the dumbbells straight up by straightening, but not hyperextending, your arms at the elbow. The dumbbells should travel in a diagonal line so that when your arms are straight the ends of the dumbbells are together. Focus on squeezing your pectorals at the top of the movement.

Remind your client

- Make sure your back is flat on the bench. Your knees should be bent and your feet should be flat on the floor to keep you from arching your back.
- Do not allow your wrists to flex or extend.
- Remember that the advantage of using dumbbells is that you are able to lower them deeper than you would be able to lower a bar and feel a better stretch in your pectorals before you begin to press the dumbbells up.
- Control the position of your forearms. Do not allow your shoulders to rotate out of the proper plane. Your wrists should stay in the same plane with your elbows and shoulders.

Trainer's pointers

- If your client seems to have trouble keeping her back down on the bench, have her put her feet on a flat bench placed at the end of the incline bench.
- If you notice that your client can't keep her elbows and wrists in the same plane with her shoulders, reduce the weight.

153

FLAT DUMBBELL PRESS

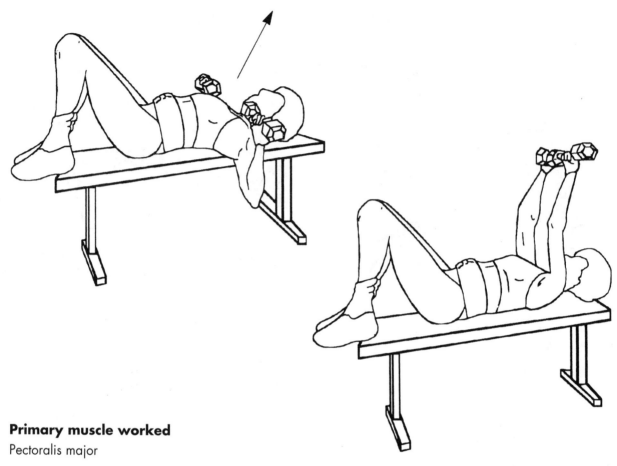

Primary muscle worked

Pectoralis major

Secondary muscles worked

Anterior deltoid, pectoralis minor, subclavius, subscapularis, triceps brachii

Objective

To straighten the arms and bring them toward the center of the body by squeezing the pectorals together

How to do it

Lie on your back on a flat bench with your feet up on the bench. Grasp one dumbbell in each hand, with palms facing forward, elbows bent, and dumbbells just to the side of your shoulders. Your elbows, shoulders, and wrists should be in the same plane. Your knuckles should face the ceiling. Press the dumbbells up by straightening, but not hyperextending, your arms. At the top of the movement, the dumbbells should be over your chin.

Remind your client

- Don't let your wrists flop around. Keep them straight.
- Control the dumbbells so that they are close to your body. When your elbows are bent, the inner part of the dumbbells should touch your shoulders.
- Control the position of your forearms. Remember to keep elbows and shoulders in the same plane.

Trainer's pointer

Watch the position of your client's forearms. If you notice that they are moving toward her pelvis so that the dumbbells are below nipple level when she lowers them, this means that her rotator cuffs can't control the resistance. Reduce the weight and review proper form.

BARBELL INCLINE PRESS

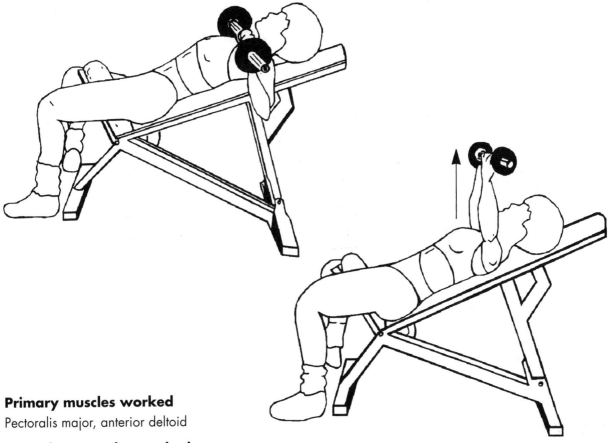

Primary muscles worked

Pectoralis major, anterior deltoid

Secondary muscles worked

Pectoralis minor, subclavius, subscapularis, triceps brachii

Objective

To press the bar upward by straightening the arms

How to do it

Lie on your back on an incline bench. Grasp a bar with an evenly spaced grip approximately 6 inches (15.2 cm) wider than shoulder width. Have your trainer or spotter help you unrack the bar. Keeping your elbows in line with your shoulders, slowly lower the bar to within 1 inch (2.5 cm) of your chest and press it back up by straightening, but not hyperextending, the arms.

Remind your client

- Keep your back flat and completely on the bench.
- Control your wrists. They should stay straight.
- Do not bounce the bar off your chest.
- Go through a full range of motion. Be sure to extend at the shoulder joint, not just flex the elbow.

Trainer's pointers

- Watch your client's back. Make sure it stays in contact with the bench. Some clients need to put their feet up on another bench to make sure the back stays flat.
- Watch the relative position of elbows and shoulders. Make sure your client keeps them in line and doesn't allow her upper body to droop toward the lower body.

PEC DECK

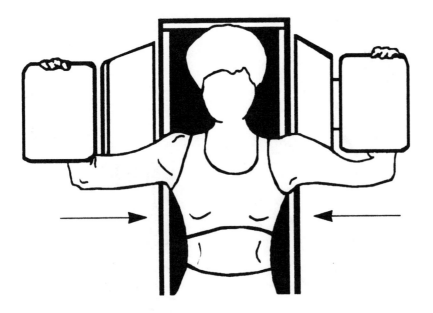 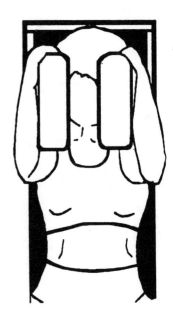

Primary muscle worked

Pectoralis major

Secondary muscles worked

Supraspinatus, infraspinatus, teres major

Objective

To squeeze the elbows together

How to do it

Sit on the chair of a pec deck machine or the pec deck attachment of a universal machine. Adjust the seat so that your elbows are at a 90-degree angle when your arms are on the pads. Place your forearms on the pads and bring the pads together by contracting your pectorals. Squeeze your pectorals at the peak of contraction. After the set is completed, release one pad at a time by turning your torso in the direction of the pad.

Remind your client

- Be *absolutely certain* that you have the weight stack under control. This exercise is one in which you should be extremely cautious about using excessive weight, since your arm is in a position of abduction and external rotation, the most vulnerable position for your rotator cuff. It is essential that you do not lose control of the weight stack. Therefore, be sure not to allow your arms to move outside the same plane as your head.
- Push through with your forearms, not with your hands. Think of trying to bring your elbows together.
- Keep your upper body relaxed. You should move only at the shoulder joint.
- Don't turtle. Your upper trapezius should be relaxed.

Trainer's pointers

- **Caution:** The beginning position, shoulder abduction and external rotation, is one of the most vulnerable positions for the rotator cuff. Be careful!
- Make sure your client does not allow her upper arms to go behind the plane her head is in. Avoid excessive external shoulder rotation.
- Make sure your client doesn't rock her body.
- Spot your client by making sure she doesn't exceed a controllable range of motion.

FLYS

Primary muscle worked

Pectoralis major

Secondary muscles worked

Supraspinatus, infraspinatus, teres major, biceps brachii, triceps brachii

Objective

To move the upper arms in toward the center of the body

How to do it

Lie on your back on a flat or incline bench. Grasp one dumbbell in each hand. Begin the exercise by positioning your arms so that they extend overhead with your elbows slightly bent and the dumbbells in a palms-together position, touching. I sometimes call this exercise the "barrel squeeze" because the idea is to squeeze the dumbbells together as if you were squeezing a barrel. Slowly, and under control, lower your upper arms until they are in line and parallel with the bench (no lower) and return them to the start position by squeezing your pectorals.

Remind your client

- Keep your upper body relaxed. You should move only at the shoulder joint.

- Keep your back down on the bench. If you are doing the exercise on an incline bench, your feet should be flat on the floor with your knees flexed. If you are doing the exercise on a flat bench, your knees should be bent and your feet should be up on the bench.

- Keep your elbows, wrists, and shoulders in the same plane at all times.

- Make sure to keep your elbow joints rigid. It is a common mistake to flex elbow joints during the exercise, which turns it into a press rather than a fly. If you feel the need to do this, reduce the amount of weight you're using.

Trainer's pointers

- Don't let your client lower her upper arms below the bench.
- Don't let your client flex or extend her elbows when she lowers the weights. If she can't keep her elbows rigid, reduce the weight and work up to something heavier.
- Warn your client of the risk of banging her fingers.
- If your client is doing this exercise on an incline bench and cannot keep her feet on the floor while keeping the knees bent, place another bench at her feet to use as a footrest.

REVERSE BARBELL CURL

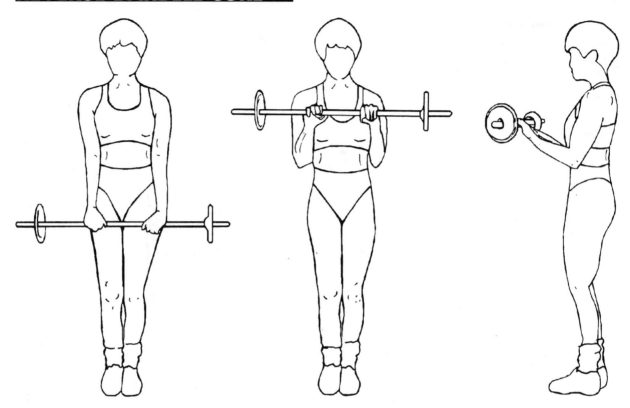

Primary muscles worked

Biceps brachii, brachialis, brachioradialis

Secondary muscles worked

Pronator quadratus, pronator teres

Objective

To lift the barbell by flexing the arm at the elbow

How to do it

Stand and hold a bar in front of you. You should have a palms-down grip with your hands approximately shoulder-width apart. Keeping your upper arms against your body, curl the bar up and toward your body. Repeat for the required number of repetitions.

Remind your client

- Keep the wrists rigid. Don't flex or extend at the wrist.
- Don't rock your body. No spinal extension, please!
- Keep the neck relaxed.
- Keep your upper arms firmly against your body.

Trainer's pointers

- If your client flexes and extends her wrists, elbow tendinitis is a distinct possibility. Watch for this.
- Discourage excessive gripping. Yes, she needs to hold onto the bar. But she doesn't need to grip it as tightly as if she were hanging from a 500-foot drop.
- Be sure your client maintains her four-finger space between the pelvis and rib cage.

REVERSE DUMBBELL CURL

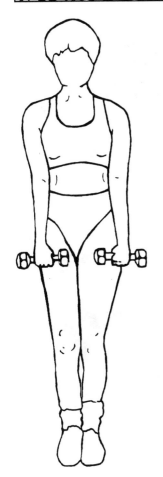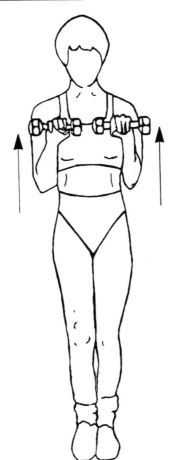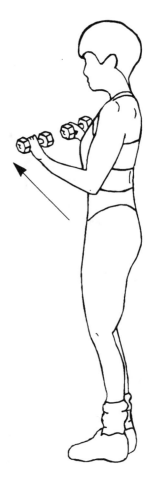

Primary muscles worked

Biceps brachii, brachialis, brachioradialis

Secondary muscles worked

Pronator quadratus, pronator teres

Objective

To lift dumbbells by flexing the arms at the elbows

How to do it

This exercise is identical to the barbell curl except that, instead of a palms-up (supinated) grip, you grasp the dumbbells with your palms down (pronated). Keep your upper arms firmly against your body and raise the weight by flexing at the elbow joint.

Remind your client

Do not rock your body during the exercise. The only action should be at the elbow joint. If you need to rock your body back and forth, reduce the amount of weight. Keep your knees soft and relaxed.

Trainer's pointer

Make sure your client keeps her knees soft and relaxed, which will help her keep her body from rocking. If she rocks her body even when her knees are relaxed, have her do the exercise with her back against the wall.

WRIST FLEXION

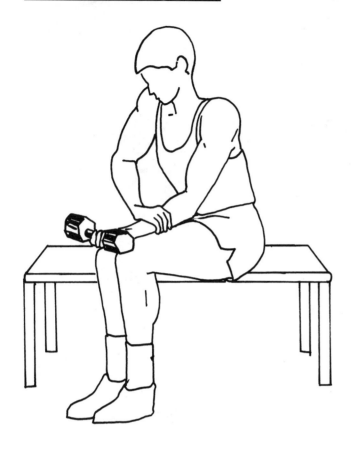

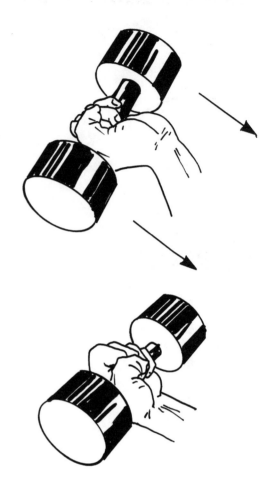

Primary muscles worked

Flexor carpi radialis, flexor carpi ulnaris

Objective

To flex the wrist

How to do it

This exercise can be done with a dumbbell or a light bar. It can be done seated with the forearms resting on the thighs, palms up with the wrists hanging over the end of your knees, or standing at a hyperextension bench with the forearms resting on the pad at about waist level. Hold the dumbbell or bar with a palms-up grip. Perform the exercise by flexing your wrists.

Remind your client

Do not allow the weight to roll off your fingers as you see the exercise performed by some athletes. The only action is at the wrist joint.

Trainer's pointer

If your client has experienced elbow tendinitis, he might find this exercise difficult to do without pain. Still, this exercise is beneficial for those with elbow tendinitis. Therefore, try having the client perform the movement with no weight. If he can do so without pain, try a half-pound (1.28 kg) or 1-pound (2.5 kg) weight and gradually work up to something more challenging.

WRIST EXTENSION

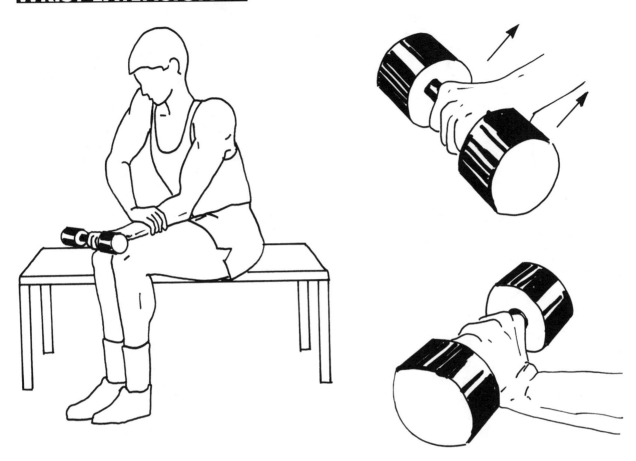

Primary muscles worked

Extensor carpi radialis longus, extensor carpi radialis brevis, extensor carpi ulnaris

Objective

To flex the wrist back

How to do it

Like wrist flexion, this exercise can be done seated with the forearms resting on the thighs, or standing at a hyperextension bench. Grasp a dumbbell or a light bar with a palms-down grip. Perform the exercise by flexing the wrists to raise the resistance.

Remind your client

- This exercise is more difficult than wrist flexion. Perform it slowly and deliberately without using momentum.
- Do not move the forearm. The only action is at the wrist joint.

Trainer's pointer

If your client has experienced elbow tendinitis, he might find this exercise difficult to do without pain. Still, this exercise is beneficial for those with elbow tendinitis. Therefore, try having the client perform the movement with no weight. If he can do so without pain, try a half-pound (1.28 kg) or 1-pound (2.5 kg) weight and gradually work up to something more challenging.

HAMMER CURL

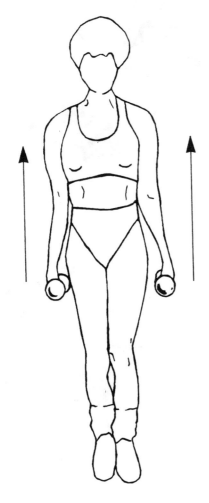 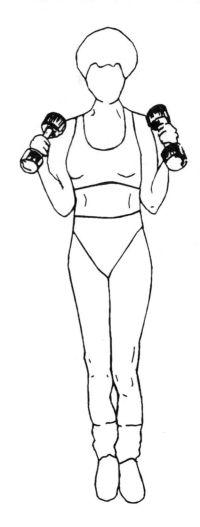

Primary muscles worked

Biceps brachii, brachialis, brachioradialis

Secondary muscle worked

Supinator

Objective

To bend the elbow

How to do it

Stand or sit on a bench with a back support and grasp a dumbbell in each hand, palms facing the body. Keeping the upper arms against your torso, curl the weight by flexing at the elbow joint. Raise the dumbbells to shoulder level. Lower and repeat. Your palms should be facing in during the entire exercise.

Remind your client

This exercise is very similar to the dumbbell curl. The difference is that you do not rotate your palms so that your little fingers are higher than your thumbs during the exercise. Rather, you maintain the palms-facing-you position throughout.

Trainer's pointer

Make sure your client keeps her upper arms firmly against her body.

LYING LEG CURL

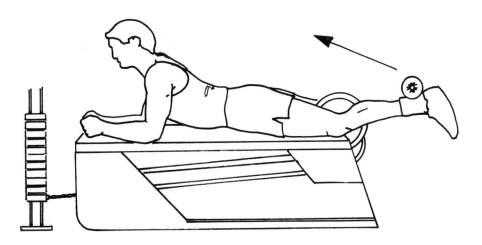

Primary muscles worked

Biceps femoris, semitendinosus, semimebranosus

Secondary muscle worked

Gastrocnemius

Objective

To lift the weight stack by flexing the knee

How to do it

Lie facedown on a leg curl machine. Adjust the machine's pads so that your knees are just off the edge of the bench and the ankle pad hits you at the Achilles tendon. Place your feet under the ankle pad. Before initiating any knee flexion, tighten your gluteus and transversus abdominis. Raise the stack by flexing your knees.

Remind your client

- Do not rest when your leg or legs are straight. Lift and lower the weight in a controlled fashion.
- Keep your hip joint out of the exercise by keeping your transversus abdominis and glutes tight and your pelvis pressed against the bench. Flex and extend only at the knee.
- Concentrate on keeping your feet from turning out. Keep them straight, with the balls of the feet in line with the knees.

Trainer's pointers

- Give your client a tactile cue for activating the glutes and transversus abdominis by placing your fingers on these muscles and having him activate them before he does the exercise. Ask him if he can feel the difference between these muscles being flexed and relaxed, and remind him that they should feel activated the whole time he's doing the exercise.
- I strongly recommend that you have your client do these one leg at a time occasionally for balanced development.
- It will be difficult for your client to keep his glutes tight, but encourage him to try.

STANDING LEG CURL

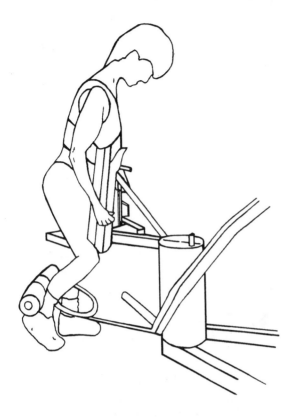 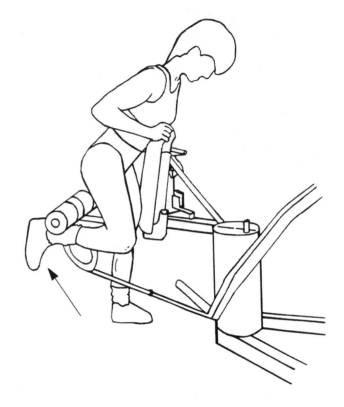

Primary muscles worked

Biceps femoris, semitendinosus, semimembranosus

Secondary muscle worked

Gastrocnemius

Objective

To flex the knee

How to do it

Stand in front of a standing leg curl machine with your ankles behind the pad. Activate your gluteus and transversus abdominis. You should keep these muscles tight the entire time you're doing the exercise. Keeping the knee of your supporting leg soft, lift the stack by flexing the knee of your working leg.

Remind your client

- This is a single-joint movement. Don't twist at the waist or rock your pelvis.
- Try to keep the foot of the working leg straight, not turned out.

Trainer's pointer

Constantly monitor the position of the pelvis and the activation of the gluteus and transversus abdominis. If you notice that your client can't execute the movement without arching her back, reduce the resistance.

BARBELL DEADLIFT

Primary muscles worked

Biceps femoris, semitendinosus, semimembranosus

Secondary muscles worked

Adductor magnus, adductor brevis, adductor longus

Objective

To bend forward at the waist by flexing the hip

How to do it

Grasp a barbell with an evenly spaced palms-down grip. Create your four-finger space by lifting your rib cage and pulling your shoulder blades in line with your spinal column. Tighten your gluteus and transversus abdominis. Keeping your head up and your back flat, bend forward at the waist until the bar is just below your knees. Return to the start position. Repeat for the required number of repetitions.

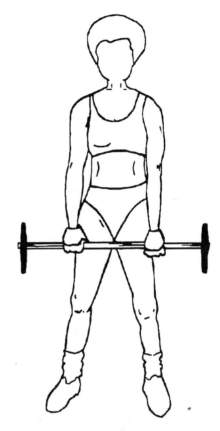

Remind your client

- Keep your back flat.
- The bar must stay extremely close to your body.
- Your knees should be soft, but don't flex or extend them.
- Keep your transversus abdominis and gluteus tight.
- Go through a full range of motion. Straighten your back completely on every repetition.

Trainer's pointers

- Watch your client's back. If it rounds, go through the posture checklist (chapter 4, p. 60) with her again.
- Make sure your client keeps the resistance close to her body. Suggest that she imagine shaving the front of her legs with the bar.
- Make sure this movement is done slowly and under control. No ballistics or jerking!
- Beginners should perform this exercise with dumbbells to avoid the risk of elbow tendinitis.
- **Caution:** This is an advanced exercise that might be risky for those with weak abdominals and/or excess abdominal weight. It is *never* appropriate for those with known low-back pathology or undiagnosed back pain. These clients need to avoid weighted forward spinal flexion.

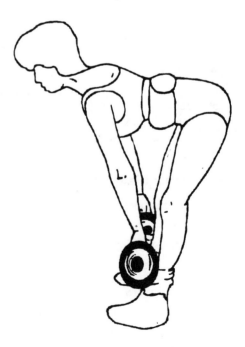

DUMBBELL DEADLIFT

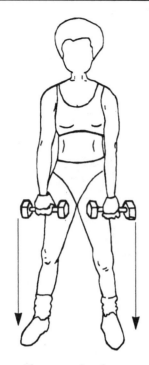
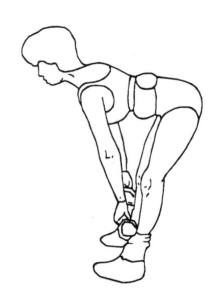

Primary muscles worked

Biceps femoris, semitendinosus, semimembranosus

Secondary muscles worked

Adductor magnus, adductor brevis, adductor longus

Objective

To bend forward at the waist by flexing the hip

How to do it

While standing, grasp two dumbbells (one in each hand). Hold the resistance in front of your thighs, palms down. Create your four-finger space between your pelvis and rib cage and pull your shoulder blades in line with your spinal column. Tighten your gluteus and transversus abdominis. Keeping your head up, bend forward at the waist until the resistance is just below your knees. Return to the start position. Repeat for the required number of repetitions.

Remind your client

- Keep your back flat. Check your posture. If it is correct, you will automatically have a flat back.
- The resistance must stay extremely close to your body.
- Do not flex or extend your elbows.
- Do not turtle.

Trainer's pointers

- Watch your client's back. If it rounds, go through the posture checklist (chapter 4, p. 60) with her again.
- Make sure your client keeps the resistance next to the body. Suggest that she imagine shaving the front of her legs with the dumbbells.
- **Caution:** This is an advanced exercise that might be risky for those with weak abdominals and/or excess abdominal weight. It should not be performed by those with pre-existing low back problems due to compressive forces on the spine.

BACK EXTENSION ON FLOOR

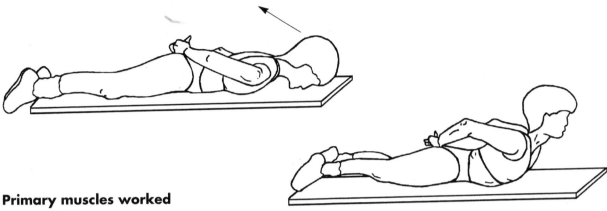

Primary muscles worked

Illiocostalis thoracis (aka illiocostalis dorsi), long-
issimus thoracis (aka longissimus dorsi), spinalis thoracis (aka spinalis thoracis), illiocostalis lumborun;
sometimes these muscles are collectively called the sacrospinalis group

Secondary muscle worked

Quadratus lumborum

Objective

To lift the chest off the mat or floor

How to do it

Lie facedown on the floor. Place your hands behind your back. Lift your chest off the mat or floor. Return to the start position.

Remind your client

- Do not hyperextend your neck. Keep your chin down so that your neck is in line with your spine.
- Do not twist your spine.
- Maintain your pace. Lift and lower your chest at a steady rate.

Trainer's pointers

- Stabilize your client's pelvis by placing your hands on her thighs.
- To make this exercise more challenging, have your client raise her arms over her head.
- To make this exercise easier, have your client place her hands at her sides, in contact with the ground, and lift her chest while straightening her arms.
- Advanced trainers can do this exercise on the leg curl machine by setting the pad so that the feet can be comfortably placed under them.
- **Caution:** While back extensions on the floor are safe for most healthy adults without pre-existing back problems, remember that an overwhelming majority of adults do eventually develop low back pain. Low back problems may be latent, lying in wait until the person engages in an activity imposing extreme compression forces on the

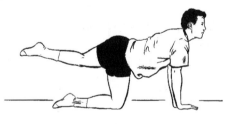

spine, and suddenly, excrutiating pain! If you have any doubt about the ability of your client to do this exercise safely, please substitute one of the exercises on the right. For more information, see chapters 12 and 13 of *Low Back Disorders* by Stuart McGill, published by Human Kinetics in 2002.

LEG EXTENSION

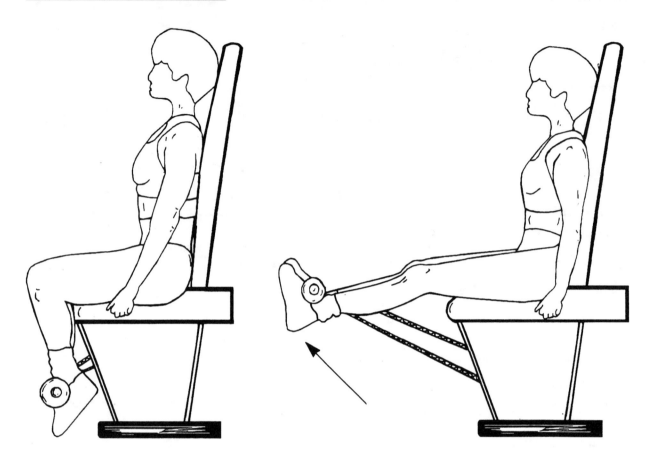

Primary muscles worked

Rectus femoris, vastus lateralis, vastus medialis, vastus intermedialis

Objective

To straighten the knee while keeping the hip relaxed

How to do it

Sit on the leg extension station of a universal or similar machine with your knees bent and your feet behind the pads of the leg extension attachment, which should hit you at the ankle joint. Extend your legs by straightening them at the knee joint. While generally done two legs at a time, this exercise can also be done one leg at a time for greater isolation and balanced development.

Remind your client

- Try to actively flex the front of your thighs when the working leg is in the extended position. One good way to focus on this is to hold the peak contraction for a count of one.
- Keep your upper body relaxed. Do not allow your body to come up out of the chair or your hips to rise.
- Make sure that the machine, chair, or bench provides adequate back support.

Trainer's pointer

Make sure your client keeps her upper body relaxed. If she's bouncing around in the chair, she's trying to use her hip flexors to move the resistance. Reduce the weight.

BARBELL SQUAT

Primary muscles worked

Gluteus maximus, biceps femoris, semitendinosus, semimembranosus, rectus femoris, vastus lateralis, vastus medialis, vastus intermedialis

Secondary muscles worked

Adductor magnus, adductor brevis, adductor longus, transversus abdominis, rectus abdominis, sacrospinalis group

Objective

To lower the body as if sitting in a chair

How to do it

Stand in front of a squat rack with the bar at the appropriate height to allow you to unrack it without rising on your toes or bending over. Go under the bar and unrack it, maintaining a palms-forward grip, holding the bar behind your head and resting it on your shoulders. Step away from the rack and stand with your feet approximately shoulder-width apart. Shift body weight back to heels. This should cause a slightly forward lean, which is fine provided the back stays flat. Bend at the knees by flexing your hips, lowering the glutes behind the heels. When your thighs are parallel to the floor and your knees are flexed at 90 degrees, immediately push back up to the starting position. Don't rest when your legs are straight. Ascend and descend at a controlled, steady pace, up to a count of two and down to a count of three or four. When you've finished the designated number of reps, come to a complete stop.

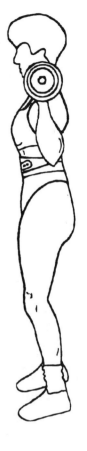

Remind your client

- Keep body weight back on the heels.
- Make sure you keep the bar firmly on the back of your shoulders. Do not allow the bar to roll down your back.
- Always squat with a spotter and understand the proper method for bailing out.
- It is suggested that you wear a weight belt during squats and lunges.
- Be sure to initiate the exercise by flexing at the hip, not the knee. Drop your hips as if you were sitting down on an imaginary bench. It may feel like you are sticking your rear end out, and if it does, you're doing it right.
- Keep your head up, back straight, and abdominals tight.
- Never go lower than the point where thighs are parallel with the floor; that is, knees should never be flexed at an angle smaller than 90 degrees.

Trainer's pointers

- Have your client activate the glutes and transversus abdominis before descending.
- Make sure your client's knees stay directly over her feet, not in front of them.
- Watch for the beginner's tendency to flex not at the hip joint, but only at the knee, which places the knee in hyperflexion. If your client's knees move in front of the balls of her feet, stop her and review form.
- Those with round-shouldered posture may be unable to achieve sufficient external rotation at the shoulder joints to hold a bar behind their heads. If this is the case, address this problem before attempting a barbell squat. Consider substituting a leg press or a dumbbell squat.
- **Caution:** The barbell squat is an advanced exercise that should not be performed until clients have sufficient strength in the low back and abdominals to hold the spine in a neutral, unbuckled position during the exercise.

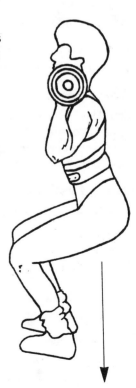

DUMBBELL SQUAT

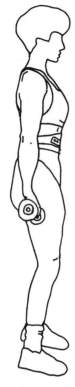
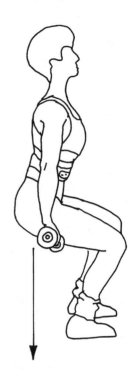

Primary muscles worked

Gluteus maximus, biceps femoris, semitendinosus, semimembranosus, rectus femoris, vastus lateralis, vastus medialis, vastus intermedialis

Secondary muscles worked

Adductor magnus, adductor brevis, adductor longus

Objective

To lower the body as if sitting in a chair

How to do it

Stand with your feet approximately shoulder-width apart and hold a dumbbell in each hand. Shift your weight back to your heels. With your arms straight and at your sides, descend by flexing at the hip and then flexing at the knee until your thighs are parallel with the ground. Return to the starting position. Repeat for the required number of repetitions.

Remind your client

- Be sure to initiate the movement at your hip joint, not the knees. Think about dropping your gluteus behind your heels.
- Keep your weight back on your heels.
- Keep the dumbbells at your sides.

Trainer's pointers

- Have your client activate the gluteus and transversus abdominis before descending.
- Make sure your client's knees stay directly over her feet, not in front of them.
- Watch for the beginner's tendency to flex not at the hip joint, but only at the knee, which places the knee in hyperflexion. If your client's knees move in front of the balls of her feet, stop her and review form.

LEG PRESS

Primary muscles worked

Vastus lateralis, vastus medialis, vastus intermedialis

Secondary muscles worked

Adductor magnus, adductor brevis, adductor longus

Objective

To press the weight stack up by straightening the leg at the knee

How to do it

Sit on the seat of a leg press machine. Before beginning, check the seat's position. It should be positioned so that you are able to place your feet flat on the machine's platform without hyperextending your knees or flexing your hips. Unrack the stack, and lower it under control until your legs are at approximately 90 degrees of flexion. Press the stack up. Do not pause at the top. Repeat for the required number of repetitions.

Remind your client

- Don't hyperextend your knees when pressing up the stack. They should retain a slight softness even when the stack is pressed up.
- Keep your upper body relaxed.
- Keep your feet on the platform.
- Make sure that the knees are aligned over the feet. They should not collapse in or flare out.
- Do not pause at the top of the movement.

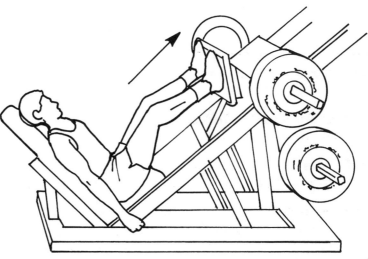

Trainer's pointers

- Advise your client to use caution when adding or removing plates from a loaded leg press machine. Alternate removing plates from each side. *Never* remove them all from one side at a time because the machine could tip over.
- Vary the width between the clients' feet to target different areas of the quadriceps.

BARBELL LUNGE

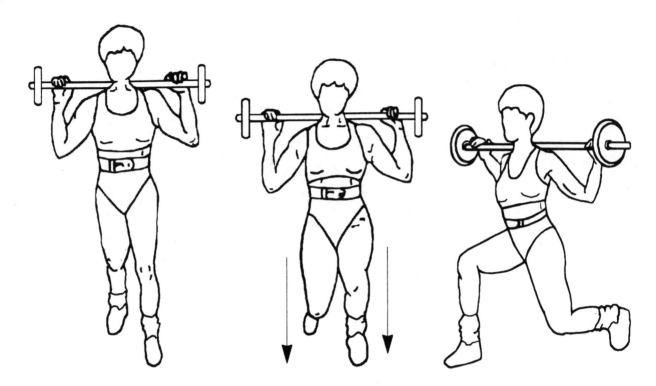

Primary muscles worked

Gluteus maximus, vastus lateralis, vastus medialis, vastus intermedialis

Secondary muscles worked

Adductor magnus, adductor brevis, adductor longus

Objective

To lower the body toward the ground by flexing both the knees and the hips

How to do it

Stand in front of a squat rack with the bar at the appropriate height to allow you to unrack it without rising on your toes or bending over. Go under the bar and unrack it. Step away from the rack. Keeping one leg slightly in front of your body, extend one leg behind and slightly (about 30 degrees) away from the center of your body with the foot flexed. Maintaining good posture, lower your body by flexing both knees 90 degrees. Return to the starting position and repeat the required number of repetitions.

Remind your client

- Be sure to flex both knees. Beginners tend to flex only the front knee, causing it to go beyond the ball of the foot, a potentially dangerous move.
- Keep the glutes tight. Think of them as a sponge and squeeze.
- Be sure to exert enough force with the arms and shoulders to keep the bar from rolling down the back.

Trainer's pointers

- Observe your client from the side to make sure she is flexing both knees. There is a tendency not to flex the back one, placing the front knee in a dangerous hyperflexed position.
- Make sure your client has her body weight distributed on her front heel and back toe.

DUMBBELL LUNGE

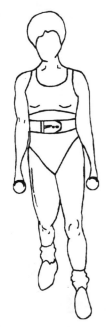 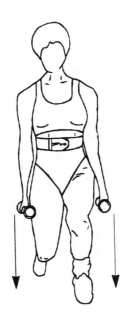 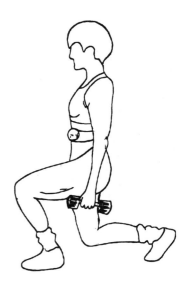

Primary muscles worked

Gluteus maximus, vastus lateralis, vastus medialis, vastus intermedialis

Secondary muscles worked

Adductor magnus, adductor brevis, adductor longus

Objective

To lower the body toward the ground by flexing both the knees and the hips

How to do it

Hold a dumbbell in each hand, palms facing your body and arms beside your body. Keep your head up and back straight. Extend your leg back and slightly to the outside (about 30 degrees away from the center of the body) with the foot flexed. Maintaining good posture, lower your body by flexing both knees 90 degrees. Return to the start position and repeat the required number of repetitions.

Remind your client

- Be sure to keep the dumbbells close to your body, in line with your ears. If you allow your arms to travel forward, this will change your center of gravity and cause you to lean forward, putting a great deal of stress on your low back.
- Flex both knees, but do not let the back knee touch the ground.
- Do not look down! If you do, you will bend forward, which stresses the low back.
- Keep your four-finger space between your pelvis and rib cage.
- The front knee should *never* go farther forward than the ball of the front foot.
- Keep the body's weight back on the front heel and rear toe.
- Keep the glutes tight throughout the exercise.

Trainer's pointers

- Watch the tendency to flex only the front leg at the knee while flexing the back leg only at the hip.
- Have your client activate her glutes and transversus abdominis before beginning the movement.
- Make sure your client keeps her scapula in line with the spinal column.

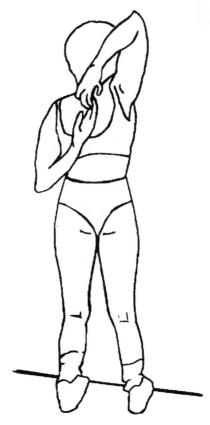

Some general notes about the rotator cuff: As noted in the text, the rotator cuff is one of the most important and most neglected groups of muscles in the body. Most weightlifters will develop rotator cuff problems unless they work on strength and flexibility in this area. As your client does the rotator cuff exercises, be aware of the following:

1. Is your client experiencing any clicking or popping at the shoulder joint? I find it helpful to place my hands on the shoulders to feel for these symptoms. If so, try to adjust the position of the scapula (by having the client pull it down) or the upper arm. If the clicking and popping continues, try reducing the weight.

2. Is your client experiencing any pain or discomfort in the shoulder or elsewhere while doing these exercises? If so, try reducing the weight or doing the exercise without any additional weight at all. If the exercise is too easy without added weight, try using some manual resistance.

3. How much range of motion does your client have at the shoulder joint? Does it differ between sides of the body? Can he touch his fingers together between his shoulder blades? (See illustration.) This information will help you refine the client's workout.

4. Is your client a lot stronger on one side than the other? If so, you need to concentrate on the weak side. You might also find it necessary to use a lighter weight on the weaker side until you and your client are able to correct this imbalance.

5. Does your client have a winging scapula? A winging scapula sticks out rather than lying flush with the back and is an extremely common condition, especially among the round-shouldered and the tight-necked. If she does have this condition, work on strengthening the serratus and the external rotators of the shoulder and stretching the internal rotators of the shoulder.

WINDMILL

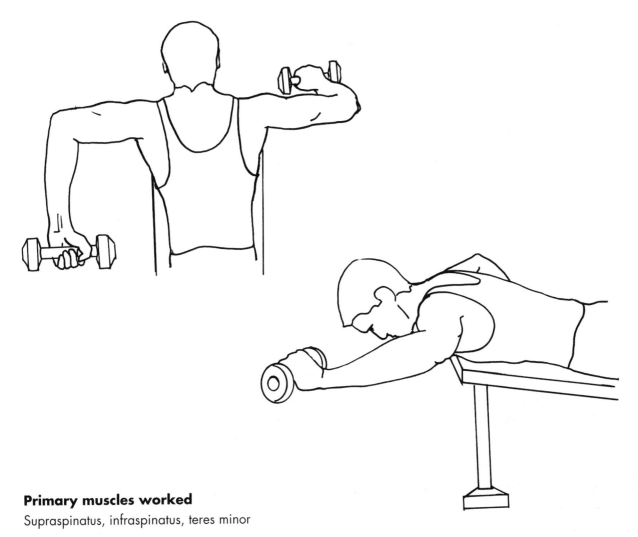

Primary muscles worked

Supraspinatus, infraspinatus, teres minor

Secondary muscle worked

Pectoralis minor

Objective

To rotate the upper arms back and forth

How to do it

Hold a light dumbbell in each hand. Lie facedown on a bench with your head hanging over the edge. With your upper arms at 90 degrees to your body and your elbows flexed 90 degrees, rotate your arms back and forth until the dumbbells are alternately level with your head and the bench. Your neck should be straight; your head should be in line with your spinal column. Your shoulder blades should be in line with your spinal column.

Remind your client

- Keep your arms and elbows at 90-degree angles.
- Keep your head up.

Trainer's pointer

This is an advanced exercise. It is helpful in correcting round-shoulder posture, but in order to do it in correct form, the client must have a little background in weight training and the body awareness that comes with it.

LYING L

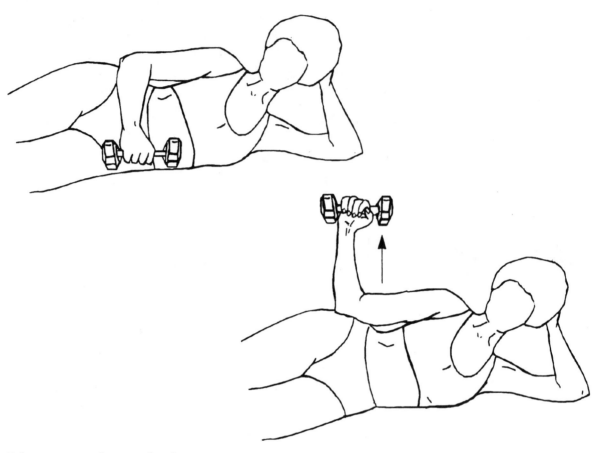

Primary muscles worked

Supraspinatus, infraspinatus, teres minor

Objective

To rotate the upper arm at the shoulder joint

How to do it

Lie on your side on the floor. Support your head with one hand (elbow bent). Hold a light dumbbell in the other hand. Place the upper arm of this hand firmly against your body with the elbow flexed at 90 degrees. Keeping your wrist straight and maintaining this 90-degree angle at the elbow joint, move the dumbbell up toward the ceiling, then back until it is in line with your body. After performing the designated number of repetitions, switch sides.

Remind your client

- Keep the wrist straight.
- Keep your neck relaxed. Don't turtle.
- Keep your scapula pulled down and in line with your spinal column.
- Keep the elbow in contact with the hipbone.

Trainer's pointers

- Make sure the client is doing this exercise slowly and under control. There is a tendency to throw the weight up and down.
- Watch the wrist for undesirable flexion and extension.

LYING INTERNAL/EXTERNAL ROTATION

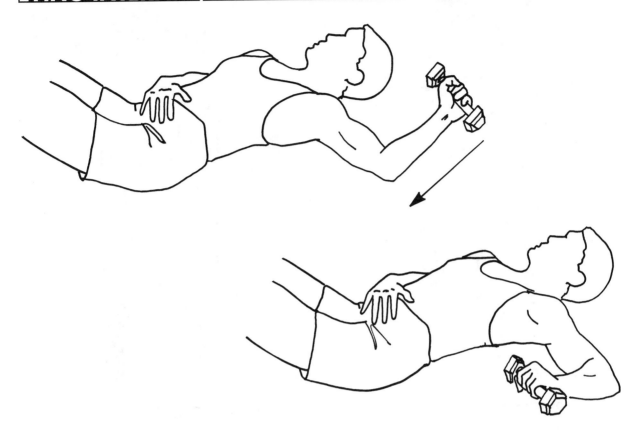

Primary muscles worked

Supraspinatus, infraspinatus, teres minor

Secondary muscle worked

Pectoralis minor

Objective

To rotate the upper arm

How to do it

Lie on your back on the floor with your knees bent. Hold a light dumbbell in one hand. Your upper arm should be at a 90-degree angle to your body, and your elbow should be flexed 90 degrees. Maintaining these two 90-degree angles, move the dumbbell as far in both directions as you can comfortably and under full control while keeping your shoulder on the ground. Do the required number of repetitions, then repeat on the other side.

Remind your client

- Keep your upper arm at a 90-degree angle. Do not allow this to straighten.
- Keep the wrist rigid.
- Keep your neck and shoulders relaxed.
- Keep your scapula in line with your spinal column.

Trainer's pointer

Each client's range of motion on this exercise will be different. Some may be able to lower the dumbbell all the way to the floor in both directions with their shoulders on the ground. Monitor the range of motion and try to work toward gradual improvement.

DUMBBELL SHOULDER PRESS

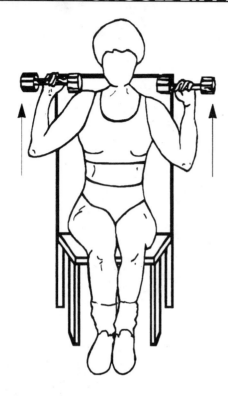
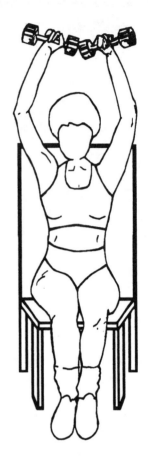

Primary muscles worked

Medial deltoid, supraspinatus

Secondary muscles worked

Trapezius (upper division), levator scapulae

Objective

To press the dumbbells overhead by straightening the arms

How to do it

Sit on a bench with a back support. Hold one dumbbell in each hand, palms facing forward. Begin with the dumbbells at shoulder level and press them up overhead. The dumbbells should come together at the top of the movement.

Remind your client

- Make sure you bring the dumbbells all the way down to your shoulders on each rep.
- The dumbbells should travel on the same plane with your head. Don't allow your upper arms to move forward during the exercise.
- Remember to control your wrists. Do not allow them to flex and extend or otherwise flop around. Keep them straight.
- Keep your back against the bench.

Trainer's pointers

- Ask your client if she is experiencing any clicking or popping in her shoulders. Place your hands on her shoulders to feel for anything unusual. If clicking or popping is a problem, have your client try doing the exercise with her hands in a neutral position (palms facing each other).
- Make sure your client keeps her neck relaxed.

BARBELL SHOULDER PRESS

Primary muscles worked
Medial deltoid, supraspinatus

Secondary muscles worked
Trapezius (upper division), levator scapulae

Objective
To press the barbell overhead by straightening the arms

How to do it
Sit on a stable chair with a back support. Grasp the bar slightly wider than shoulder-width apart with palms facing forward. On a count of three, have your trainer or spotter give you a lift off. Lower the bar under control to about ear level in front of your head. Press the bar up by straightening your arms.

Remind your client

- This is a multijoint exercise. Be sure to lower the upper arms as well as flexing and extending at the elbows.
- Keep the wrists as straight as possible.
- Don't turtle!

Trainer's pointers

- Be sure that your client maintains good posture (for example, keeping the four-finger space between the pelvis and rib cage).
- Watch for uneven arm extension. It's not uncommon for the weaker side to lag behind.
- While it is extremely important that your client go through a full range of motion, there is little to be gained, and much potential harm to the shoulder, from lowering the bar below ear level.

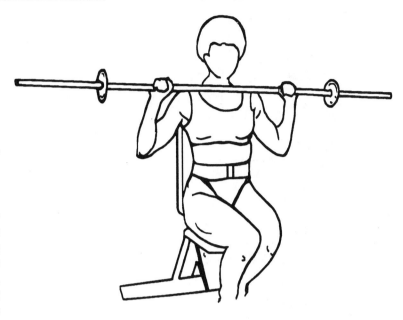

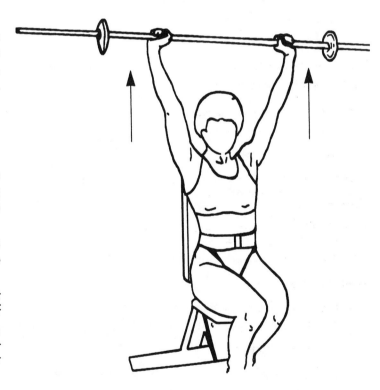

DUMBBELL SIDE RAISE

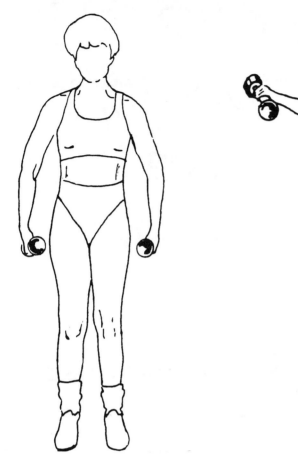
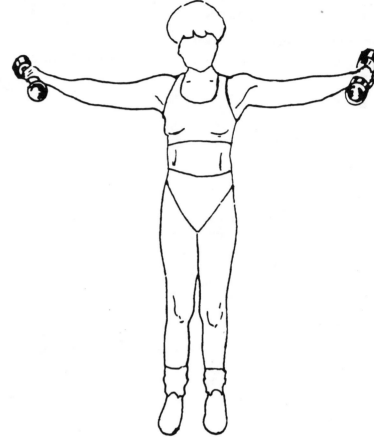

Primary muscles worked

Medial deltoid, supraspinatus

Objective

To lift the upper arms away from the body

How to do it

This exercise may be done seated or standing. Hold one dumbbell in each hand, palms facing your sides. Lift your arms out to your sides until they are at shoulder level. Lower and repeat.

Remind your client

- Keep your elbow joints soft, but straight. The action is only at the shoulder joint.
- Do not turtle. Your upper trapezius should stay relaxed.

Trainer's pointer

Be alert for clicking and popping in the shoulder joint. Ask your client if there's any clicking or popping and place your hands on the shoulder to check. If you find any, try adjusting the position of the upper arms by moving them forward or back. Having your client depress her scapula might help. You should also reduce the weight. If this doesn't work, eliminate this exercise until your client's neck and shoulder flexibility improves and it can be done without the snap, crackle, and pop.

DUMBBELL FRONT RAISE

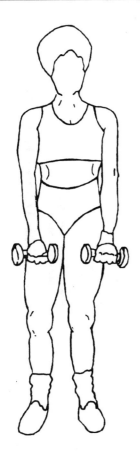 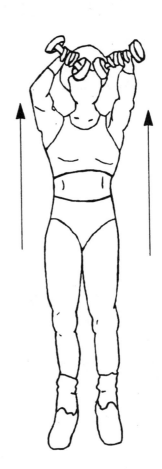

Primary muscles worked

Anterior deltoid, coracobrachialis

Objective

To lift the arms in front of the body

How to do it

Stand holding a dumbbell in each hand with palms down and directly in front of your thighs. Keeping your good posture, with your elbows slightly bent, raise your arms in front of your body.

Remind your client

- Don't rock or twist your body. Your spine should stay still and relaxed. The shoulder is the only axis of rotation.
- Keep the wrist rigid.
- Do not flex or extend the elbow. Keep it frozen.
- Keep the knees soft and relaxed.

Trainer's pointers

- Be sure your client maintains good posture (for example, keeping the four-finger space between the pelvis and rib cage).
- If your client begins rocking her body, suggest that she soften the knees.
- This exercise may also be done by alternating the arms.

BENT DUMBBELL RAISE

Primary muscle worked
Posterior deltoid

Secondary muscle worked
Rhomboids

Objective
To lift the arms at a 45-degree angle to the body

How to do it
Sit on a chair or a bench. Hold one dumbbell in each hand. Bend forward at the waist. With your upper arms at approximately a 45-degree angle to your head and your elbows slightly bent, place the front ends of the dumbbells together. Lift your arms out to your sides. Concentrate on keeping your upper arms in the proper plane. Lower and repeat. When viewed from above, you should resemble the letter Y, not the letter T.

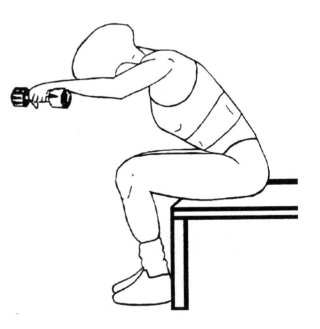

Remind your client

- Keep your elbows slightly bent but rigid. The action is at the shoulder joint.
- Do not allow your wrists to flop around.
- Do not move your body at the spine or neck. Keep your body relaxed and move only at the shoulder joint.
- If you feel the need to rock your body up and down during the exercise, the weight you are using is too heavy.
- Lift your upper arms until they are in line with your head and no higher.
- Never do this exercise standing, unless your back is supported.
- Maintain your four-finger space between your pelvis and rib cage—don't slouch!

Trainer's pointers

- Watch the tendency to move the upper arms back in line with the shoulders rather than the ears. When viewed from above, the client should look like a Y. Place your hands on the upper arms if necessary to keep them in the proper plane.
- Make sure your client keeps her scapula depressed and her rib cage lifted.
- The challenges here are to keep the back flat and straight and to keep the neck relaxed. Pay particular attention to these critical form points.

CABLE SIDE RAISE

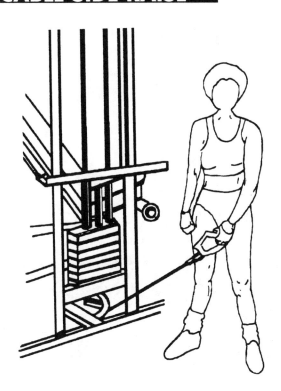 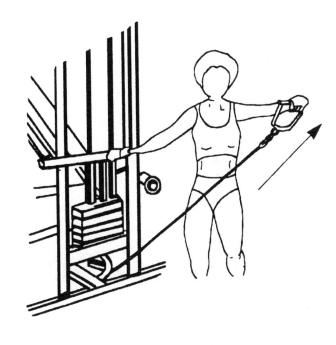

Primary muscles worked

Medial deltoid, supraspinatus

Objective

To lift the upper arm out to the side

How to do it

Stand with your right side facing a machine with a low pulley. Grasp the handle with your left hand. Stand up straight with the handle in front of your body. Bend your left elbow slightly. Keeping the shoulder blades pulled down and the left elbow rigid, lift the left arm out to the side until it is at shoulder level. Repeat for the required number of repetitions. Turn and work the right shoulder with the handle in the right hand.

Remind your client

- Keep the spine straight and relaxed. Don't rock back and forth, twist, or rotate.
- Don't turtle. Keep the shoulder blades pulled down.
- Don't flex or extend the elbow. Keep it rigid to keep the focus on the shoulder.
- Keep the wrist rigid.

Trainer's pointers

- Make sure that your client maintains the four-finger space and keeps the shoulder blades pulled down.
- Check for clicking and popping in the working shoulder. If you detect it, suggest that your client readjust the shoulder blade by pulling it down.
- If your client rocks her body, suggest that she soften the knees more.
- Watch for and strongly discourage turtling.

CABLE FRONT RAISE

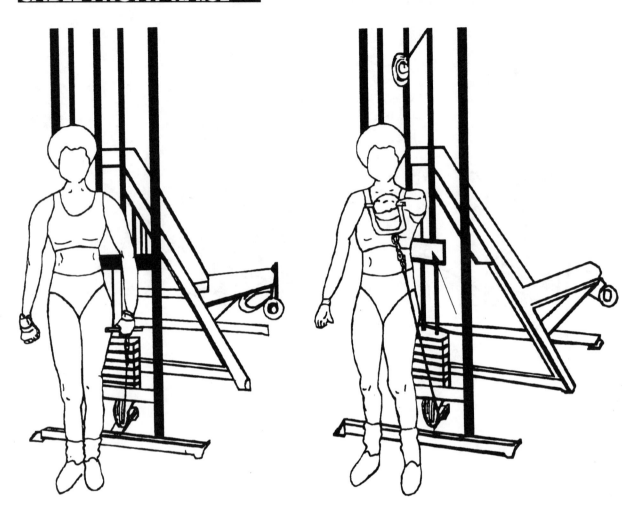

Primary muscles worked

Anterior deltoid, coracobrachilis

Objective

To lift the arm in front of the body

How to do it

Stand with your back to a machine with a low handle. Grasp the handle with your palm down. Keeping your posture correct and your elbows slightly bent, raise your arm in front of your body.

Remind your client

- Don't rock or twist your body. Your spine should stay still and relaxed.
- Keep the wrist rigid.
- Do not flex or extend the elbow.

Trainer's pointers

- Make sure that the shoulder, elbow, and wrist are in the same plane.
- If your client begins rocking her body, suggest that she soften the knees more.

BENT CABLE RAISE

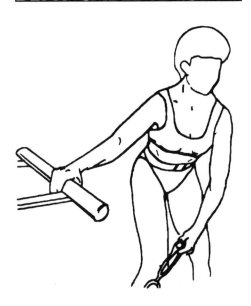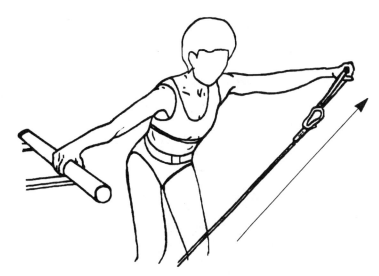

Primary muscle worked

Posterior deltoid

Objective

To lift the upper arm out to the side while bending forward at the hip and keeping the elbow rigid

How to do it

Stand with your right side facing a machine with a low pulley. Grasp the handle with your left hand. Flex the knees and bend forward at the waist. Support your body weight by placing your right hand on the machine. Grasp the handle in front of your body. Bend your left elbow slightly. Keeping the shoulder blades pulled down and the left elbow rigid, lift the left arm out to the side until it is at shoulder level. Repeat for the required number of repetitions. Turn and work the right shoulder with the handle in the right hand.

Remind your client

- Keep the spine straight and relaxed. Don't rock back and forth, twist, or rotate. The spine should stay rigid.
- Don't turtle.
- Don't flex or extend the elbow. Keep it rigid and focus on the shoulder.
- Keep the wrist rigid.
- Keep the knees soft.

Trainer's pointers

- Make sure that your client maintains both good posture and her forward stance.
- Check for clicking and popping in the working shoulder. If you detect it, suggest that your client readjust her shoulder blade by pulling it down.
- If your client rocks her body, suggest that she soften the knees.
- Watch for and strongly discourage turtling.
- Elbow flexion and extension can be a major problem. If your client can't do the exercise without flexing her elbow, reduce the amount of weight.

UPRIGHT ROW

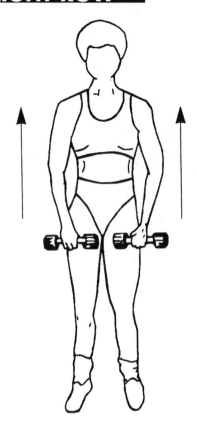
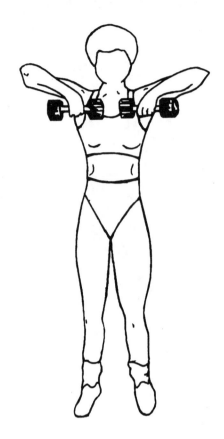

Primary muscles worked
Medial deltoid, supraspinatus, trapezius (upper division)

Secondary muscles worked
Levator scapulae, biceps brachii, pronator quadratus, pronator teres

Objective
To lift the upper arms, leading with the elbows

How to do it
Grasp a bar or dumbbells with a palms-down grip. Place your hands about shoulder-width apart or closer, whichever is more comfortable. Stand with your back straight and knees soft. Keeping the bar or dumbbells very close to your body, pull the resistance up until it is under your chin. At this point, your elbows should be just below ear level. Lower back to the start position.

Remind your client
- Do not swing your upper body. It should remain still.
- Use moderate amounts of weight for this exercise.
- Lead with your elbows. Do not shrug your shoulders toward your ears.
- Keep your knees soft and relaxed.

Trainer's pointer
Some clients who have trouble doing this exercise with a bar can do it successfully with dumbbells because the weight is lighter and dumbbells allow more adjustment in the plane of motion. Also, they place less stress on the wrists and forearms.

BARBELL SHRUG

Primary muscles worked

Trapezius (upper division), levator scapulae

Secondary muscles worked

Rhomboid

Objective

To pull the shoulders up toward the ears while keeping the arms straight

How to do it

Stand while holding a bar in front of you. Your hands should be approximately shoulder-width apart. Keeping your elbows frozen, shrug your shoulders up toward your ears.

Remind your client

- Don't flex or extend the elbows.
- Don't roll the shoulders back and forth. The shoulders should elevate, not rotate.
- Keep the knees soft and relaxed.
- Keep the bar extremely close to the body.

Trainer's pointers

- Be sure that your client maintains good posture.
- Watch for elbow flexion or extension.

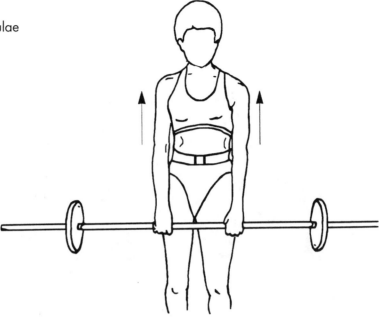

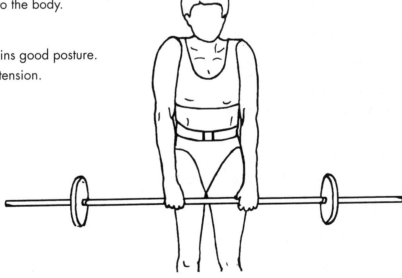

DUMBBELL SHRUG

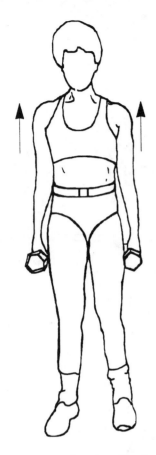 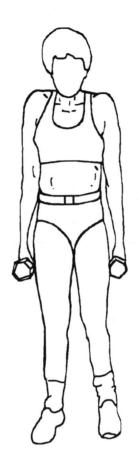 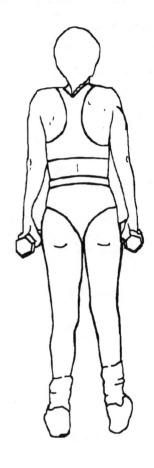

Primary muscles worked

Trapezius (upper division), levator scapulae

Secondary muscle worked

Rhomboid

Objective

To elevate the shoulders up toward the ears while keeping the arms straight

How to do it

Stand while holding a pair of dumbbells, one in each hand, at your sides. Keeping your elbows rigid, shrug your shoulders up toward your ears.

Remind your client

- Don't flex or extend the elbows.
- Don't roll the shoulders back and forth. The shoulders should elevate, not rotate.
- Keep the knees soft and relaxed.
- Keep the dumbbells close to the body.

Trainer's pointers

- Be sure that your client maintains good posture.
- Watch for elbow flexion or extension.
- Dumbbell shrugs may also be done with the dumbbells in front of your body.

LYING SIDE RAISE (HORIZONTAL ABDUCTION)

Primary muscle worked

Posterior deltoid

Secondary muscles worked

Rhomboid, trapezius (lower division)

Objective

To lift the arm out to the side until it is in line with the body while keeping the elbow stationary

How to do it

Lie on your right side on a bench or on the floor with your knees slightly bent and your upper body resting on your right forearm. Your pelvis should be facing squarely forward. Hold a dumbbell in your left hand, palm down. Your left elbow should be slightly bent, approximately in line with your shoulder and facing out. Keeping the scapula depressed and the elbow stationary, lift your arm until the elbow is in line with your head. Return to the beginning position and repeat for the specified number of repetitions. Switch positions so that you are lying on your left side. Perform the same number of repetitions on the right side.

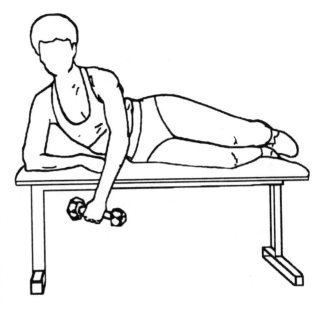

Remind your client

- Don't allow your body to roll toward one side or the other.
- Your entire body should be facing forward.
- Keep the wrist rigid.
- Keep the neck relaxed.
- Keep the shoulder blades pulled down.

Trainer's pointers

- Be sure that your client maintains good posture. There should be no forward spinal flexion.
- Watch carefully for elbow flexion and extension. If it isn't possible for your client to do the exercise without bending the elbow, reduce the weight.
- Suggest that your client visualize her arm moving back and forth like a wing in a flying motion.
- Check for clicking and popping in the working shoulder. If clicking and popping are present, adjusting the position of the arm with relation to the body might help.

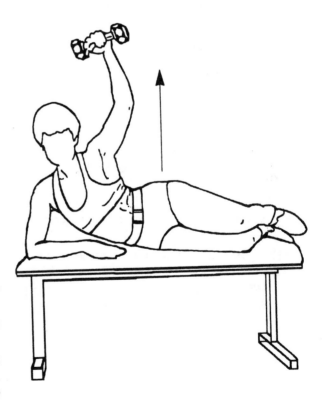

- Large or less experienced clients will find this exercise easier to do on the floor for stability.

LYING SIDE RAISE (FRONTAL ABDUCTION)

Primary muscles worked

Medial deltoid, supraspinatus

Secondary muscles worked

Trapezius (upper division), levator scapulae

Objective

To lift the arm away from the side and toward the head

How to do it

Lie on your right side on a bench or on the floor with your knees slightly bent. Your pelvis should be facing squarely forward. Hold a dumbbell in your left hand, palm down. Your elbow should be slightly bent. Begin with your left arm on top of your left thigh. Lift your arm up until the dumbbell is over your head. Return to start position and repeat for the specified number of repetitions. Switch positions so that you are lying on your left side. Perform the same number of repetitions on the right side.

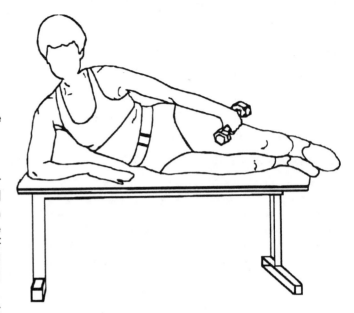

Remind your client

- Don't allow your body to roll toward one side or the other.
- Your entire body should be facing forward.
- Keep the wrist rigid.
- Keep the neck relaxed.
- Keep the shoulder blades pulled down.

Trainer's pointers

- Be sure that your client maintains good posture.
- Suggest that your client think of her arm moving up like the hand of a clock in reverse.
- This exercise is more difficult than it looks and is recommended only for advanced clients.
- Larger or less experienced clients will find this exercise easier to do on the floor.

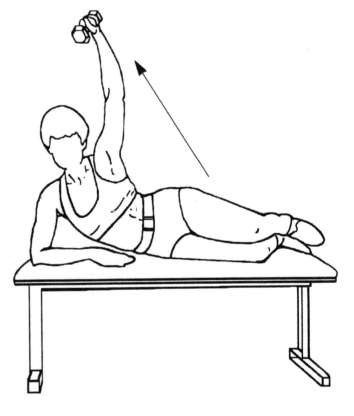

TRICEPS PUSH-DOWN

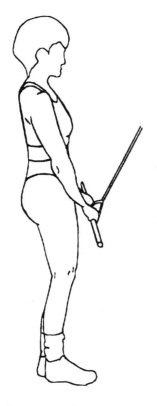 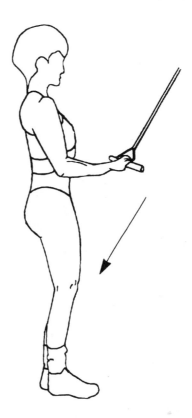

Primary muscle worked

Triceps brachii

Secondary muscle worked

Anconeus

Objective

To bend and straighten the arms at the elbow while keeping the upper arm against the body

How to do it

Stand in front of a machine with a high pulley. Grasp the overhead bar attached to the cable with palms down and thumbs on top. Keeping the upper arms firmly against and slightly in front of the center of the body, push the bar down by straightening the elbows. Allow your elbows to flex 90 degrees and no more. Repeat for the required number of repetitions.

Remind your client

- *Do not* allow your upper arm to move during the exercise. Keep your upper arm glued to the side of your body!
- Do not shrug your shoulders up toward your ears. Try to keep your neck relaxed.
- Focus on flexing and extending your elbows.

Trainer's pointers

- Make sure your client moves the resistance by flexing and extending at the elbow. Some people have a tendency to try to use the shoulder during this exercise.
- A V-shaped bar is easier on the forearms and wrists than a straight bar.
- Watch for the tendency to bend the wrist at the top of the movement. Bending the wrist should be avoided.

SINGLE TRICEPS PULL-DOWN

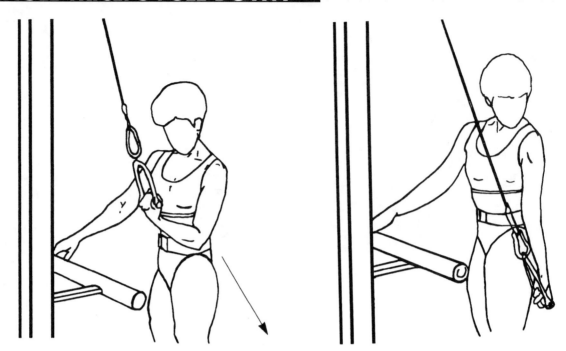

Primary muscle worked

Triceps brachii

Secondary muscle worked

Anconeus

Objective

To straighten the arm at the elbow joint while keeping the upper arm against the body

How to do it

Stand facing a machine with a high pulley. Attach the small handle. Grasp the handle with your left hand in a palms-up grip. Keeping the upper arm firmly against the body, straighten the arm at the elbow. Return to the beginning position (90 degrees of elbow flexion). Repeat for the required number of repetitions. Switch arms and perform the same number of repetitions on the right arm.

Remind your client

- Don't rock your body. The only axis of rotation is the elbow.
- Keep the upper arm firmly against your body.
- Keep your neck relaxed.
- Don't flex or extend the wrist.
- Don't rotate at the spine.

Trainer's pointers

- The angle at the elbow joint should not be less than 90 degrees to maintain pressure on the triceps.
- You might suggest that your client place the hand of her nonworking arm on her working triceps to increase focus and activation.
- This exercise may also be done with a palms-down grip.
- Watch for the tendency to bend the wrist at the top of the movement. Bending the wrist should be avoided.

LYING BARBELL TRICEPS EXTENSION

Primary muscle worked

Triceps brachii

Secondary muscles worked

Anconeus, anterior deltoid, subscapularis, pectoralis minor, latissimus dorsi, pectoralis major, subclavius

Objective

To bend and straighten the arms at the elbow

How to do it

Lie faceup on a flat bench. Your knees should be bent and your feet should be flat on the bench. Grasp a straight or curled bar in your hands. Straighten your arms so that the weight is over your head and your upper arms are at about nipple level. Your upper arms should be at a 90-degree angle to your body and to the bench. Keeping your upper arms stationary, lower the weight to your forehead by flexing your elbows. Straighten your arms and repeat.

Remind your client

- Do not move your upper arms. Concentrate on moving at the elbow joint and flexing the triceps. This exercise is sometimes called a "skull crusher."
- Keep your elbows in line and in the same plane with your shoulders.
- Do not arch your back. Make sure your feet are up on the bench.

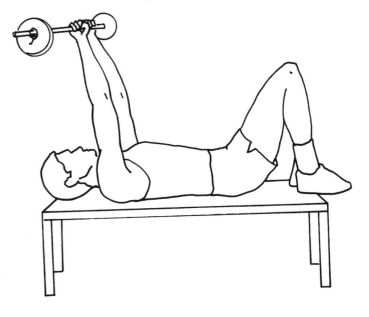

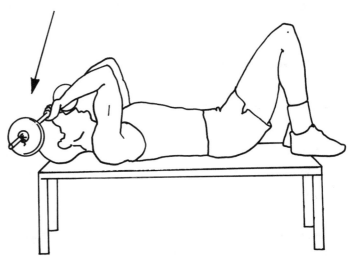

Trainer's pointers

- Reassure your client by placing your hands just above and to the sides of his head. Constantly monitor the position of the elbows to make sure they are in line with the shoulders.
- Watch for the tendency to flex or extend the wrists.
- A curled bar is easier on the wrists and forearms than a straight bar.
- To keep his elbows in line with his shoulders, have your client visualize holding a ball between his elbows.

LYING DUMBBELL TRICEPS EXTENSION

Primary muscle worked

Triceps brachii

Secondary muscles worked

Anconeus, anterior deltoid, subscapularis, pectoralis minor, latissimus dorsi, pectoralis major, subclavius

Objective

To bend and straighten the arms at the elbow

How to do it

Lie on your back on a flat bench with your feet up on the bench. Grasp one dumbbell in each hand. Straighten your arms with your palms in and your elbows in the same plane as your shoulders. Your arms should be at a 90-degree angle to your body and the bench. Lower the dumbbells to ear level by flexing at the elbow. Return to the start position by straightening, but not hyperextending, your elbows.

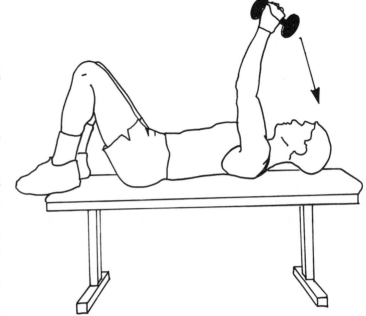

Remind your client

- Do not move your upper arms. Keep them at a 90-degree angle to your upper body.
- Keep your elbows in line with your shoulders. Do not allow them to flare out away from your body.
- Do not flex, extend, or deviate the wrist.

Trainer's pointers

- Spot the client by placing your hands on the ends of the dumbbells. Don't take resistance off, but rather reassure your client that you will be there to take the dumbbells if he needs you to.

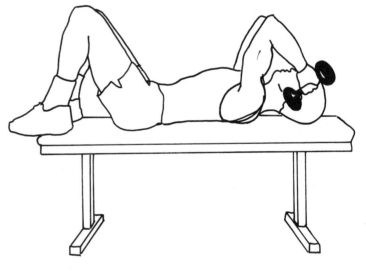

- Watch for the tendency to bend the wrist at the top of the movement. Bending the wrist should be avoided.
- To keep his elbows in line with his shoulders, have your client visualize holding a ball between his elbows.

SEATED DUMBBELL TRICEPS EXTENSION

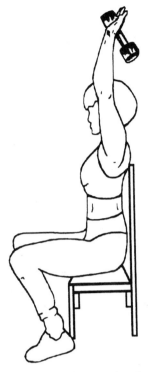 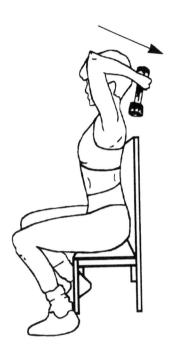 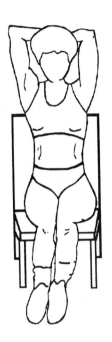

Primary muscle worked

Triceps brachii

Secondary muscles worked

Anconeus, anterior deltoid, trapezius (upper division), levator scapulae

Objective

To bend and straighten the arms at the elbow

How to do it

Sit on a chair or on a bench with a back support. Grasp one dumbbell in both hands with your fingers around the plate at one end. Straighten your arms so the weight is over your head and your upper arms are next to your ears. Keeping your upper arms stationary, lower the weight behind your head to the back of your neck by flexing only at your elbow joints. Straighten your arms and repeat.

Remind your client

- Do not move your upper arms. Concentrate on flexing the triceps.
- The only action should be at the elbow joint.
- Keep your elbows next to your head.
- If your upper arms move forward, you might whack yourself in the head.

Trainer's pointers

- Your client should go through a full range of motion. Make sure she lowers the weight all the way to the base of her neck and completely straightens the elbows on each rep.
- Some clients have insufficient range of motion in the shoulder joint to do this exercise correctly.
- Watch for the tendency to bend the wrist at the top of the movement. Bending the wrist should be avoided.
- To keep her elbows in line with her shoulders, have your client visualize holding a ball between her elbows.

DOUBLE SEATED TRICEPS KICKBACK

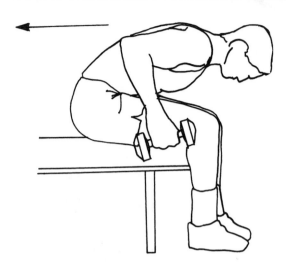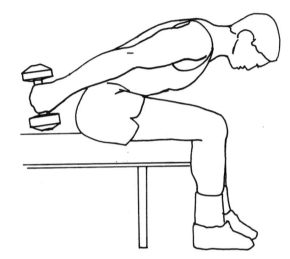

Primary muscle worked

Triceps brachii

Secondary muscles worked

Anconeus, latissimus dorsi, teres major, posterior deltoid

Objective

To straighten the arm at the elbow

How to do it

Sit on the end of a bench and bend forward at the waist. Grasp a dumbbell in each hand, palms in. Flex your elbows to 90 degrees and place your upper arms against your body. Your upper arms should be parallel with the ground. Straighten your arms at the elbows. Pause a moment when your arms are straight before returning them to 90 degrees of elbow flexion.

Remind your client

- Do not move at the shoulder joint! Keep your upper arms parallel to the ground and next to your body.
- Do not rock your body.
- Maintain the four-finger space between your pelvis and rib cage—don't slouch!

Trainer's pointers

- Make sure your client completely straightens his arms and goes through a full range of motion.
- Watch the position of the upper arms. They tend to move forward out of the horizontal position as the client fatigues.
- Make sure your client keeps his scapula in line with his spinal column.
- Watch for the tendency to bend the wrist at the top of the movement. Bending the wrist should be avoided.

SINGLE SEATED TRICEPS KICKBACK

Primary muscle worked

Triceps brachii

Secondary muscles worked

Anconeus, latissimus dorsi, teres major, posterior deltoid

Objective

To bend and straighten the arm at the elbow

How to do it

Your body should be in the same position as it is for the dumbbell row. The upper part of the working arm should be parallel with the ground. Grasp a dumbbell in one hand, bend your arm at the elbow, and place the upper arm against your body. You should begin with your elbow flexed 90 degrees and your palm facing your body. Straighten the working arm by extending at the elbow joint. Pause, then return the elbow to the flexed position. After you have completed the designated number of repetitions, switch arms.

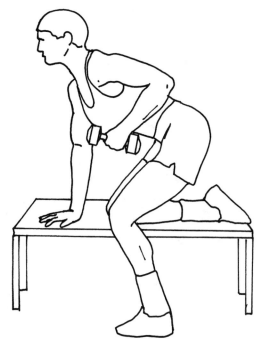

Remind your client

- You must not allow the upper arm to move during this exercise. There is only one axis of rotation in this exercise, the elbow joint.
- Do not do this exercise without supporting your back.
- Keep your weight on your leg, not on your wrist.
- Maintain the four-finger space between your pelvis and rib cage. Keep your back flat.

Trainer's pointers

- Watch for the tendency for the upper arm to drop. It should stay parallel to the ground at a 90-degree angle.
- Make sure your client fully extends his elbow. There is a tendency to cheat by not straightening the arm completely.
- Make sure your client keeps his scapula in line with the spinal column, that is, keeps the four-finger space.
- Check that your client keeps his weight on the leg, not the wrist.
- Watch for the tendency to bend the wrist at the top of the movement. Bending the wrist should be avoided.

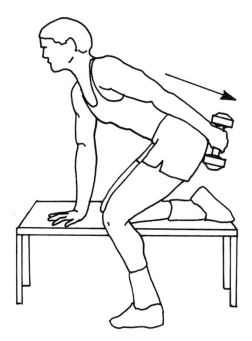

BENCH DIP

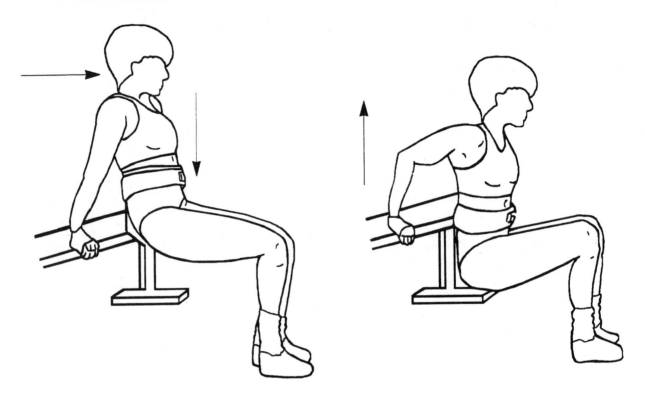

Primary muscle worked

Triceps brachii

Secondary muscles worked

Anconeus, rhomboid, latissimus dorsi, teres major, posterior deltoid

Objective

To bend and straighten the arms at the elbow

How to do it

Sit on a bench with your hands next to your hips. With your knees bent, lift your body off the bench. Your weight should be resting on your arms, which should be straight. Lower your body by flexing at the elbows. Flex your elbows to 90 degrees. Return to the start position by straightening your arms at the elbows.

Remind your client

- Do not move excessively at the knee or hip joints. Remember, the main axis of rotation is the elbow, not the shoulder.
- Flex the elbows to 90 degrees.
- Keep the upper trapezius and neck relaxed.

Trainer's pointers

- If the exercise is easy for the client with her knees bent, have her straighten them.
- Make sure your client flexes her elbows to about 90 degrees and doesn't cheat by trying to move only at the shoulder.
- Before the client begins, make sure her hands are not too far apart! The hands should be right next to her hips.

CLOSE-GRIP PUSH-UP

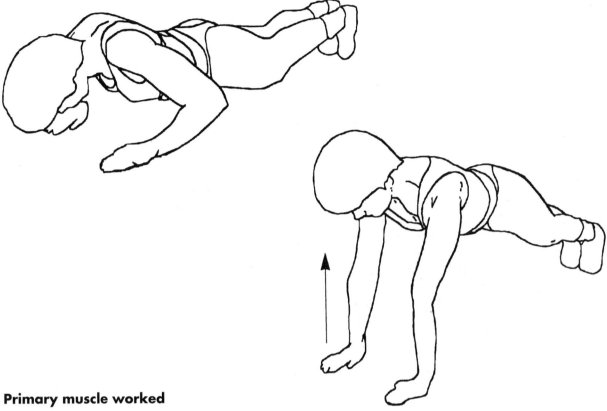

Primary muscle worked
Triceps brachii

Secondary muscles worked
Anterior deltoid, subscapularis, pectoralis minor, latissimus dorsi, pectoralis major, subclavius

Objective
To push the body up by straightening the arms at the elbow

How to do it
Begin on the floor or on a mat on all fours. Keeping the hands directly under the shoulders, straighten the spine by straightening the knees and tucking the toes under. The abdominals should be contracted to keep the spine firm and straight. Keeping the knees rigid, flex the elbows and lower the body as a single unit until the chest is approximately 2 inches (5.1 cm) from the floor.

Remind your client
- Don't flex or extend the body at the hips or knees. Both must stay rigid.
- Keep the neck relaxed. Don't turtle!
- Don't rest all of the body's weight on the wrist. Try to distribute it across all of the fingers.
- Go through a full range of motion.

Trainer's pointers
- Beginners can do this exercise on the knees (easy), on an incline (easier), or against the wall (easiest). If your client cannot complete the exercise through a full range of motion, have her perform an easier version.
- Spot your client by kneeling next to her and placing one hand on the front of her body at pelvic level. Use your other hand to cue her to relax the neck if needed.

CLOSE-GRIP BENCH PRESS

Primary muscle worked

Triceps brachii

Secondary muscles worked

Anterior deltoid, subscapularis, pectoralis minor, latissimus dorsi, pectoralis major, subclavius

Objective

To press the bar up by straightening the arms

How to do it

Lie on your back on a bench with bar supports. Your knees should be bent and your feet should be resting on the bench. Grasp the bar with a shoulder-width (and no wider) grip. With the help of your trainer or spotter, lift the bar off the supports. Beginning with your arms straight, lower the bar until it is an inch (2.5 cm) away from your chest. Press it up slowly and under control. Repeat for the required number of repetitions.

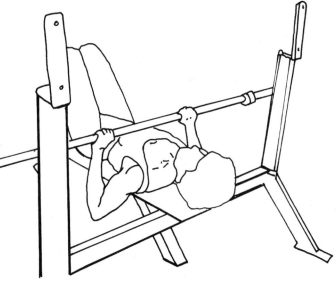

Remind your client

- Keep the wrists rigid.
- Unlike the regular bench press, during the down phase of the repetition, your upper arms should stay close to the upper body. The elbows should point down, not out.

Trainer's pointers

- Watch for uneven arm elevation.
- The bar should be at about the mid-point of the sternum throughout the exercise.
- If your client is tall or has a long torso, place another bench or step at the end of the bench for her to put her feet on.

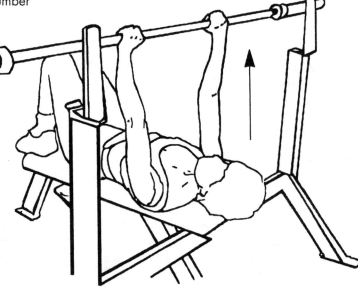

HIP FLEXOR STRETCH

How to do it

Kneel with one knee on the ground and the opposite foot on the ground. Keeping the front foot stationary, slide the rear foot back until the instep rests on the ground. Gently try to push the rear foot toward the floor.

Form points

- Make sure that the knee of the front foot doesn't move forward past the instep of the foot.
- Do not rotate the spine.

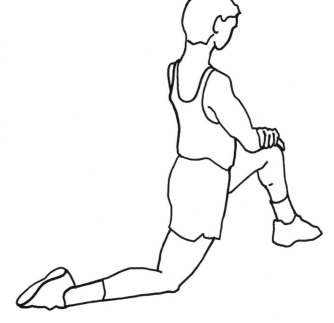

LYING HIP ABDUCTOR STRETCH

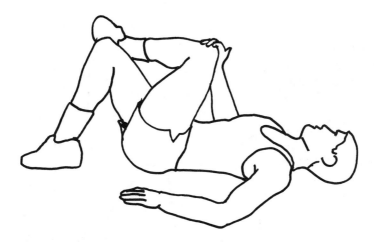

How to do it

Lie on your back with your knees bent. Place your left ankle on your right knee. Place your right hand on the outside of your left knee and gently press it toward your right shoulder. Feel the stretch deep in the left glute. Hold the stretch for 30 to 40 seconds. Repeat with the other side.

Note that this stretch **effectively targets the piriformis muscle** (a deep muscle that laterally rotates the femur at the hip), often a sore spot.

QUADRICEPS STRETCH

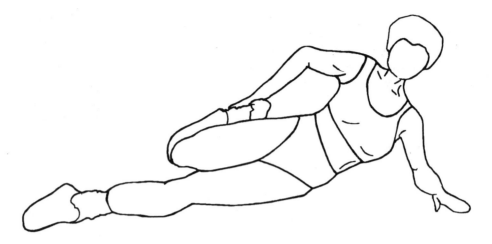

How to do it

Lie on your side on the floor. Keeping the bottom leg straight, flex the knee so that you can grasp the ankle of the top leg. Gently pull the heel of this leg toward your gluteus to stretch the quadriceps. Repeat with the other leg.

Form points

- Make sure you don't overstretch your knee.
- Don't let your body roll.

LYING HAMSTRING STRETCH

How to do it

Lie on your back with your knees bent. Straighten one leg. Place your hands behind the thigh of this leg. Keeping your gluteus down, try to bring the thigh as close to your chest as you can while keeping the leg straight. Repeat with the other leg.

Form point

Make sure that the gluteus stays down on the floor.

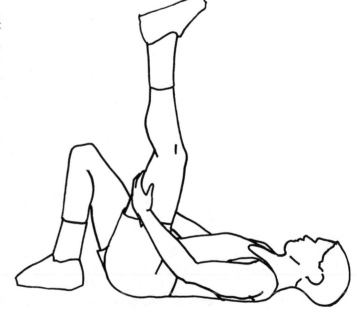

LYING GLUTEUS STRETCH

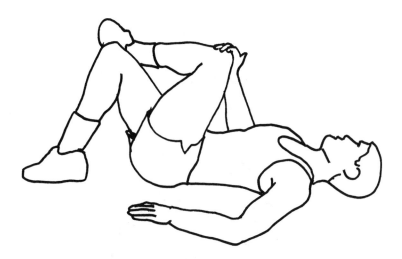

How to do it

Lie on your back with your knees bent. Place the left ankle on the right knee. Keep the right foot on the floor. Gently pull the right knee toward the left shoulder. Repeat on the other side.

Form points

- Keep the shoulders on the floor.
- Keep the neck relaxed.

LOW BACK STRETCH

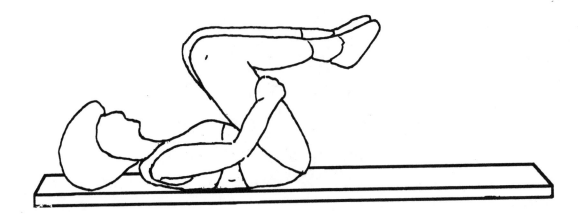

How to do it

Lie on your back. Bend both knees and lift your feet off the ground. Place your hands behind your knees and hug them into your chest while pressing your low back into the floor.

Form point

Keep the neck relaxed.

SEATED GLUTEUS AND HIP STRETCH

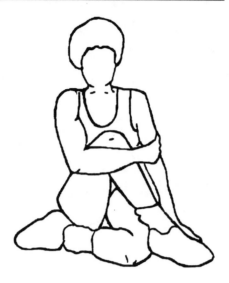

How to do it

Sit with your left leg extended at a 45-degree angle from your body. Bend the knee of the right leg and place the right foot outside the left thigh. Place your right hand behind you and the left hand on the right knee. Bend the left knee. Gently pull the bent knee toward your shoulder. Repeat on the opposite side.

Form point

Make sure your weight is evenly distributed on each hipbone. Don't lean.

GROIN STRETCH

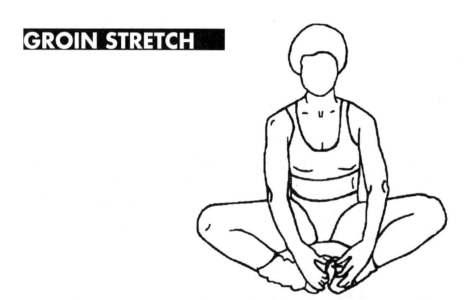

How to do it

Sit with your knees bent and the bottoms of your feet together. Create a space between your rib cage and your pelvis by lifting your chest and pulling in your low abdominals. Try to push your knees to the floor. Leading with your chest, lean forward at the waist.

Form points

- Relax your neck.
- Keep your chest elevated—don't lose your four-finger space.

PECTORALS AND ANTERIOR DELTOID STRETCH

How to do it

Stand with your fingers interlocked behind you. Pull your shoulder blades together and down.

Form points

- Don't turtle.
- Don't pull excessively on the wrists. The objective is to pull the shoulder blades together.

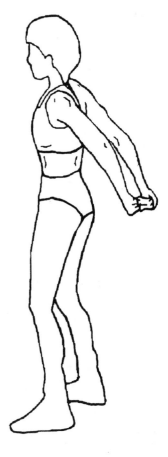

SUPERMAN STRETCH

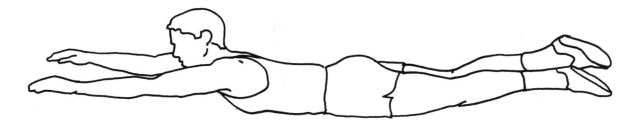

How to do it

Lie on the floor facedown with your legs and arms outstretched. Lift your chest, arms, and legs simultaneously and hold.

Form points

- Keep the neck relaxed.
- This is an advanced stretch that helps strengthen the low back. It might not be appropriate for beginners or those with very weak low backs, and is definitely not appropriate for those with known low-back pathology. If in doubt about its safety for any client, try modifying it by having the client keep the legs on the floor and just lifting the chest and arms. Progress to arms plus one leg, then opposite arm and leg, and finally the version shown.

QUADRATUS LUMBORUM SIDE STRETCH

How to do it

Sit with your right leg extended at a 45-degree angle to your body and the left knee bent. The right toe should point toward the ceiling. Create the four-finger space between your pelvis and rib cage by lifting the chest and pulling in the lower abdominals. Slide the right hand next to the right calf. Straighten the left arm and reach to the ceiling. (The left arm should be next to your head.) Keeping your chest forward and your scapula in line with the spinal column, lean sideways toward the right leg. Try to get the right elbow down to the floor. Repeat on the other side.

Form points

- Make sure the shoulder blade of the out-stretched arm stays in line with the spinal column.

- Make sure the torso stays in the frontal plane.

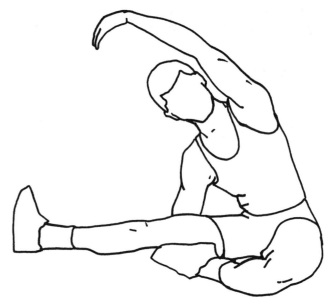

GASTROCNEMIUS STRETCH

How to do it

Stand about 12 inches (30.5 cm) away from a wall. Place the left foot forward and extend the right foot back. Place your forearms against the wall. Lean into the wall and keep the right leg straight with the heel down to stretch its gastrocnemius. Repeat on the other side.

Form points

- It's important to keep the heel down. If you can't, move the left leg closer to the wall. As the stretch gets easier, you can move the right leg farther away from the wall.
- Keep the pelvis straight and facing forward.
- Make sure the left knee does not extend past the foot.

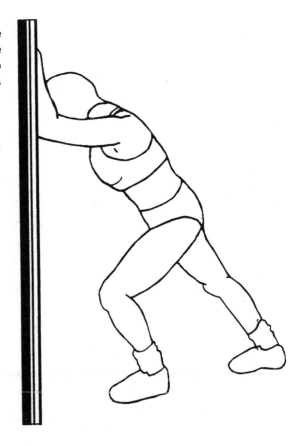

SOLEUS STRETCH

How to do it

Same as gastrocnemius stretch, except that you bend the knee of the extended leg.

Form point

Same as gastrocnemius stretch.

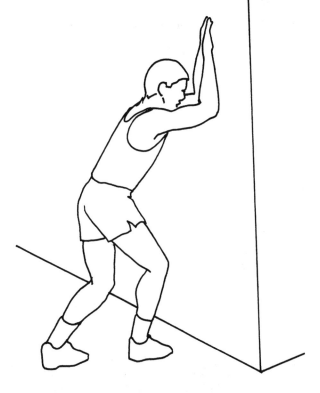

DOOR STRETCH

How to do it

Stand in a doorway. Flex your elbows 90 degrees and place your forearms against the door frame. With your feet behind the doorway, lean into the door space.

Form points

- Make sure that forearms stay against the door frame.
- Don't turtle.

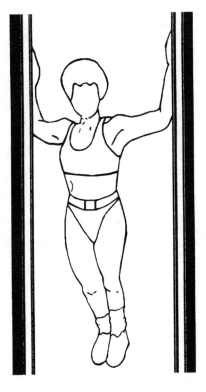

POSTERIOR DELTOID STRETCH

How to do it

Place one hand just above the elbow of one arm. Gently pull the upper arm toward your chest. Switch sides.

Form points

- Keep your scapulae pulled down and in line with each other.
- Don't turtle.

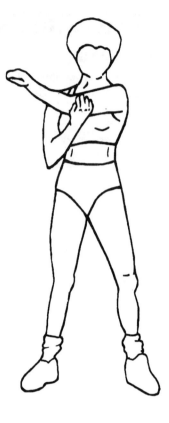

INTERNAL/EXTERNAL ROTATOR CUFF STRETCH

How to do it

Standing or seated, straighten your right arm up next to your head. The upper portion of the arm should be next to your head and the forearm should be behind your back, with the palm of the hand and fingers resting on your back between the shoulder blades. Reaching down with the right arm and up with the left, try to touch a finger from each hand together between your shoulder blades. Then reverse arms.

Form point

If it's impossible for you to get your fingers together, use a towel and try to get a little closer together each time by inching your fingers up and down the towel.

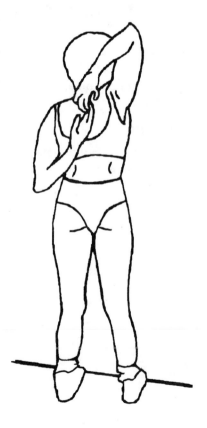

TRICEPS AND LATERAL FLEXION STRETCH

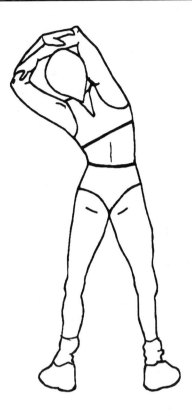

How to do it

Stand. Lift both arms up next to your head. Flex your elbows and place each hand on the opposite arm. Exert gentle pressure on the left elbow while leaning slightly to the right. Switch sides.

Form points

- This exercise can also be done seated.
- Do not hyperextend your neck. Keep your chin down so that your neck is in line with the spine.

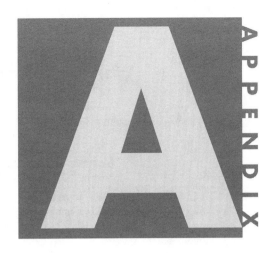

Sample Forms

Waiver, Release, and Assumption of Risk

Waiver and Assumption of Risk (Home Workouts)

Letter of Agreement

Health History Questionnaire

Medical Clearance and Physician's Consent to Participate in Fitness Assessment and Exercise Program

Injury Report

Goal Inventory

Lifestyle Questionnaire

Notes on Using the Workout Record Form

Workout Record

Waiver, Release, and Assumption of Risk

This form is an important legal document. It explains the risks you are assuming by beginning an exercise program. It is critical that you read and understand it completely. After you have done so, please print your name legibly and sign in the spaces provided at the bottom.

Waiver, Informed Consent, and Covenant Not to Sue

I,_____, have volunteered to participate in a program of physical exercise under the direction of **(your business's name),** which will include, but may not be limited to, weight and/or resistance training. In consideration of **(your business's name)** agreement to instruct, assist, and train me, I do here and forever release and discharge and hereby hold harmless **(your business's name),** and their respective agents, heirs, assigns, contractors, and employees from any and all claims, demands, damages, rights of action, or causes of action, present or future, arising out of or connected with my participation in this or any exercise program including any injuries resulting therefrom. THIS WAIVER AND RELEASE OF LIABILITY INCLUDES, WITHOUT LIMITATION, INJURIES WHICH MAY OCCUR AS A RESULT OF (1) EQUIPMENT THAT MAY MALFUNCTION OR BREAK; (2) ANY SLIP, FALL, DROPPING OF EQUIPMENT; AND (3) OUR NEGLIGENT INSTRUCTION OR SUPERVISION.

Assumption of Risk

I,_____, recognize that exercise might be difficult and strenuous and that there could be dangers inherent in exercise for some individuals. I acknowledge that the possibility of certain unusual physical changes during exercise does exist. These changes include abnormal blood pressure; fainting; disorders in heartbeat; heart attack; and, in rare instances, death.

I understand that as a result of my participation in an exercise program, I could suffer an injury or physical disorder that could result in my becoming partially or totally disabled and incapable of performing any gainful employment or having a normal social life.

I recognize that an examination by a physician should be obtained by all participants prior to involvement in any exercise program. If I,_____, have chosen not to obtain a physician's permission prior to beginning this exercise program with **(your business's name),** I hereby agree that I am doing so at my own risk.

In any event, I acknowledge and agree that I assume the risks associated with any and all activities and/or exercises in which I participate.

I acknowledge and agree that no warranties or representations have been made to me regarding the results I will achieve from this program. I understand that results are individual and may vary.

I ACKNOWLEDGE THAT I HAVE THOROUGHLY READ THIS WAIVER AND RELEASE AND FULLY UNDERSTAND THAT IT IS A RELEASE OF LIABILITY. BY SIGNING THIS DOCUMENT, I AM WAIVING ANY RIGHT I OR MY SUCCESSORS MIGHT HAVE TO BRING A LEGAL ACTION OR ASSERT A CLAIM AGAINST (YOUR BUSINESS NAME) FOR YOUR NEGLIGENCE OR THAT OF YOUR EMPLOYEES, AGENTS, OR CONTRACTORS.

_____   _____
Participant's signature   Date

_____
Please print name

Waiver and Assumption of Risk (Home Workouts)

Please note: This form is to be used in addition to, and not in lieu of, the general Waiver, Release, and Assumption of Risk.

This Agreement, dated this _____ day of _____, 200___, by and between _____ ("Client") and **(your business's name)** ("Consultant").

Recitals

1. I, _____, have requested that Consultant, through its authorized agents or contractors, conduct our training sessions in my home.

2. I will provide the equipment to be used in connection with our workouts, including but not limited to benches, dumbbells, barbells, and similar items (the "Equipment"), and I will have control over the area in which we perform our workouts.

In consideration of Consultant's agreeing to conduct our training sessions in my home, I hereby agree as follows:

1. I acknowledge and agree that (i) Consultant (or, if applicable, any independent contractor employed by Consultant) has not inspected the Equipment, and that (ii) I have sole custody and control of the area in my home in which workouts will be conducted and that I am solely responsible for the condition of the Equipment.

2. I hereby agree to hold Consultant, and their respective agents, assigns, employees, and contractors, harmless from any loss or damage resulting from or connected with any injury that I sustain as a result of any defect, latent or apparent, in the design or condition of the Equipment, and/or the condition of the area in which we work out, and I hereby assume any and all risks connected with the condition or design of the Equipment and the condition of such area.

3. I hereby assume any and all risks arising from or connected with any hazardous condition in my home, in the specific area in which the workouts are conducted or otherwise, that may result in my injury during any workout with Consultant or Consultant's agents, employees, or contractors.

4. This waiver and release of liability includes, without limitation, injuries which may occur as a result of (i) equipment that may malfunction or break; (ii) any slip, fall, dropping of equipment; (iii) any improper maintenance of equipment or facilities; (iv) any hazardous condition that may exist on the premises, including the specific workout area, my home, and the surrounding property; and (v) your negligent instruction or supervision.

5. I acknowledge that I have thoroughly read this waiver and release and fully understand that it is a release of liability. By signing this document, I am waiving any right I or my successors might have to bring a legal action or assert a claim against **(your business's name)** for your negligence or that of your employees, agents, or contractors.

AGREED AND ACCEPTED THIS _____ DAY OF _____, 200___.

_____
Client's signature

_____
Please print name

Letter of Agreement

This Agreement made and entered into this _____ day of _____, 200___, by and between _____ ("Client") and _____ ("Trainer").

In consideration of the mutual promises exchanged herein and other good and valuable consideration, the parties agree as follows:

1. Client and Trainer have agreed that Trainer will conduct ___ one-hour workout sessions. Each session will begin at a mutually convenient, agreed-upon time and shall be subject to the policies attached hereto as "Exhibit A."

2. Client will pay Trainer, in advance, the sum of $_____ for these workout sessions. Client acknowledges and agrees that no credit or refund shall be due for sessions canceled by Client, except as provided in the Policies attached hereto as Exhibit A.

3. Concurrently with the execution of this Agreement, Client has executed and delivered to Trainer a Waiver and Assumption of Risk Agreement and a Waiver for Home Workouts Agreement (if applicable) (these agreements herein collectively referred to as the "Waiver Agreements"), in which Client assumes the risk of participating in an exercise program and agrees that Trainer and his or her agents, employees, or contractors, if any, shall have no liability for any injury, illness, or similar difficulty that Client may suffer arising out of or connected with Client's participation in Trainer's program. Client hereby acknowledges and agrees that the execution and delivery of the Waiver Agreements are material inducements to Trainer's permitting Client to participate in Trainer's program and agrees to be bound by same.

4. Client and Trainer may agree to conduct additional sessions at such times and locations as they may agree upon, and in such event (i) the provisions of this Agreement, including the Policies attached hereto as Exhibit A, shall be deemed to apply to such additional sessions and (ii) Client will pay Trainer, in advance, the sum of $_____. Client acknowledges and agrees that no credit or refund shall be due for sessions canceled by Client, except as provided in the Policies attached hereto as Exhibit A.

IN WITNESS WHEREOF, Client and Trainer have caused this Agreement to be executed on the day and year first above written.

by: _____
Trainer's signature

_____
Trainer, please print name

by: _____
Client's signature

_____
Client, please print name

Exhibit A

Policies

1. Sessions last about one hour. Please be *ready to begin* at your scheduled time.

2. Time slots are available on a "first-come, first-served" basis by appointment. Clients who train on a monthly basis will usually have priority since they can schedule regular standing times (for example, Monday, Wednesday, and Friday at 5:30 P.M.).

3. About cancellations:

   a. During the period of your first _____ sessions ("Initial Training Period"), you will receive no credit for canceled or missed workouts, *regardless of the reason*, unless we cancel, in which case you'll receive a free workout for each session canceled.

   b. If you continue as a client after your Initial Training Period, you will pay the monthly rate and receive credit for canceled sessions as follows:

   $_____ per session, subject to paragraphs c–g below

   c. You will not receive credit for any workout unless it was canceled with at least 24 hours' advance notification. Cancellations must be given by calling _____ to be deemed effective.

   d. You will not receive credit for more than one (1) canceled workout per month unless we cancel, in which case you will receive credit for each canceled workout.

   e. If you receive credit for a missed workout, you must use the credit within 60 days of the missed workout, or it will be waived.

   f. If you are entitled to credit in accordance with this paragraph, such credit will appear on the following month's invoice and shall not be deducted from the current month's invoice.

   g. No credit shall be due if a session is canceled due to any of the following: floods, fires, earthquakes, tornadoes, power failure, or similar severe weather conditions or acts of God making travel extremely difficult or impossible; automobile accidents involving you or resulting in your inability to arrive at your scheduled workout; or any event of similar magnitude, beyond the control of the parties. (You will still get credit if we cancel because we are involved in an accident, illness, or other difficulty.) See the following paragraph for holiday credits.

   _____
   Client's initials

4. Payment is due in advance of the first session. If you are training on a monthly basis, you will receive a statement on or about the first of the month, which is due and payable on or before the fifth of the month. If you want to train on a monthly basis but your start date is on a date other than the first of the month, you will be billed a prorated amount for the month that you start. Then you will receive an invoice on the first of the next month. If a regularly scheduled session occurs on one of the following holidays, no credit is due: President's Day, Memorial Day, the Fourth of July, Labor Day, Thanksgiving Day, Christmas Day, New Year's Day. Sometimes holidays necessitate schedule modifications. For example, the gym may close early on Christmas Eve or New Year's Eve. If you are unavailable to modify your schedule to fit in a workout under these circumstances, no credit will be due.

5. You will be required to sign and return the following forms to me before taking a fitness evaluation or beginning any program:

   a. Waiver, Release, and Assumption of Risk

   b. Waiver and Assumption of Risk (Home Workouts), if applicable

   c. Health History Questionnaire

   d. Goal Inventory

6. If you have any of the following physical conditions, you will be required to have a Medical Clearance and Physician's Consent Form:

   a. Hypertension (>145/95 mm Hg)

   b. Hyperlipidemia (cholesterol >220 mg/dl or a total cholesterol-to-HDL ratio of >5.0)

   c. Diabetes

   d. Family history of heart disease prior to age 60

   e. Smoking

   f. Abnormal resting EKG

   g. Any other condition that I in my sole discretion may deem to present an unreasonable risk to your health, were you to participate in a fitness evaluation or program.

7. Clients will be required to keep a food diary for 2 weeks at the beginning of the program. After 2 weeks, the diary will be analyzed for nutritional content, and I will make suggestions to help you improve your diet.

8. Clients are required to observe any and all rules of the gym or facility where workouts take place.

9. Shirts and shoes are required at all times during sessions. I suggest that you also bring a towel and a lock, since these are not supplied at the gym.

10. Clients have the right to terminate a particular exercise or workout at any time. **You are in control of your workouts!** If an exercise is uncomfortable or painful, or if you want to stop for any reason, you may do so. If a particular exercise is painful for you to do or you have an injury or other limitation that makes it difficult for you to do, I can probably substitute another exercise to work that particular muscle group.

11. Clients are encouraged to drink plenty of water during the workout. You do not need my permission to get a drink or go to the bathroom.

12. You will get from your workouts what you put in. I will show you how to work your muscles correctly and encourage you to go to your safe limit, but whether you reach your goal is ultimately up to you. You are the only one who can make sure you work out consistently (missing workouts is a guarantee to get nowhere!), eat properly, rest enough, and live a healthful lifestyle.

_____

Client's signature

 From Teri S. O'Brien. 2003. *The Personal Trainer's Handbook, Second Edition*. Champaign, IL: Human Kinetics.

Health History Questionnaire

Name _____ Date _____

Street address _____ City _____

Phone (home) _____ (work) _____

Email address _____ (cell phone) _____

Person to contact in case of emergency: Date of birth_____

Name_____ Phone _____

For most people, physical activity should not pose any problem or hazard. The following questions are designed to identify the small number of adults for whom physical activity might be inappropriate or those who should have medical advice concerning the type of activity most suitable for them.

Common sense is your best guide in answering these questions. Please read them carefully and check the "Yes" or "No" response opposite the question if it applies to you.

Yes   No

___   ___   1. Has your doctor ever said you have heart trouble? If yes, please describe the problem and state when it was diagnosed.

_____

_____

___   ___   2. Do you frequently have pain in your heart or chest?

___   ___   3. Do you often feel faint or have spells of severe dizziness?

___   ___   4. Has a doctor ever told you that your blood pressure was too high?

___   ___   5. Has your doctor ever told you that you have a bone or joint problem, such as arthritis, that has been aggravated by exercise or might be made worse by exercise?

___   ___   6. Is there a good physical reason not mentioned here why you should not follow an activity program even if you wanted to do so?

___   ___   7. Are you over age 65 and/or not accustomed to vigorous exercise?

___   ___   8. Are you or have you ever been a diabetic?

___   ___   9. Are you now pregnant, or have you been pregnant within the last 3 months?

___   ___   10. Have you had any surgery in the last 3 months?

___   ___   11. Have you been hospitalized in the last 2 years? If so, when and why?

_____

___   ___   12. Have you ever seen a chiropractor, acupuncturist, or other alternative medicine practitioner? If so, when and why?

_____

Please check the box if you have ever experienced any of the following symptoms:

	When first experienced	Treatment used
❑ Pain or discomfort in the chest	_____	_____
❑ Unaccustomed shortness of breath	_____	_____
❑ Dizziness	_____	_____
❑ Labored or uncomfortable breathing, with or without pain	_____	_____
❑ Swollen ankles	_____	_____
❑ Heart palpitations	_____	_____
❑ Heart murmur	_____	_____
❑ Limping	_____	_____

❑ Yes ❑ No   Do you have high blood pressure? If yes, what is your current blood pressure without medication?

_____

❑ Yes ❑ No   Are you taking any medication for hypertension? If so, what medication?

_____

❑ Yes ❑ No   Is your total serum cholesterol level over 240?

❑ Yes ❑ No   Do you smoke?

❑ Yes ❑ No   Have you ever smoked? If so, when did you quit?

❑ Yes ❑ No   Do you have diabetes?

❑ Yes ❑ No   Do you have a family member who has had coronary or atherosclerotic disease before age 55?

❑ Yes ❑ No   Do you have pain or discomfort in your back?

❑ Yes ❑ No   Do you have pain or discomfort in your knee?   If so, ❑ right or ❑ left?

❑ Yes ❑ No   Do you have pain or discomfort in your shoulder?   If so, ❑ right or ❑ left?

❑ Yes ❑ No   Do you have pain or discomfort in your elbow?   If so, ❑ right or ❑ left?

❑ Yes ❑ No   Do you have pain or discomfort in your wrist?   If so, ❑ right or ❑ left?

❑ Yes ❑ No   Do you have pain or discomfort in your ankle?   If so, ❑ right or ❑ left?

If you checked "Yes" above, please describe your pain. On a scale of 1 to 10, with 1 being almost nonexistent and 10 being excruciating, how severe is it? Does it get more or less severe as the day goes on? When do you notice it? What really aggravates it?

_____

_____

_____

_____

❑ Yes ❑ No   Have you ever torn ligaments or cartilage in your knee? If so, when? _____

Did you have surgery on this knee? If so, when? _____

❑ Yes ❑ No   Have you ever dislocated your shoulder? If so, when?

_____

❑ Yes ❑ No   Have you ever had shoulder surgery? If so, which shoulder? When?

_____

❑ Yes ❑ No   Have you ever had a neck injury, such as whiplash? If so, when?

_____

❑ Yes ❑ No   Have you ever been treated for a spinal disk injury? If so, when?

_____

❑ Yes ❑ No   Do you ever experience tingling or numbness in your elbows or hands?

_____

What is the present state of your general health? _____

What regular physical activities do you do now? _____

How often? _____ For how long each session? _____

I, _____, certify that I understand the foregoing questions and my answers are true and complete. I also understand that this information is being provided as part of my initial consultation and may not be periodically updated.

I, _____, assume the risk for any changes in my medical condition that might affect my ability to exercise.

_____   _____
Signature   Date

If you answered yes to one or more questions and you have not recently consulted with your doctor, do so before beginning an exercise program. Tell your doctor which questions you answered yes to and explain that you plan to undergo an exercise program that may include, but may not be limited to, weight and/or resistance training. After medical evaluation, ask your doctor

1. which activities you may safely participate in, and
2. what specific restrictions, if any, should apply to your condition and which activities and/or exercises you should avoid.

I, _____, acknowledge that I have read the foregoing statements and understand the content thereof.

_____   _____
Signature   Date

Medical Clearance and Physician's Consent to Participate in Fitness Assessment and Exercise Program

To: **(your name, address, city, state, and zip)**

Dear Personal Trainer:

My patient, _____, has advised me that he or she intends to participate in (1) a fitness assessment, including body composition assessment, muscular endurance and flexibility tests, a blood pressure reading, and cardiovascular fitness assessment; and (2) an exercise program, which will include, but not be limited to, resistance training. The sessions will last approximately 1 hour and will begin at a very moderate, submaximal level.

Please be advised that my patient, _____, should be subject to the following restrictions in the fitness assessment and/or in his or her exercise program:

_____

_____

_____

In addition, under no circumstances should he or she do the following:

_____

_____

I have discussed the foregoing restrictions and limitations with my patient, _____, and, with these specific restrictions, he or she has my permission to participate in a fitness assessment and pursue an exercise program under your guidance.

Very truly yours,

_____
Please sign name here

_____
Please print name here

Date: _____

Phone number: _____

 From Teri S. O'Brien. 2003. *The Personal Trainer's Handbook, Second Edition.* Champaign, IL: Human Kinetics.

Injury Report

(This report would be used only for serious injuries. Note day-to-day aches or pains in the client's workout record form, and monitor them. If they don't get better, you'll need to refer to a physician.)

Name of injured person _____

Date _____   Time _____ ❑ A.M. or ❑ P.M.

Location

_____

_____

What happened? (describe the event, and the mechanism of injury)

_____

_____

Anatomical area involved (be sure to specify left or right side)

_____

_____

Witnesses

_____

_____

Action taken (first aid administered, EMS involvement if any)

_____

_____

Referral action? ❑ yes or ❑ no

If yes, to whom referred? _____

_____

Trainer's signature

Goal Inventory

Client _____   Date _____

1. What I want to accomplish.
   These are my outcome goals for the next 8 weeks:

   _____

   _____

   _____

2. Why I want to accomplish these goals.
   These goals are very important to me because:

   _____

   _____

   _____

3. I'll do almost anything except this.
   I am willing to do anything within reason to reach these goals, other than (please be as specific as possible):

   _____

   _____

   _____

4. "I think that my exercising at least 4 days a week, every week, is highly likely." Please circle the number of the answer that best describes your response to this statement.
   1   Strongly agree
   2   Agree
   3   Disagree
   4   Strongly disagree

   If you circled 3 or 4, why? (Please be as specific as possible.)

   _____

   _____

   _____

5. When I reach this goal, here's what I will get and how I will feel:

   _____

   _____

   _____

 From Teri S. O'Brien. 2003. *The Personal Trainer's Handbook, Second Edition*. Champaign, IL: Human Kinetics.

Lifestyle Questionnaire

Your Attitude Toward Food

Diets

Have you ever been on a diet? If so, please answer the following questions:

How many diets have you been on in the last 2 years? _____

Describe any diets you've been on. Did you go to a commercial weight-loss service (Jenny Craig, Diet Center, etc.)? Did you follow a diet from a book or article? If so, which one?

_____

_____

Describe your experience with diets. Did you lose weight? Did you gain any of it back?

_____

_____

Food

❏ Yes ❏ No   Do you eat breakfast?

❏ Yes ❏ No   Typically, do you eat after 8 P.M.? If so, what do you usually eat?

_____

How many times a day do you eat?

_____

❏ Yes ❏ No   Can you recall ever eating to avoid doing something? If so, when was this?

_____

❏ Yes ❏ No   Do you ever eat when you aren't hungry? If so, when?

_____

How often do you read food labels?

_____

❏ Yes ❏ No   Do you ever "treat" yourself with food? If so, when?

_____

What sources of information about nutrition have you found most helpful?

_____

❏ Yes ❏ No   Has someone ever encouraged you to eat something that is not in your best interest? If yes, did you do it? Why?

_____

Your Attitude Toward Exercise: What's the Point of All of This, Anyway?

You need to create a clear, tangible image in your mind of the benefits of staying on your fitness program. It must be vivid and powerful enough to sustain you through difficult times when you feel your self-discipline and motivation slipping. This exercise will help you create that image.

Complete this sentence: "Doing three cardiovascular exercise sessions and two to three resistance training sessions per week will . . ."

	Not likely				Very likely	
Improve my appearance	1	2	3	4	5	6
Allow me to cope with stress better	1	2	3	4	5	6
Help me avoid getting sick	1	2	3	4	5	6
Give me a powerful sense of personal achievement	1	2	3	4	5	6
Increase my self-esteem	1	2	3	4	5	6
Improve my physical strength	1	2	3	4	5	6
Make me more independent	1	2	3	4	5	6
Improve my ability to concentrate	1	2	3	4	5	6
Take up too much time	1	2	3	4	5	6
Cause pain, soreness, and discomfort	1	2	3	4	5	6
Make me very tired	1	2	3	4	5	6
Cause me to get injured	1	2	3	4	5	6

Please rewrite this sentence and complete it in your own words.

Doing three cardiovascular sessions and two to three resistance training sessions per week will . . .

_____

_____

Do you need support from others (friends, family, etc.) to stay consistent with your exercise and nutrition program?
❑ Yes ❑ No   Do you have this type of support? ❑ Yes   ❑ No

On a scale of 1 to 10 (with 10 being the ultimate nurturing, supportive group), how would you rate your support from others? _____

Are there people in your life who either intentionally or unintentionally discourage you or interfere with your staying consistent in your exercise and/or nutrition program? ❑ Yes   ❑ No   If yes, how do they interfere? How do you deal with it?

_____

_____

Has someone else ever interfered with your choice to exercise? ❑ Yes ❑ No   If yes, what happened?

_____

If you answered yes to questions 3 or 4, how have you dealt with these situations in the past? What are your thoughts about how to improve these responses in the future?

_____

_____

_____

	Not likely				**Very likely**	
I think it is very likely that I will exercise five times a week.	1	2	3	4	5	6
I think exercise is a waste of time for me.	1	2	3	4	5	6
I know that I will be consistent with my fitness and nutrition program for six months.	1	2	3	4	5	6
When I exercise, I look like a dork.	1	2	3	4	5	6
When I exercise, I always feel beat up afterward.	1	2	3	4	5	6

Notes on Using the Workout Record Form

1. Record the day and date of the session. While it might not seem important, sometimes you will see a pattern that will be helpful in your planning. For example, you might start to notice that a client's energy level on Mondays is distinctly lower than it is during your Wednesday workouts. Then you learn that her work schedule dictates that she be in at 6 A.M. on Mondays for a weekly staff meeting. You can use this information to adjust the intensity of Monday and Wednesday workouts.

2. Write down the time.

3. Record notes on the general warm-up.

4. Refocus your attention on what you and your client are working on during the current phase. A phase can last anywhere from 3 weeks to 4 months, depending on the client's fitness level, goals and objectives, and similar considerations.

5. Record any special needs or concerns affecting this client, such as back problems, shoulder problems, and so forth.

6. Record the order in which the exercises are performed. The reason for this should be obvious. If, for example, you are not able to do the exercises in the order you planned, your client's strength could be affected. Say you planned deadlift then leg curl, but because someone was using the power rack, you reversed the order. This change might affect the difficulty of the leg curl. Then again, it might not, but it's good to know.

7. Record the seat position or other adjustable components of any machine you use.

8. Write down the subjective intensity rating (SIR) for each exercise.

9. Review the workout after it's completed. Consider the client's SIR and your impression of the quality of his form and decide whether to increase the number of repetitions (+#), decrease the rest interval (−↓), increase the amount of weight (+↑), or leave things status quo (↔).

10. Make notes about anything significant that happens during the workout.

11. Abdominals have their own section because you will probably work on them every workout.

12. Record the muscle or muscle groups stretched by checking the appropriate box and, where necessary, writing in the name of the stretch.

13. Record any aches, pains, or problems your client reports. Be as specific as possible.

14. Note any matters you want to talk to your client about.

15. Record your client's most recent weight.

16. Record your client's energy level. How do you know? You ask her at the beginning of the workout.

 From Teri S. O'Brien. 2003. *The Personal Trainer's Handbook, Second Edition.* Champaign, IL: Human Kinetics.

Workout Record

Client's name: _____

1. Day and date	3. Warm-up	4. Goals this phase	Grade of this workout
2. Time		5. Client's limitations, if any	

6. Order Exercise		W	1st Goal	1st Actual	2nd Goal	2nd Actual	3rd Goal	3rd Actual	9.	10. Notes
7. Machine position	Wt								+ # ☐ – ↓ ☐ + ↑ ☐ ↔ ☐	8. SIR
	Reps									
	Rest									
Machine position	Wt								+ # ☐ – ↓ ☐ + ↑ ☐ ↔ ☐	SIR
	Reps									
	Rest									
Machine position	Wt								+ # ☐ – ↓ ☐ + ↑ ☐ ↔ ☐	SIR
	Reps									
	Rest									
Machine position	Wt								+ # ☐ – ↓ ☐ + ↑ ☐ ↔ ☐	SIR
	Reps									
	Rest									
Machine position	Wt								+ # ☐ – ↓ ☐ + ↑ ☐ ↔ ☐	SIR
	Reps									
	Rest									
Machine position	Wt								+ # ☐ – ↓ ☐ + ↑ ☐ ↔ ☐	SIR
	Reps									
	Rest									
Machine position	Wt								+ # ☐ – ↓ ☐ + ↑ ☐ ↔ ☐	SIR
	Reps									
	Rest									
Machine position	Wt								+ # ☐ – ↓ ☐ + ↑ ☐ ↔ ☐	SIR
	Reps									
	Rest									
Machine position	Wt								+ # ☐ – ↓ ☐ + ↑ ☐ ↔ ☐	SIR
	Reps									
	Rest									
Machine position	Wt								+ # ☐ – ↓ ☐ + ↑ ☐ ↔ ☐	SIR
	Reps									
	Rest									

11. Abdominals

Exercise					
Reps	Rest	Reps	Rest	Reps	Rest
Reps	Rest	Reps	Rest	Reps	Rest

12. Flexibility
- ☐ Hamstrings
- ☐ Upper back
- ☐ Neck
- ☐ Hips
- ☐ Groin
- ☐ Biceps
- ☐ Pectorals
- ☐ Low back
- ☐ Calf
- ☐ Triceps
- ☐ Shoulder
- ☐ Hip abduction/adduction
- ☐ Internal/external shoulder rotators

13. Aches, pains, problems:

14. Discuss with client:

15. Weight _____ on _____ (date)

16. Energy level:

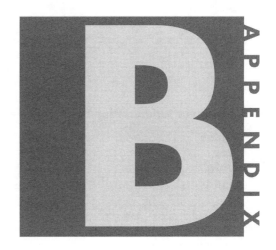

Fitness Testing

Body Composition

Sit-and-Reach Test for Hamstring Flexibility

Finger-Touch Test for Rotator Cuff Flexibility

Three-Minute Step Test

Curl-Up Test for Abdominal Strength

Body Composition

Percent Fat Estimates for Three Sites—Men

Sum of three skinfolds (in mm)	\multicolumn{9}{c}{Age}								
	18-22	23-27	28-32	33-37	38-42	43-47	48-52	53-57	>58
8-12	1.8	2.6	3.4	4.2	4.9	5.7	6.5	7.3	8.1
13-17	3.6	4.4	5.2	6.0	6.8	7.6	8.4	9.1	9.9
18-22	5.4	6.2	7.0	7.8	8.6	9.3	10.1	10.9	11.7
23-27	7.1	7.9	8.7	9.5	10.3	11.1	11.9	12.6	13.4
28-32	8.8	9.6	10.4	11.2	12.0	12.8	13.5	14.3	15.1
33-37	10.4	11.2	12.0	12.8	13.6	14.4	15.2	15.9	16.7
38-42	12.0	12.8	13.6	14.4	15.2	15.9	16.7	17.5	18.3
43-47	13.5	14.3	15.1	15.9	16.7	17.5	18.3	19.0	19.8
48-52	15.0	15.8	16.6	17.4	18.1	18.9	19.7	20.5	21.3
53-57	16.4	17.2	18.0	18.8	19.6	20.3	21.1	21.9	22.7
58-62	17.8	18.5	19.3	20.1	20.9	21.7	22.5	23.3	24.1
63-67	19.1	19.9	20.6	21.4	22.2	23.0	23.8	24.6	25.4
68-72	20.3	21.1	21.9	22.7	23.5	24.3	25.1	25.8	26.6
73-77	21.5	22.3	23.1	23.9	24.7	25.5	26.3	27.0	27.8
78-82	22.7	23.5	24.3	25.0	25.8	26.6	27.4	28.2	29.0
83-87	23.8	24.6	25.3	26.1	26.9	27.7	28.5	29.3	30.1
88-92	24.8	25.6	26.4	27.2	28.0	28.8	29.6	30.3	31.1
93-97	25.8	26.6	27.4	28.2	29.0	29.8	30.5	31.3	32.1
98-102	26.7	27.5	28.3	29.1	29.9	30.7	31.5	32.3	33.1
103-107	27.6	28.4	29.2	30.0	30.8	31.6	32.4	33.2	33.9
108-112	28.5	29.3	30.1	30.8	31.6	32.4	33.2	34.0	34.8
113-117	29.3	30.0	30.8	31.6	32.4	33.2	34.0	34.8	35.6
118-122	30.0	30.8	31.6	32.4	33.1	33.9	34.7	35.5	36.3
123-127	30.7	31.5	32.2	33.0	33.8	34.6	35.4	36.2	37.0
128-132	31.3	32.1	32.9	33.7	34.4	35.2	36.0	36.8	37.6
133-137	31.9	32.7	33.4	34.2	35.0	35.8	36.6	37.4	38.2
138-142	32.4	33.2	34.0	34.8	35.5	36.3	37.1	37.9	38.7
143-147	32.9	33.6	34.4	35.2	36.0	36.8	37.6	38.4	39.2
148-152	33.3	34.1	34.8	35.6	36.4	37.2	38.0	38.8	39.6
153-157	33.6	34.4	35.2	36.0	36.8	37.6	38.4	39.2	39.9
158-162	33.9	34.7	35.5	36.3	37.1	37.9	38.7	39.5	40.3
163-167	34.2	35.0	35.8	36.6	37.4	38.1	38.9	39.7	40.5
168-172	34.4	35.2	36.0	36.8	37.6	38.4	39.1	39.9	40.7
173-177	34.6	35.3	36.1	36.9	37.7	38.5	39.3	40.1	40.9
178-182	34.7	35.4	36.2	37.0	37.8	38.6	39.4	40.2	41.0

Percent Fat Estimates for Three Sites—Women

Sum of three skinfolds (in mm)	Age								
	18-22	**23-27**	**28-32**	**33-37**	**38-42**	**43-47**	**48-52**	**53-57**	**>58**
8-12	8.8	9.0	9.2	9.4	9.5	9.7	9.9	10.1	10.3
13-17	10.8	10.9	11.1	11.3	11.5	11.7	11.8	12.0	12.2
18-22	12.6	12.8	13.0	13.2	13.4	13.5	13.7	13.9	14.1
23-27	14.5	14.6	14.8	15.0	15.2	15.4	15.6	15.7	15.9
28-32	16.2	16.4	16.6	16.9	17.0	17.1	17.3	17.5	17.7
33-37	17.9	18.1	18.3	18.5	18.7	18.9	19.0	19.2	19.4
38-42	19.6	19.8	20.0	20.2	20.3	20.5	20.7	20.9	21.1
43-47	21.2	21.4	21.6	21.8	21.9	22.1	22.3	22.5	22.7
48-52	22.8	22.9	23.1	23.3	23.5	23.7	23.8	24.0	24.2
53-57	24.2	24.4	24.6	24.8	25.0	25.2	25.3	25.5	25.7
58-62	25.7	25.9	26.0	26.2	26.4	26.6	26.8	27.0	27.1
63-67	27.1	27.2	27.4	27.6	27.8	28.0	28.2	28.3	28.5
68-72	28.4	28.6	28.7	28.9	29.1	29.3	29.5	29.7	29.8
73-77	29.6	29.8	30.0	30.2	30.4	30.6	30.7	30.9	31.1
78-82	30.9	31.0	31.2	31.4	31.6	31.8	31.9	32.1	32.3
83-87	32.0	32.2	32.4	32.6	32.7	32.9	33.1	33.3	33.5
88-92	33.1	33.3	33.5	33.7	33.8	34.0	34.2	34.4	34.6
93-97	34.1	34.3	34.5	34.7	34.9	35.1	35.2	35.4	35.6
98-102	35.1	35.3	35.5	35.7	35.9	36.0	36.2	36.4	36.6
103-107	36.1	36.2	36.4	36.6	36.9	37.0	37.2	37.3	37.5
108-112	36.9	37.1	37.3	37.5	37.7	37.9	38.0	38.2	38.4
113-117	37.8	37.9	38.1	38.3	39.2	39.4	39.6	39.8	39.5
118-122	38.5	38.7	38.9	39.1	39.4	39.6	39.8	40.0	40.0
123-127	39.2	39.4	39.6	39.8	40.0	40.1	40.3	40.5	40.7
128-132	39.9	40.1	40.2	40.4	40.6	40.8	41.0	41.2	41.3
133-137	40.5	40.7	40.8	41.0	41.2	41.4	41.6	41.7	41.9
138-142	41.0	41.2	41.4	41.6	41.7	41.9	42.1	42.3	42.5
143-147	41.5	41.7	41.9	42.0	42.2	42.4	42.6	42.8	43.0
148-152	41.9	42.1	42.3	42.8	42.6	42.8	43.0	43.2	43.4
153-157	42.3	42.5	42.6	43.0	43.0	43.2	43.4	43.6	43.7
158-162	42.6	42.8	43.0	43.1	43.3	43.5	43.7	43.9	44.1
163-167	42.9	43.0	43.2	43.4	43.6	43.8	44.0	44.1	44.3
168-172	43.1	43.2	43.4	43.6	43.8	44.0	44.2	44.3	44.5
173-177	43.2	43.4	43.6	43.8	43.9	44.1	44.3	44.5	44.7
178-182	43.3	43.5	43.7	43.8	44.0	44.2	44.4	44.6	44.8

From Teri S. O'Brien. 2003. *The Personal Trainer's Handbook, Second Edition*. Champaign, IL: Human Kinetics. **231**
Reproduced by permission of the YMCA of the USA from *The Y's Way to Physical Fitness* by Lawrence Golding, Clayton Myers, and Wayne Sinning, Copyright © 1989 (Champaign, IL: Human Kinetics Publishing).

Sit-and-Reach Test for Hamstring Flexibility

The most widely used test for low-back and hamstring flexibility is the sit-and-reach. It certainly has its deficiencies, the principal one being that it fails to take into account individual differences in torso and arm length. Someone with very long arms or a long torso will get a higher score because of these structural characteristics that have nothing to do with flexibility in the hamstrings and low back. That having been said, these deficiencies are problematic only when you view the test as a means for comparison of one person to another. Where you are comparing Client A on day 1 versus day 60, these deficiencies disappear. The test is 100% valid for comparing changes in an individual client's flexibility.

You can do this test either with a commercial flexibility box or with a yardstick and tape measure. If you choose the latter, which is more portable, tape the yardstick to the ground (tape perpendicular to the yardstick) at the 15-inch (38 cm) mark. Have your client sit with the yardstick between his legs and heels at the 15-inch (38 cm) mark. His feet should be 10 to 12 inches (25.4 to 30.5 cm) apart. Have him bend at the waist, drop his head forward, and reach with one hand on top of the other as far as he can. It's important that he keep his knees straight and not rotate at the torso, which is the reason you ask him to place one hand on top of the other. Do the test three times and take the best result.

Rating	Females						Males					
Age	46+		36-45		35 and less		46+		36-45		35 and less	
	Inches	Cm	Inches	Cm	Inches	Cm	Inches	Cm	Inches	Cm	Inches	Cm
Excellent	22	55.9	23	58.4	23	58.4	20	50.8	22	55.9	21	53.3
Good	19	48.0	21	53.3	21	53.3	17	43.2	19	48.0	19	48.0
Above average	18	45.7	19	48.0	20	50.8	15	38.0	16	40.6	17	43.2
Average	15	38.0	17	43.2	18	45.7	13	33.0	14	35.5	15	38.0
Below average	14	35.5	14	35.5	15	38.0	11	28.0	12	30.5	12	30.5
Fair	11	28.0	12	30.5	14	35.5	8	20.3	10	25.4	9	22.8
Poor	9	22.8	10	25.4	11	28.0	5	12.7	5	12.7	7	17.8

 From Teri S. O'Brien. 2003. *The Personal Trainer's Handbook, Second Edition.* Champaign, IL: Human Kinetics. Adapted by permission of the YMCA of the USA from *The Y's Way to Physical Fitness* by Lawrence Golding, Clayton Myers, and Wayne Sinning, Copyright © 1989 (Champaign, IL: Human Kinetics Publishing).

Finger-Touch Test for Rotator Cuff Flexibility

The subject should be wearing a tank top or be shirtless. After the general warm-up and a brief specific warm-up (arm circles), have her stand with her back to you. Have her reach up toward the ceiling with her left arm next to her head, then, keeping the left upper arm stationary, flex the left elbow and place her left hand against her upper back. Place the right hand behind the back and reach up with the back of the hand against the back. The objective is to touch the fingers behind the back. Measure and record the distance between the fingers. Perform the test of the opposite side by reversing the hand and arm positions.

Scoring

(Distance between fingers in inches and centimeters)

	Males		Females	
	Inches	**Cm**	**Inches**	**Cm**
Excellent	0 - 1	0 - 2.5	0 - .5	0 - 1.28
Good	1 - 3	2.5 - 7.6	.5 - 2.5	1.28 - 6.3
Average	3 - 4	7.6 - 10.2	2.5 - 4	6.3 - 10.2
Poor	4 - 10	10.2 - 25.4	4 - 10	10.2 - 25.4

Author's note: This table is derived from my measurements of a variety of individuals of all ages. It's less important where your client falls on the scale than whether he or she is improving from test to test.

Three-Minute Step Test

Equipment needed: 12-inch-high (30.5 cm) box or bench, Metronome, stopwatch

This test was developed by the YMCA. While it does not test $\dot{V}O_2$max, it does give a rough estimate of cardiovascular fitness by measuring the heart's rate of recovery.

How to do it: Set the metronome to 96 beats (24 steps) per minute and the stopwatch to 3 minutes.

Demonstrate this technique to your client: Keeping pace with the metronome, step up with your right foot, up with your left, down with your right, and down with your left. Allow your client to practice by stepping in time. You can keep track of the client's heart rate in one of two ways—either locate your client's radial pulse (I suggest you mark it with a felt-tip pen) and take it manually, or have your client wear a heart monitor during the test. Advise your client that he should feel free to stop stepping any time he feels dizziness, light-headedness, chest pain, or nausea, or for any other reason. Have your client begin stepping and start the timer. After time expires, have your client sit down and take his pulse for 1 minute. His score is his resting pulse after 1 minute.

Many unconditioned middle-aged people can't complete the full 3 minutes, either because of orthopedic problems (knee or back pain) or because their heart rates climb like a NASA booster rocket and they are too exhausted to continue. You will notice that the client is no longer able to keep up with the metronome and can no longer speak. In this case, you should stop the test, then record the ending pulse rate and the amount of time completed. On the retest, your goal will be to complete the full 3 minutes, or at least a greater percentage than he completed the last time.

Norms for 3-Minute Step Test

(1-Minute Recovery Heart Rate)

	Women			Men		
	18-35	**36-55**	**56-85**	**18-35**	**36-55**	**56-85**
Excellent	72-90	74-95	74-82	70-82	72-88	72-88
Good	91-102	96-105	83-103	83-88	89-98	89-96
Above average	103-111	106-116	104-116	81-100	99-108	97-103
Average	112-120	117-120	117-122	101-108	108-117	104-113
Below average	121-128	121-126	123-128	109-117	118-123	114-121
Fair	129-135	127-137	129-134	118-129	124-134	122-132
Poor	136-154	136-152	135-151	130-164	135-158	133-152

 From Teri S. O'Brien. 2003. *The Personal Trainer's Handbook, Second Edition*. Champaign, IL: Human Kinetics. Adapted by permission of the YMCA of the USA from *The Y's Way to Physical Fitness* (3d ed.) by Lawrence Golding, Clayton Myers, and Wayne Sinning, Copyright © 1989 (Champaign, IL: Human Kinetics Publishing).

Curl-Up Test for Abdominal Strength

Most of us remember that sit-up test from when we were kids. We paired up with a partner who held our feet while we attempted to do as many sit-ups as possible within a given number of minutes. As many of you know, the problem with this test is that the hip flexors, not abdominals, do most of the work when the feet are anchored. The curl-up test was developed in an attempt to make the test more specific to abdominals.

The client lies on his back, arms by the sides, palms down on the floor, elbows rigid, fingers straight, knees flexed at 90 degrees. Measure 3 inches (7.6 cm) away from the longest fingertip of each hand and mark this spot with tape. The client performs the test by curling his head and shoulders up while keeping the feet and fingers on the floor for 1 minute.

Keep in mind that this test is less a matter of quantitative precision than it is a rule of thumb to see if your client is getting stronger. More curl-ups in 1 minute with good form demonstrates that your program is strengthening his power core.

Scoring

Excellent	>48
Good	36-48
Average	24-35
Below average	16-23
Poor	<16

acetyl CoA—The compound that results from the breakdown of carbohydrate and free fatty acids and enters the Krebs cycle to produce more energy.

actin—Cellular protein that makes up one of the filaments essential to muscular contraction.

acute—Occurring as a result of a brief event, as opposed to *chronic*, which is the result of repeated and long-term exposure to the cause; generally used to distinguish types of injuries.

adenosine triphosphate (ATP)—The high-energy molecule that provides energy for cellular function.

adipose tissue—Fat.

aerobic—In the presence of oxygen.

anaerobic—Without oxygen.

anatomy—The study of the structure of the body and the relationships of the body parts to one another.

angina—Chest pain caused by inadequate blood flow and thus oxygen supply to the heart. Often aggravated or induced by exercise. Often a sign/symptom of *coronary artery disease.*

angiotensin-converting enzyme (ACE) inhibitor—Medication used to control or decrease blood pressure by reducing vasoconstriction; very effective in treating *congestive heart failure.* May cause postexercise hypotension. Look for the suffix *pril,* as in Capotoril, a commonly prescribed ACE inhibitor.

anthropometric measurement—Pertaining to the measurement of the size, weight, and proportions of the human body.

apparently healthy—Showing no signs or symptoms of disease and no known disease.

arrythymia—Abnormal heart rhythm or beat.

arteriosclerosis—Loss of elasticity, narrowing, and hardening of the arteries.

atherogenic lipoprotein profile (ALP)—A metabolic milieu that contributes to atherosclerosis; increases cardiovascular risk by three times; characterized by small, dense LDL particles (LDL pattern B).

atherosclerosis—Plaque accumulation in the lining of the arteries; leads to arteriosclerosis.

beta blockers—Medications used to treat hypertension and angina; commonly prescribed examples include Inderal(proprinal), Lopressor (metropolol), Ternomin (atenolol). May blunt effects of hypoglycemia in insulin-dependent diabetics.

beta oxidation—The breakdown of free fatty acids to acetyl CoA.

bioelectric impedance (BIA)—A method of determining body composition by measuring resistance to electric current.

biomechanics—The laws of physics applied to the body.

body mass index (BMI)—A relative measure of body height to body weight used to determine the degree of obesity.

bradycardia—Slowness of the heartbeat as evidenced by a pulse rate of less than 60 bpm.

breach—Failure to fulfill a legal duty; negligence.

cardiac output (Q)—Heart rate multiplied by stroke volume; when a dot appears above Q, total blood pumped per minute.

cardiopulmonary resuscitation (CPR)—External support of the circulation and ventilation systems for a victim of cardiac or respiratory arrest, providing oxygen to the brain, heart, and other vital organs until appropriate medical treatment can restore normal heart and ventilatory action.

cardiorespiratory fitness—The ability to sustain an activity for an extended period while the lungs maintain their ability to provide oxygen to the blood and circulatory system for transporting blood and its nutrients to tissues.

cardiovascular (or heart rate) drift—An increase in heart rate that occurs without increase in intensity the longer exercise continues; it results from the body's need to compensate for decreased stroke volume and still maintain cardiac output.

cardiovascular risk factor—A condition, behavior, or disease that increases one's risk for cardiovascular disease.

catabolism—Breakdown.

causation—An act or omission of action that causes an injury.

center of gravity—The point at which all of a body's mass is concentrated; that is, the point at which all the mass of the body is balanced because it is equally distributed around this point.

chronic—Occurring as a result of long-term and frequent exposure.

citric acid cycle—see *Krebs cycle.*

client motivation—Ability to focus on something the client values and educate her about her ability to achieve it by continuing the program.

closed-chain exercise—An exercise in which the terminal, or distal, end of the kinetic chain is in contact with the ground, wall, or floor, as opposed to an open-chain exercise in which the terminal end swings freely. For example, a leg press is a closed-chain exercise; a leg extension is an open-chain exercise.

commitment—Your pledge to uphold your duty and honor your responsibility as a personal trainer.

congestive heart failure (CHF)—A clinical syndrome due to heart disease characterized by shortness of breath and sodium and water retention resulting in edema. The congestion can occur in the lungs, in peripheral circulation, or both. Chronic hypertension is one cause.

contract—A legally binding agreement; for our purposes, a written agreement signed by the participant and the personal trainer that states the goals to be achieved over a given period.

coronary artery disease (CAD)—Almost always a result of atherosclerosis. Includes hypertension, stroke, congestive heart failure, peripheral vascular disease, and valve disease.

coronary heart disease risk factors—Behavioral and genetic conditions that increase one's chances for coronary heart disease.

customer service—Your ability to provide to your clients the service that they need, in the way that they want it.

delayed-onset muscular soreness (DOMS)—Muscle soreness that results 24 to 48 hours after heavy exercise.

diabetes mellitus—A disease of carbohydrate metabolism in which an absolute or relative deficiency of insulin results in an inability to metabolize carbohydrates normally.

diastole—The phase of the cardiac cycle when the left ventricle is filling with oxygenated blood.

dual-energy X-ray absorptiometry (DEXA or DXA)—A technique using X rays to assess bone density or body composition.

duty—A legal obligation to do or refrain from doing something.

dyspnea—Difficult or labored breathing; a feeling of "air hunger."

eccentric—Describes a muscle working against resistance while lengthening; the "negative" part of a repetition of a resistance exercise.

edema—Swelling as a result of the collection of body fluids within the body tissues.

ejection fraction—The fraction of blood ejected out of the left ventricle with each ventricular contraction.

electron transport chain—A process that occurs deep inside the mitochondria in which electrons are passed by a "bucket brigade" of electron carriers and ATP is produced.

enzymes—Proteins that accelerate and facilitate chemical reactions.

ethical behavior—Conduct indicative of a highly skilled professional with a high level of personal and professional integrity, honesty, and trust.

eustress—Good stress that results in challenge and improvement.

exculpatory clause—A clause in a waiver in which the person gives up the right to sue.

exercise-associated cardiovascular complication (ECVC)—Sudden loss of consciousness or similar serious incident during exercise; can result in death. Risk is reduced by screening and by recognizing high-risk scenarios.

exercise physiology—The study of how the body's systems respond and adapt to different forms of exercise.

exercise prescription—The successful integration of exercise science with behavior techniques that result in long-term program compliance and attainment of the individual's goals.

fat-free mass—The part of the body containing no lipids.

FIT—Frequency (how often), intensity (how hard), and time (how long). Used to describe aerobic exercise prescription.

flexibility—A joint's ability to move freely in every direction or through a full and normal range of motion.

Frank-Starling mechanism—A mechanism by which an increased amount of blood in the left ventricle causes a stronger ventricular contraction and increased amount of blood ejected.

fungible—Interchangeable; the same as any other; what you want to avoid being if you want to command top dollar as a personal trainer.

gluconeogenesis—The production of glucose from protein.

glucose—A simple sugar, the simplest form in which all carbohydrates are used by the body for energy production.

glycogen—The chief carbohydrate storage material. It is formed in the liver and stored in the liver and muscle.

glycolysis—The breakdown of glucose.

health history questionnaire—A written form containing questions to identify individuals for whom physical activity is inappropriate and if medical advice concerning the type of activity is necessary.

health screening—A means for the personal trainer to (1) identify medical conditions that may place the client at risk when participating in certain activities, (2) identify possible contraindicated activities, (3) design exercise programs that include safe activities and appropriate modifications, and (4) fulfill legal and insurance requirements for the personal trainer or health club.

heart-rate reserve (HRR)—The reserve capacity of the heart; the difference between maximal heart rate and resting heart rate.

helping—Process of advising, informing, correcting, and directing, ultimately facilitating the client to take more control over his health and wellness and become self-sufficient.

high-density lipoprotein (HDL)—A plasma of complex lipids and proteins that contains relatively more protein and less cholesterol and triglycerides. High HDL levels are associated with a low risk of coronary heart disease because they carry *low-density lipoprotein* (LDL) back to the liver instead of allowing it to clog arteries.

homeostasis—The state of balance that the body strives to achieve by maintaining appropriate temperature, hydration, and pH.

hydrostatic weighing—A method of determining body composition by weighing an individual underwater.

hyperglycemia—An abnormally high content of glucose in the blood.

hypertension (HTN)—High blood pressure.

hypertrophic cardiomyopathy (HCM)—A congenital heart defect that is the leading cause of

sudden death during exercise in people under 30 years old.

hypoglycemia—A deficiency of glucose in the blood commonly caused by too much insulin, too little glucose, or too much exercise.

hyponatremia—Water intoxication; an imbalance in electrolytes that can result in cardiac arrhythmia. Typically occurs during ultraendurance events in hot, humid weather.

impingement syndrome—A common and painful orthopedic problem causing pain in the shoulder and upper arm; results from imbalance in the rotator cuff and poor posture.

increased risk—Two or more risk factors, or one or more signs or symptoms.

indemnification—Protection against loss or damage.

informed consent—The process in which a person learns about the risks and benefits of a proposed action or procedure involving him, and knowingly and voluntarily agrees to participate.

insulin insensitivity—Deficient target cell response to insulin; common in obese and sedentary people.

interval training—Short, high-intensity exercise periods alternated with periods of rest or lower-intensity exercise.

Karvonean method—A method of determining target heart rate that uses heart rate reserve (maximal heart rate minus resting heart rate).

kilocalorie—The amount of heat needed to increase the temperature of 1 kilogram of water 1 degree Celsius.

kinesiology—The study of movement.

kinetic chain—A series of joints involved in a body movement.

known disease—Known cardiac, pulmonary, or metabolic disease.

Krebs cycle—A series of chemical reactions in which energy is produced.

lactate—The by-product of anaerobic metabolism; results when hydrogen accumulates and combines with pyruvate; can be used for fuel because the liver can use it to make glucose (gluconeogenesis).

lactate threshold—During exercise of increasing intensity, the point at which blood lactate begins to accumulate.

LDL pattern A—One of two types of low-density lipoprotein patterns in which large LDL particles are predominant; "good" bad cholesterol. It is probably genetically determined.

LDL pattern B—Small, dense LDL particles that are more likely to clog arteries are predominant; more likely to cause CAD.

lean body mass—The part of the body composed of fat-free mass and essential fat, which is the amount of fat necessary for survival (approximately 2% to 3% lipids for men and 5% to 8% for women).

lordosis—Swayback; often caused by tightness in the hamstrings and weak abdominal muscles.

low-density lipoprotein (LDL)—A plasma complex of lipids and proteins that contains relatively more cholesterol and triglycerides and less protein than HDL. High LDL levels are associated with an increased risk of coronary artery disease.

maximal heart rate (MHR)—The highest heart rate attainable during an all-out effort to exhaustion; varies among individuals of the same age, size, and gender.

maximal oxygen consumption ($\dot{V}O_2max$)—The point at which oxygen consumption plateaus with an additional workload; represents a person's capacity for the aerobic synthesis of ATP.

medical clearance—Physician's written approval to participate in physical activity and identification of any required limitations.

metabolic equivalent (MET)—A unit used to estimate the metabolic cost (oxygen consumption) of physical activity; 1 MET = 3.5 milliliters of oxygen per kilogram of body weight per minute.

mitochrondria—Organelles inside the cells where most energy is produced.

moderate exercise—Exercise well within an individual's capacity that can be sustained for a prolonged period (60 minutes), has a gradual initiation and progression, and is noncompetitive.

multijoint exercise—Exercise where more than one joint allows for movement around its axis of rotation, thus involving more muscles being targeted for work.

muscular endurance—The capacity of a muscle to exert force repeatedly against a resistance, or to hold a fixed contraction over time.

muscular strength—The maximum force that a muscle can produce against resistance in a single, maximal effort.

myocardial infarction (MI)—An interruption in the blood supply to the heart muscle resulting in tissue death.

myosin—A protein critical to muscular contraction; its head contacts the actin filament, causing the two to slide together.

negligence—Failure to perform as a reasonable and prudent person (or professional) would under similar circumstances.

neuropathy—A general term denoting functional disturbances in the peripheral nervous system. In diabetes it results in a decreased ability to sense pain or discomfort in the extremities, especially the feet.

non-insulin-dependent diabetes (NIDDM)—Also known as adult-onset diabetes; 90% of diabetes is this largely preventable type.

nutrition—Eating well and making wise food choices to ensure appropriate amounts of essential nutrients are ingested.

officious intermeddler—A person who sticks his nose into a situation without having been invited; as a result, no one likes him, and he may be sued.

one repetition max (1 RM)—The amount of resistance that can be moved through the range of motion one time before the muscle is temporarily fatigued.

open-chain exercise—Exercise in which the distal (far) end of the body segment is not fixed to a ground-based surface; for example, leg extension.

osteoarthritis—Degenerative joint disease occurring chiefly in older persons and characterized by degeneration of articular cartilage, hypertrophy of the bones, and changes in the synovial membrane.

osteoporosis—A disorder, affecting primarily but not exclusively postmenopausal women, in which bone density decreases and susceptibility to fractures increases.

overtraining—Consistently doing more physical activity than the body can tolerate without recovery.

overtraining syndrome—A condition characterized by overtraining, poor performance, lack of improvement, and diminished motivation.

perceived value—What a consumer believes something is worth, and therefore an extremely individual and subjective concept.

periodization—A logical phasic method of manipulating variables in order to increase the potential for achieving specific performance goals; helps prevent overtraining.

personal training—The art and science of improving the health, fitness, and overall well-being of a client through effective, individualized program design; personal attention; and professionalism.

pH—The concentration of hydrogen in a substance; the acid-base balance.

program design—The creation of individualized, personally tailored workouts to meet the needs and desires of the client.

pulse pressure—The difference between systolic and diastolic blood pressure.

range of motion (ROM)—The number of degrees of movement of a joint.

rate of perceived exertion (RPE)—A scale to provide a standard means for evaluating a person's perception of his or her physical exertion. The scale was developed by Borg and goes from 0 to 10, with 0 representing the least exertion and 10 the greatest exertion.

recommended dietary allowance (RDA)—Recommended vitamin and mineral intake for practically all healthy people to obtain optimum health.

respiratory chain—See *electron transport chain.*

resting heart rate (RHR)—A person's heart rate at rest.

rheumatoid arthritis—An autoimmune disease that attacks healthy tissue and damages the joint.

safety—A system of minimizing the risk of injury by recommending exercise appropriate to the client's fitness level, instructing in proper methods and modes of exercise, monitoring immediate space and correcting performance, recognizing symptoms of overtraining, and properly applying biomechanical principles.

scope of practice—The range and limit of responsibilities normally associated with a specific job or profession.

self-efficacy—A person's perception of his ability to change or perform specific behavior (e.g., exercise).

Sherpas—Essential guides who through their commitment and sense of mission make it possible for people to climb Mount Everest but who can't do it *for* them; in this way they provide a model for coaches and trainers.

single-joint exercise—Exercise in which only one joint is allowing movement around the axis of rotation, making muscle involvement specific.

slander—Malicious, untrue statements that injure somebody's reputation.

standard of care—The standard to which professionals must adhere to avoid committing malpractice and possibly being sued; the standard by which professional conduct will be judged in the event of a lawsuit.

steady state—The plateau of heart rate and oxygen consumption eventually achieved shortly after exercise begins and maintained at submaximal levels when work rate stays constant.

stroke volume (SV)—The amount of blood ejected from the left ventricle during systole.

syncope—Fainting.

syndrome X—A high-risk scenario in which an individual exhibits the following symptoms: insulin insensitivity, elevated triglycerides, low HDL cholesterol, high blood pressure, and excessive abdominal fat. Also known as metabolic syndrome.

systole—The phase of the cardiac cycle when the heart contracts and the left ventricle expels blood to the body.

tachycardia—Rapid heartbeat.

target heart rate (THR)—Also known as training heart rate. A heart rate goal used to set exercise intensity.

testing and evaluation—Process of gathering information related to a client's current level of physical fitness for the following: to aid in the development of an exercise program, identify areas of health/injury risk, establish goals, provide motivation, and evaluate progress.

torque—A turning force; the amount of force needed to cause rotation.

tort law—The branch of law dealing with enforcing rights and obligations between private citizens.

United States Recommended Dietary Allowance (USRDA)—Used in food labeling; expresses nutrients of the RDA in percentages.

Valsalva maneuver—Holding the breath during exercise, especially resistance training; causes blood pressure to spike.

visionary—A person who can see a desired outcome and therefore can help to create it.

$\dot{V}O_2$max—See *maximal oxygen consumption.*

waiver—Voluntary abandonment of a right to file a lawsuit; not always legally binding.

As terrific as this book is, I didn't have time or space to include all the information you should digest to be a truly professional personal trainer. Fortunately, both you and I can benefit from the knowledge, wisdom, and experience of the following authors. I encourage you to read these books. Not only will your knowledge increase dramatically, but you will be reminded of the complexity and miraculousness of the human body and the importance of your calling.

Alter, Michael. *Science of Flexibility.* Champaign, IL: Human Kinetics, 2000.

Alter, Michael. *Sport Stretch,* 2d ed. Champaign, IL: Human Kinetics, 1997.

Very useful books with illustrations of stretches for every part of the body.

American College of Sports Medicine. *Guidelines for Exercise Testing and Prescription,* 6th ed. Baltimore: Williams & Wilkins, 1996.

A manual for professionals from the premier certifying organization, this guide contains information about testing and programming for the general population and those with special needs.

Anderson, Bob. *Stretching* (20th anniversary edition). Bolinas, CA: Shelter, 2000.

One of the first and most popular books about stretching, this contains basic physiology about stretching, as well as some specifics on stretching for a variety of conditions.

Anderson, Kristen, and Ron Zemke. *Delivering Knock Your Socks Off Service.* New York: American Management Association, 1998.

Personal training is a service business, and this little book will give you invaluable tips about being a customer service star.

Baechle, Thomas R., and Barney R. Groves. *Weight Training: Steps to Success,* 2d ed. Champaign, IL: Human Kinetics, 1998.

A wonderful book that takes you through each step of designing an effective and safe weight training program. Contains formulas and charts to help you select appropriate weights, reps, sets, and rest periods.

Bryant, Cedric X., James A. Peterson, and Jason Conviser. "High-Protein, Low-Carbohydrate Diets: Fact v. Fiction." Fitness Management, December 2001, pp. 40-44.

Clarkson, Priscilla. "Oh, Those Aching Muscles: Causes and Consequences of Delayed Onset Muscle Soreness." ACSM Health and Fitness Journal, vol. 1, no. 3, May/June 1997, pp. 12-17.

Cooper, Kenneth. The Aerobics Program for Total Well-Being. New York: Bantam Doubleday, 1991.

As the cover proclaims, Dr. Cooper is "the man who started America running." In this book, he identifies three components of total well-being: exercise, diet, and emotional balance. He explains his point system for comparing various aerobic activities, which is quite useful for clients who cross-train. Contains many useful references.

Corbin, Charles B., Gregory J. Welk, William R. Corbin, Gregory Welk, and Ruth Lindsey. *Concepts of Physical Fitness,* 11th ed. Boston: McGraw Hill, 2002.

This book stresses health-related fitness. It explains each concept with factual information, graphs, tables, and a glossary of terms for each chapter. In addition, it contains more than 25 labs for studying everything from physical activity to being an informed fitness consumer. Contains information on measuring body composition. This edition also comes with an activity CD-ROM.

Delavier, Frederic. *Strength Training Anatomy.* Champaign, IL: Human Kinetics, 2001.

Contains full-color anatomical drawings of every major muscle group being worked during exercises. The author combines his skill as an artist with a vast knowledge of anatomy. Beautiful to look at, and practical, too!

Eickhoff-Shemek, Jo-Ann, and Frank S. Forbes. "Waivers Are Usually Well Worth the Effort."

ACSM Health and Fitness Journal, vol. 3, no. 4, July/August 1999, pp. 24-29.

A great explanation of how waivers work and how, when written and administered correctly, they can protect you from paying out damages.

Fleck, Steven J., and William J. Kraemer. *Designing Resistance Training Programs,* 2d ed. Champaign, IL: Human Kinetics, 1997.

A very serious book from two of the leading authorities on resistance training. It contains a lot of heavy, scientifically based information that you can use in program design. An essential addition to your professional library.

Gavin, James. *The Exercise Habit.* Champaign, IL: Human Kinetics, 1992.

This book approaches exercise motivation by analyzing the fitness incentives that push different individuals' buttons. Is it concern for appearance? Sociability? What is the role of self-esteem? The book contains questionnaires for figuring out what motivates your client.

Gavin, James, and Nettie Gavin. *Psychology for Health Fitness Professionals.* Champaign, IL: Human Kinetics, 1995.

A little gem. A book that will help you understand your clients, support them, and effectively communicate with them.

Griffin, John C. *Client-Centered Exercise Prescription.* Champaign, IL: Human Kinetics, 1998.

I wish this book had been available when I started my personal training business. What a treasure! Loaded with case studies on everything from motivation to program design. Contains some extremely useful information on musculoskeletal assessment and prescription for muscular imbalance.

Justice, Greg. "The Numbers Game." *IDEA Personal Trainer,* July/August 1996.

Katahn, Martin, and Jamie Pope. *The T-Factor Diet 2000.* New York: W.W. Norton, 1999.

Commonsense advice on safe, permanent weight management. A good book to recommend to clients who ask, "What's so bad about those high-protein diets?"

Manore, Melinda, and Janice Thompson. *Sport Nutrition for Health and Performance.* Champaign, IL: Human Kinetics, 2000.

An excellent reference that will help you sort out the fact from fiction and give clients good, solid information about nutrition.

McArdle, William, Frank I. Katch, and Victor Katch. *Essentials of Exercise Physiology,* 2d ed. Baltimore: Lippincott, Williams and Wilkins, 2000.

I used this text when I taught exercise physiology and often refer to it to answer both simple and complex questions. A readable, well-illustrated text, with a number of useful appendices. Includes information on measuring body composition.

McGill, Stuart. *Low Back Disorders: Evidence-Based Prevention and Rehabilitation.* Champaign, IL: Human Kinetics, 2002.

Given that approximately 80% of adults experience low-back pain during their lives, chances are one of your clients may. This book will tell you everything you need to know to work with them, including the functional anatomy of the spine, myths and realities about back pain, and how to develop a safe and effective exercise program for low-back rehabilitation.

McGinnis, Peter. *Biomechanics of Sport and Exercise.* Champaign, IL: Human Kinetics, 1999.

I wish Peter McGinnis' book had been around when I was taking biomechanics. Fortunately for me and my students, it was when I taught the course. The most user-friendly explanation of the laws of physics and their effects on the body that I've ever seen. In addition, very useful information on understanding the forces that can create injuries.

National Strength and Conditioning Association. *Essentials of Strength Training and Conditioning,* 2d ed. Champaign, IL: Human Kinetics, 2000.

Thomas Baechle, executive director of the Certified Strength and Conditioning Specialist Agency, the certifying body for the National Strength and Conditioning Association (NSCA), edited this book. He is also a veteran competitive weightlifter and power lifter. In short, this guy knows his stuff. He and a group of highly qualified contributors have created an extremely valuable resource for the fitness professional who wants to help clients achieve optimal performance safely and effectively. This is one of the most comprehensive references around. It contains information on physiology, biomechanics, tissue adaptation, technique, and fitness assessment, including body fat measurement. It even has information on setting up and managing a fitness facility. An excellent, very useful book!

O'Brien, Teri. *Principles for Personal Trainers: 88 Essential Rules of Excellence.* Monterey, CA: Coaches' Choice, 2000.

Bite-sized morsels of advice that will take you to the top of your game as a professional.

Paulson, Edward. *The Complete Idiot's Guide to Starting Your Own Business.* Indianapolis: Alpha, 2000.

As much as I dislike this modern trend of taking pride in being a "complete idiot" or a "dummy," I did find this book interesting and helpful. I think that you will, too. Contains all the basic information you need to start your own business, written in an entertaining, humorous style.

Pearl, Bill, and Gary Moran. *Getting Stronger.* Bonias, CA: Shelter, 2001.

A comprehensive illustrated manual of weight training. Contains useful sections on popular sports and suggests exercises to improve performance in each.

Rejeski, Jack W., and Elizabeth A. Kenney. *Fitness Motivation: Preventing Participant Dropout.* Champaign, IL: Human Kinetics, 1988.

This book summarizes current information from the fields of psychology and sociology about motivation and compliance. It will help you answer the questions "Why don't they do what they know they're supposed to?" and "How can I help them do better?"

Roitman, Jeffrey L., Moira Kelsey, Thomas P. LaFontaine, Douglas R. Southard, Mark A. Williams, and Tracy York. *ACSM'S Resource Manual for Guidelines for Exercise Testing and Prescription,* 3d ed. Baltimore: Williams and Wilkins, 1998.

This extremely useful and comprehensive manual contains 80 individual chapters covering everything you need to know to take your ACSM certification exam. I am certain that you will use it often after you've passed the exam. Contains information on measuring body fat.

Sewell, Carl, and Paul B. Brown. *Customers for Life.* New York: Pocket Books, 1992.

The message seems obvious: Give the customer what she wants. Obvious or not, you will learn a lot about serving your clients from this book.

Watkins, James. *Structure and Function of the Musculoskeletal System.* Champaign, IL: Human Kinetics, 1999.

This excellent reference book explains complex anatomical and mechanical concepts clearly and simply so that you can understand the relationship between anatomy and biomechanics. It features chapters on all the joints in the body, describing the structure, function, movements, and anatomy of each one. Concludes with an explanation of the etiology of musculoskeletal injuries. Highly recommended.

Westcott, Wayne. *Building Strength and Stamina.* Champaign, IL: Human Kinetics, 1996.

Another winner from Westcott. Contains lots of information on using Nautilus equipment, but also a terrific, well-illustrated explanation on the effects of limb length and muscle insertion points on strength.

Westcott, Wayne. *Strength Fitness: Physiological Principles and Training Techniques.* Dubuque, IA: Brown and Benchmark, 1994.

This book is more technical than *Be Strong.* It appears to be written for a professional or academic audience. One of the best parts is the chapter on research in the area of strength training.

Westcott, Wayne. *Be Strong.* Dubuque, IA: Brown and Benchmark, 1993.

Wayne Westcott is one of the leading experts in the field of strength and resistance training. This well-written book contains illustrations of all the joint movements, and some very useful information about understanding your client's potential strength by understanding the effect of muscle length and tendon insertion points.

Wilmore, Jack H., and David L. Costill. *Physiology of Sport and Exercise,* 2d ed. Champaign, IL: Human Kinetics, 1999.

A comprehensive college text on exercise physiology. An essential for your professional library. Filled with tables and illustrations that make complex concepts come to life. Readable, well-researched, and definitely highly recommended.

REFERENCES

ACSM Code of Ethics, www.acsm.org/code_of_ethics.htm

Brownlee, Shannon. 2000. "Did a Drugstore Diet Pill Kill His Wife?" *Redbook* (March), 140.

Bryant, Cedric X., James A. Peterson, and Jason Conviser. 2001. "High-Protein, Low-Carbohydrate Diets: Fact v. Fiction." *Fitness Management* (December), 40-44.

Chase, Marilyn. 1999. "Workout Fatality Puts Focus on Gyms and Supplements." *Wall Street Journal* (June 28), B1.

City of Madeira vs. Furtner, Court of Appeals of Ohio, First Appellate District, Hamilton County, 1994 Ohio App. (Lexis 3056).

Covey, Stephen R., A. Roger Merrill, and Rebecca R. Merrill. 1994. *First Things First.* New York: Simon and Schuster, 140.

Davis, Peter. 2002. "A Closer Look: IDEA Health and Fitness Association." *Personal Fitness Professional* 4 (1) (January), 21.

Eickhoff-Shemek, Jo-Ann, and Frank S. Forbes. 1999. "Waivers Are Usually Well Worth the Effort." *ACSM Health and Fitness Journal* 3 (4) (July/August), 24-29.

Helliker, Kevin. 1999. "They Left Professions for a True Calling as Personal Trainers." *Wall Street Journal* (February 25), A-1.

Herbert, David. 2000. "Law Notes: Litigation Frenzy Predicted for Fitness Industry." *Fitness Management* (December), 20.

Hilgenkamp, Kathryn. 1998. "Ethical Behavior and Professionalism in the Business of Health and Fitness." *ACSM Health and Fitness Journal* 2 (6) (November/December), 24-27, 44.

IDEA Health and Fitness Association and American Sports Data. 2000. Personal Fitness Survey: The Consumer Perspective. *IDEA Personal Trainer* 11, 44-45.

Illinois Dietetic and Nutrition Services Practice Act, 225 ILCS 30/1 et seq.

International Health, Racquet and Sportsclub Association. 2001. "Number of Americans Working Out With a Personal Trainer Jumps by Nearly One Third in 2000." IHRSA Press Release, October, 10, 2001.

Justice, Greg. 1996. "The Numbers Game." *IDEA Personal Trainer*, July/August, 37-39.

Katahn, Martin, and Jamie Pope. 1999. *The T-Factor Diet 2000.* New York: W.W. Norton, 35-37.

Manore, Melinda, and Janice Thompson. 2000. *Sport Nutrition for Health and Performance.* Champaign, IL: Human Kinetics, 375.

McArdle, William, Frank I. Katch, and Victor Katch. 2000. *Essentials of Exercise Physiology,* 2d ed., Baltimore: Lippincott, Williams and Wilkins, 141.

McGinnis, Peter M. 1999. *Biomechanics of Sport and Exercise.* Champaign, IL: Human Kinetics, 44-45.

Payback, Letters to the Editor, *Club Industry Magazine*, February 1, 2002.

Physician and Sports Medicine. 2000. "Referring Patients to Personal Trainers: Benefits and Pitfalls." News Briefs, *Physician and Sports Medicine,* 28 (1) (January).

Pope, R.P., R.D. Herbert, J.D. Kirwan, et al. 2000. "A Randomized Trial of Preexercise Stretching for Prevention of Lower-Limb Injury. *Medicine and Science in Sports and Exercise* 32 (2): 271-77.

Roitman, Jeffrey L., Moira Kelsey, Thomas P. LaFontaine, Douglas R. Southard, Mark A. Williams, and Tracy York. 1998. *ACSM's Resource Manual for Guidelines for Exercise Testing and Prescription,* 3d ed. Baltimore: Williams and Wilkins, 443-47.

Sewell, Carl, and Paul Brown. 1998. *Customers for Life.* NY: Pocket Books.

United States Department of Health and Human Services. 2000. *Healthy People 2010: National Health Promotion and Disease Prevention Objectives.* Washington, DC: U.S. Department of Health and Human Services.

Watkins, James. 1999. *Structure and Function of the Musculoskeletal System.* Champaign, IL: Human Kinetics.

Wilmore, Jack H., and David L. Costill. 1999. *Physiology of Sport and Exercise,* 2d ed. Champaign, IL: Human Kinetics.

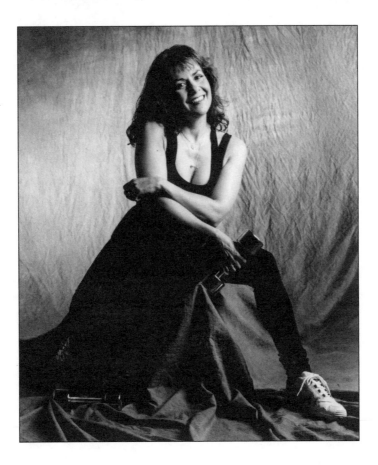

Teri O'Brien is an author, speaker, radio personality, and founder and president of Teri O'Brien Fitness Systems, Inc., a fitness consultation firm located in the Chicago area. Since starting the company in 1991, shortly after completing her master's degree in exercise science at the University of Illinois at Chicago, she has designed optimum performance programs for people of all ages and conditions. A variety of women's and professional groups have enjoyed her entertaining talks and workshops on effective exercise programming, personal effectiveness, successful aging, and optimum performance.

Teri is not your usual fitness expert. Coaching and motivational speaking are a second career for this self-described recovering (as in nonpracticing) lawyer, who practiced law for seven years. She received her bachelor of arts degree from Arizona State University (ASU), where she graduated summa cum laude and Phi Beta Kappa. She discovered the energy-boosting and stress-busting powers of exercise while she was in law school at ASU. To relieve her anxiety from school pressures, Teri began running and continued for nearly 10 years, completing five marathons and dozens of 10K races. After abandoning running in favor of weight training, Teri competed in several bodybuilding competitions, including the Gateway Classic, where she placed fourth in the lightweight class.

Teri is certified as a health fitness instructor by both the American College of Sports Medicine and the American Council on Exercise. In addition, she is a member of the National Strength and Conditioning Association.

She hosted a popular radio talk show on health and wellness on a major Chicago radio station and was featured twice in *Shape* magazine's "One on One" column. Teri also wrote and was featured in eight videos for fitness professionals in the American College of Sports Medicine's Healthy Learning series.

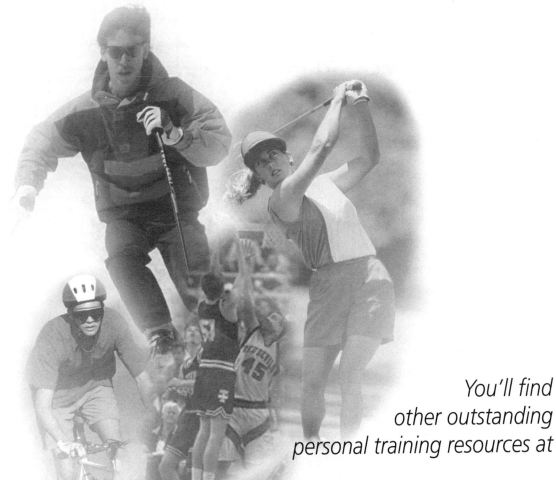

CD-ROM for The Personal Trainer's Handbook, Second Edition
MSR and install instructions

CD-ROM for The Personal Trainer's Handbook, Second Edition, can be installed on either a Windows®-based PC or a Macintosh computer. Please note that appendix A is available in Word, RTF, and PDF formats to allow for the greatest number of readers possible to access the forms in it. The forms can be modified as you choose in both Word and RTF. If you cannot access them in either of those formats, you can at least print them out from the PDF version.

Minimum System Requirements

Microsoft Windows®

- IBM PC compatible with Pentium® processor
- Windows® 95/98/NT 4.0/ME/XP or Windows® 2000
- Adobe Acrobat Reader®
- At least 4 MB RAM with 8 MB recommended
- 2x CD-ROM drive
- Printer (optional)
- Mouse

Macintosh®

- System 7.x/8.x/9.x
- Adobe Acrobat Reader®
- At least 4 MB RAM with 8 MB recommended
- 2x CD-ROM drive
- Printer (optional)
- Mouse

Windows® and Microsoft® are registered trademarks of Microsoft Corporation.

Installing *CD-ROM for The Personal Trainer's Handbook, Second Edition*

Microsoft Windows®

1. Insert the *CD-ROM for The Personal Trainer's Handbook, Second Edition,* into the CD-ROM drive.
2. Select the My Computer icon.
3. Select the O'Brien CD-ROM drive.
4. Open the PDF folder or the TEXT folder and select the document you wish to view or print.

Macintosh®

1. Insert the *CD-ROM for The Personal Trainer's Handbook, Second Edition,* into the CD-ROM drive.
2. Double-click the O'Brien CD icon on the desktop.
3. Open the PDF folder or the TEXT folder and select the document you wish to view or print.

For product information or customer support:
E-mail: support@hkusa.com
Phone: 217-351-5076
Fax: 217-351-2674
Web site: **www.HumanKinetics.com**